AF750542

Clinical Implementation of Bone Regeneration and Maintenance

Edited by Mike Barbeck,
Nahum Rosenberg, Patrick Rider,
Željka Perić Kačarević and Ole Jung

Published in London, United Kingdom

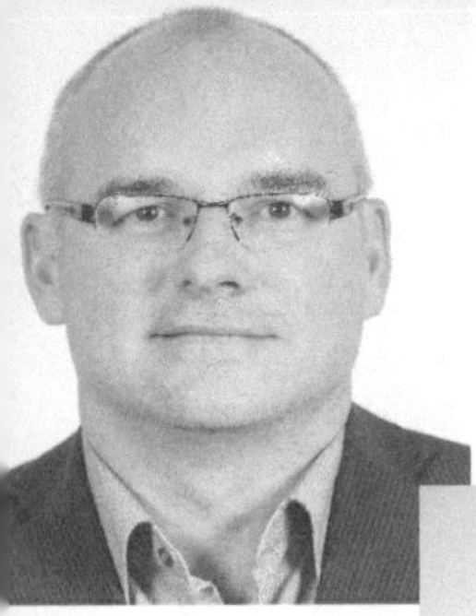
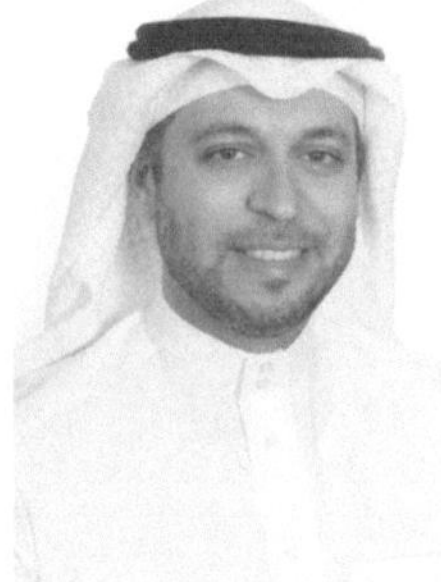
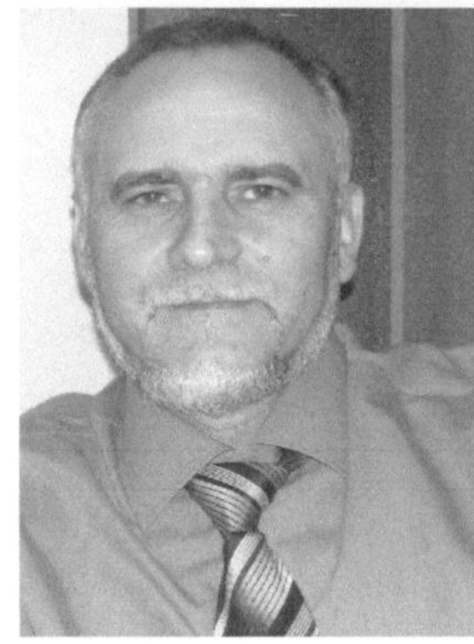
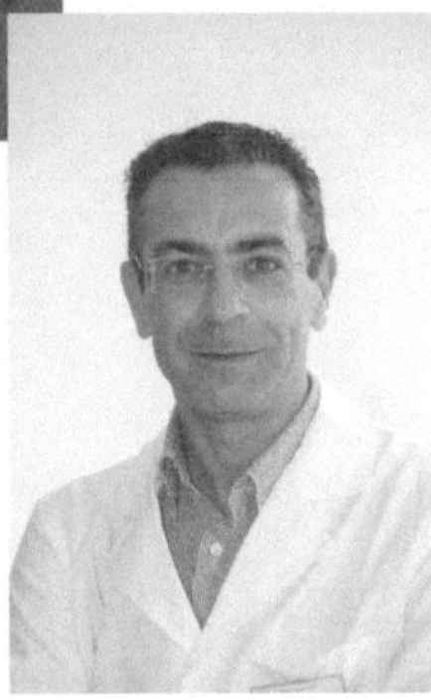
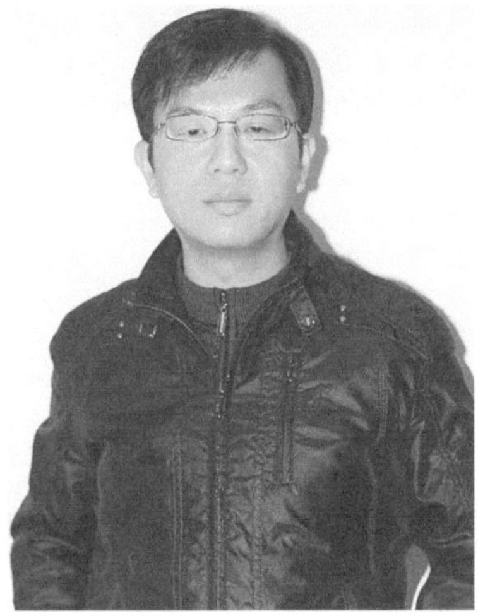
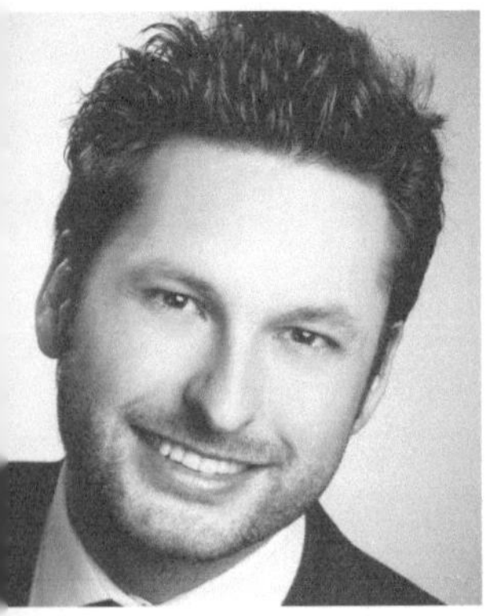
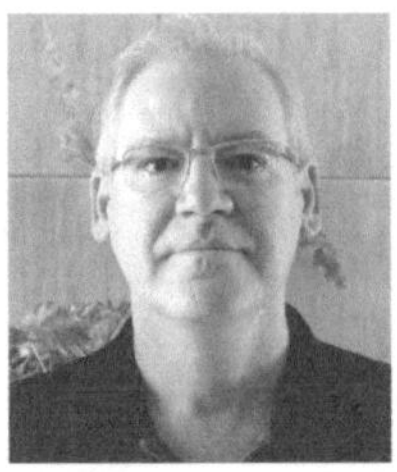

IntechOpen

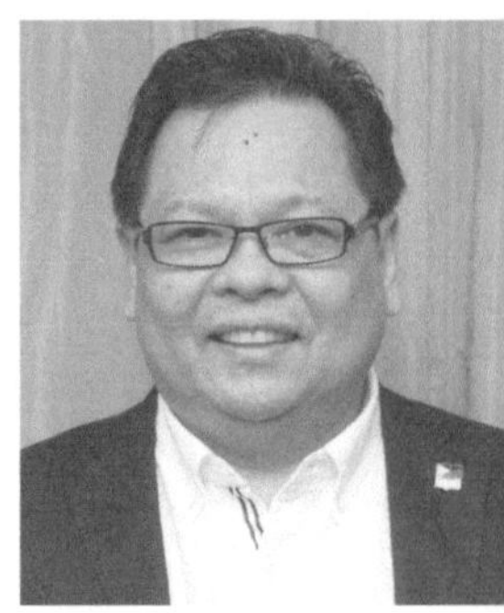
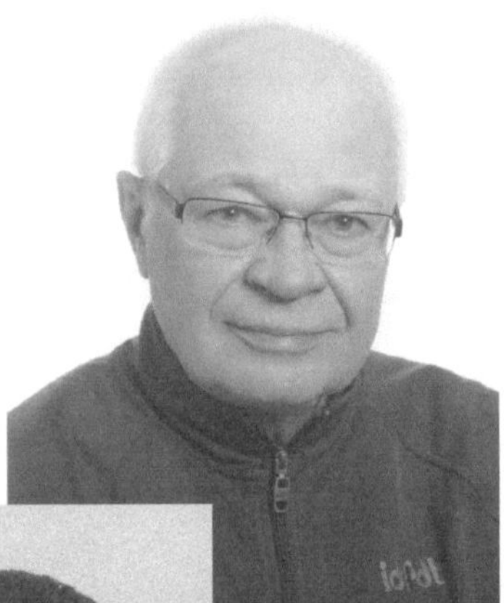
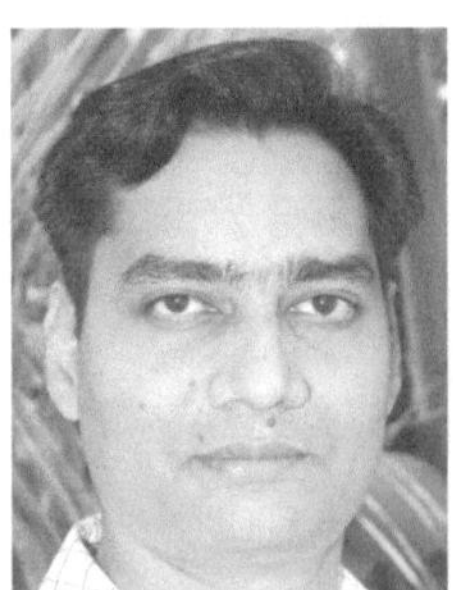
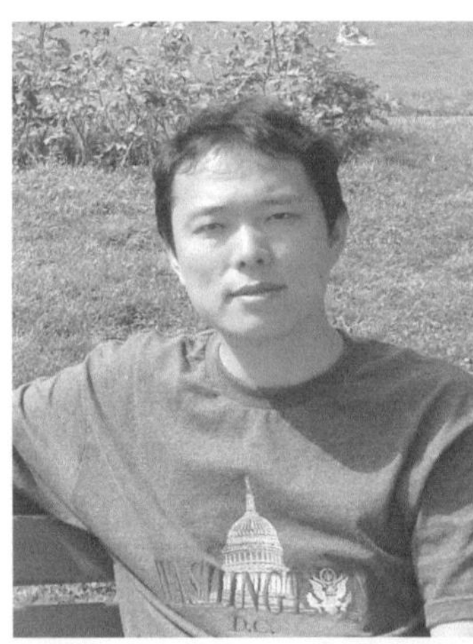
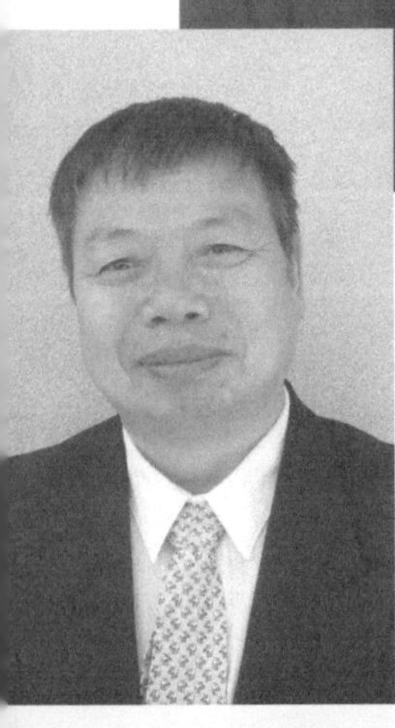
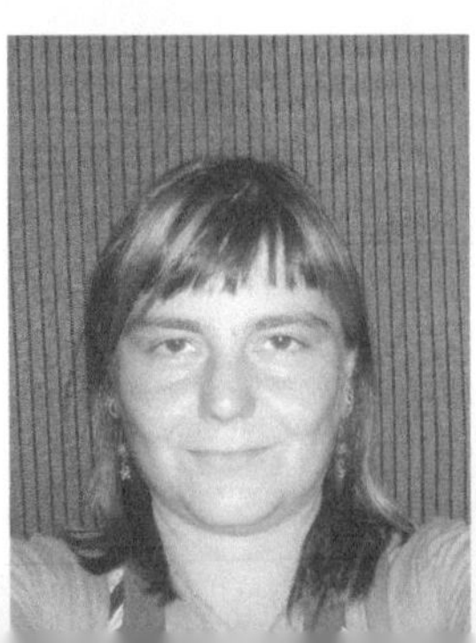

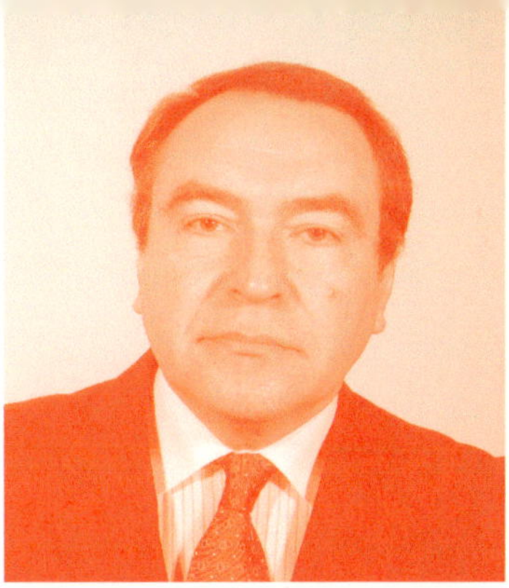

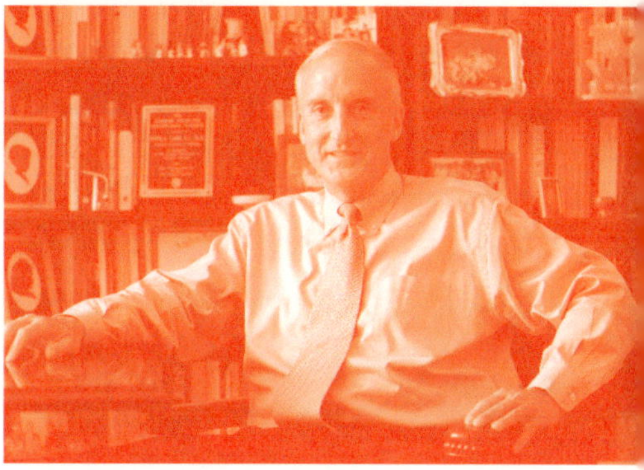

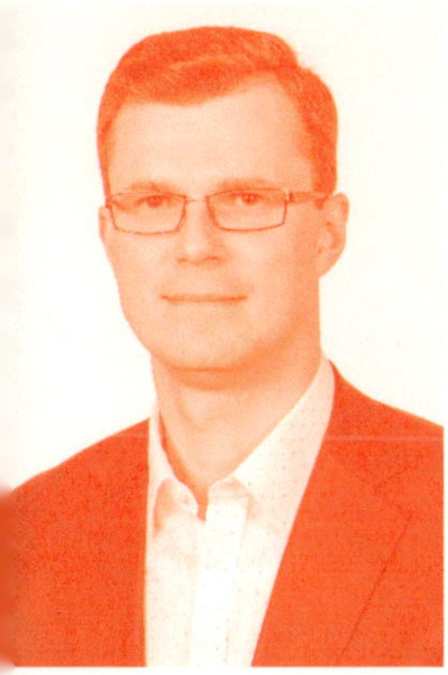

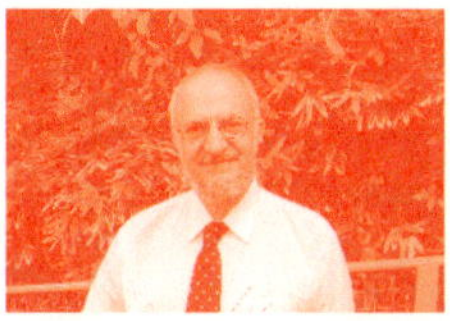

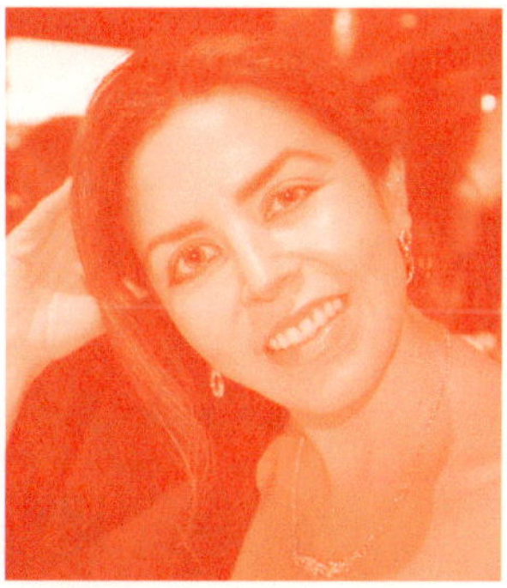

Supporting open minds since 2005

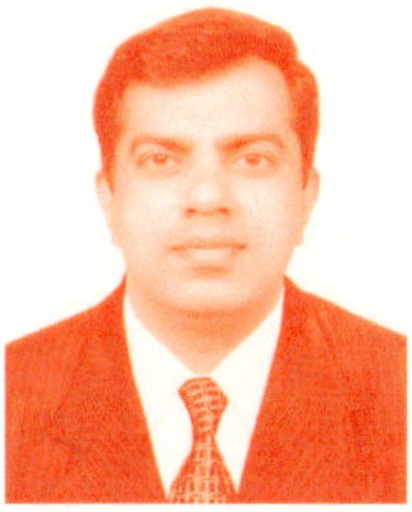

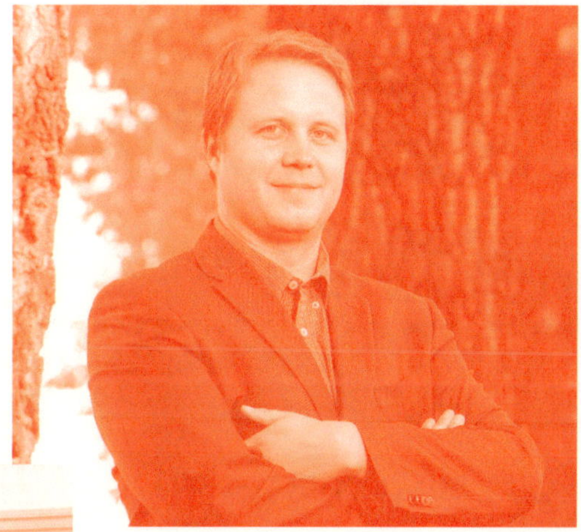

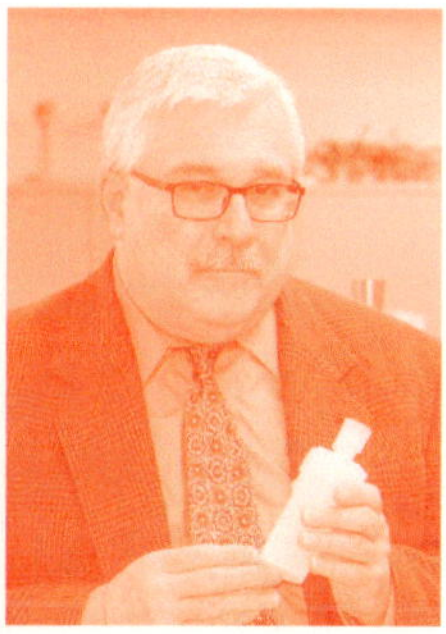

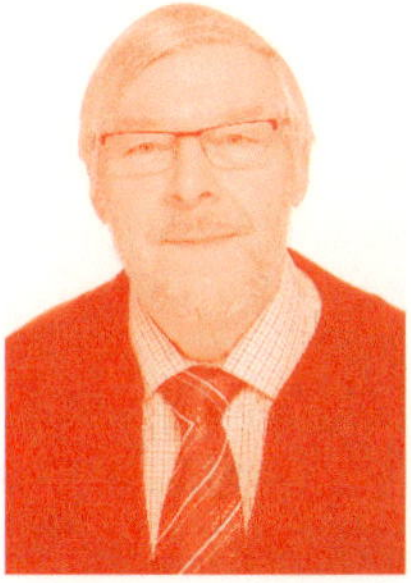

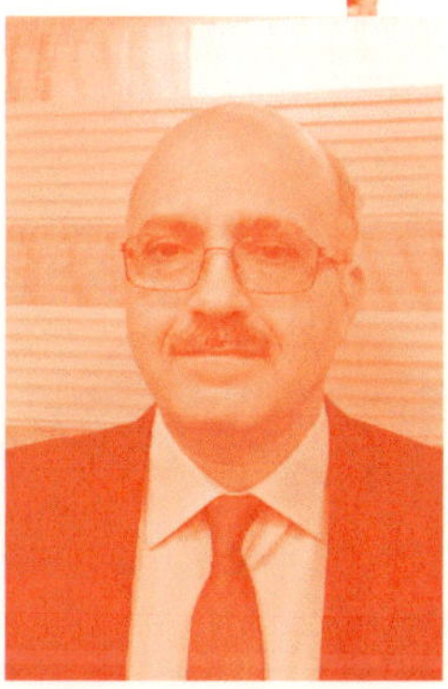

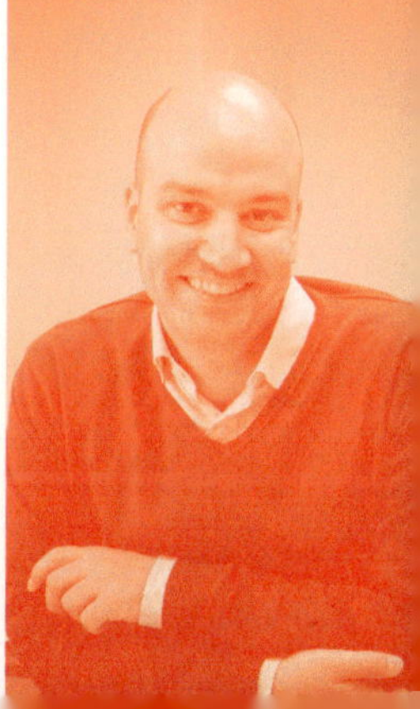

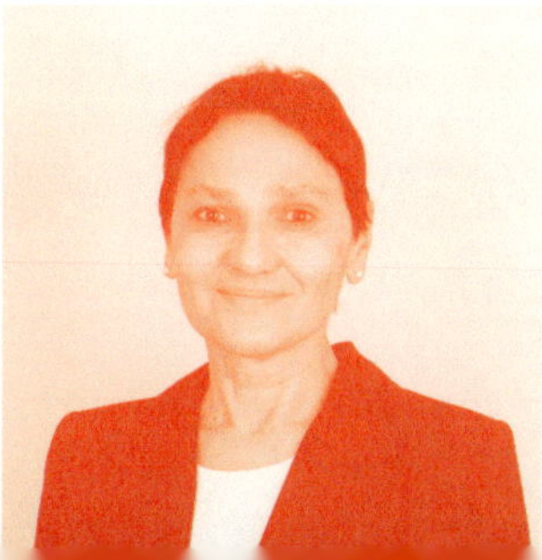

Clinical Implementation of Bone Regeneration and Maintenance
http://dx.doi.org/10.5772/intechopen.85328
Edited by Mike Barbeck, Nahum Rosenberg, Patrick Rider, Željka Perić Kačarević and Ole Jung

Contributors
Ayotunde Oladunni Oladunni Ale, Sawsan Jaghsi, Elaf Akram Abdulhameed, Marzuki Omar, Ab. Rani Samsudin, Morgan P. Lorio, Jeffrey G. Marx, Mark A. Moore, Nigeste Carter, Elena C. Gianulis, Julie McLean, Payal Sohoni, Joao Filipe Requicha, Maria Dias, Carlos Viegas, Henrique Armés, Guilherme Domingos, Antônio Lourenço Severo, Marcelo Lemos, Ivânio Tagliari, Danilo Barreto Filho, Osvandre L. C. Lech, Paulo C. F. Piluski, Carlos Castillo, Taruneet Kaur, Suman Kapila, Rajeev Kapila, Archil Tsiskarashvili, Stevo J Najman, Vladimir Cvetković, Jelena Najdanović, Olga Viktorovna Viktorovna Berdyugina, Kirill Alexandrovich Berdyugin, Daniel Paulo Strack, Nikolay Zagorodny, Svetlana Rodionova, Dmitry Gorbatyuk

© The Editor(s) and the Author(s) 2021
The rights of the editor(s) and the author(s) have been asserted in accordance with the Copyright, Designs and Patents Act 1988. All rights to the book as a whole are reserved by INTECHOPEN LIMITED. The book as a whole (compilation) cannot be reproduced, distributed or used for commercial or non-commercial purposes without INTECHOPEN LIMITED's written permission. Enquiries concerning the use of the book should be directed to INTECHOPEN LIMITED rights and permissions department (permissions@intechopen.com).
Violations are liable to prosecution under the governing Copyright Law.

Individual chapters of this publication are distributed under the terms of the Creative Commons Attribution 3.0 Unported License which permits commercial use, distribution and reproduction of the individual chapters, provided the original author(s) and source publication are appropriately acknowledged. If so indicated, certain images may not be included under the Creative Commons license. In such cases users will need to obtain permission from the license holder to reproduce the material. More details and guidelines concerning content reuse and adaptation can be found at http://www.intechopen.com/copyright-policy.html.

Notice
Statements and opinions expressed in the chapters are these of the individual contributors and not necessarily those of the editors or publisher. No responsibility is accepted for the accuracy of information contained in the published chapters. The publisher assumes no responsibility for any damage or injury to persons or property arising out of the use of any materials, instructions, methods or ideas contained in the book.

First published in London, United Kingdom, 2021 by IntechOpen
IntechOpen is the global imprint of INTECHOPEN LIMITED, registered in England and Wales, registration number: 11086078, 5 Princes Gate Court, London, SW7 2QJ, United Kingdom
Printed in Croatia

British Library Cataloguing-in-Publication Data
A catalogue record for this book is available from the British Library

Additional hard and PDF copies can be obtained from orders@intechopen.com

Clinical Implementation of Bone Regeneration and Maintenance
Edited by Mike Barbeck, Nahum Rosenberg, Patrick Rider, Željka Perić Kačarević and Ole Jung
p. cm.
Print ISBN 978-1-78985-831-0
Online ISBN 978-1-78985-832-7
eBook (PDF) ISBN 978-1-78984-398-9

We are IntechOpen, the world's leading publisher of Open Access books

Built by scientists, for scientists

5,200+
Open access books available

127,000+
International authors and editors

150M+
Downloads

156
Countries delivered to

Our authors are among the
Top 1%
most cited scientists

12.2%
Contributors from top 500 universities

CLARIVATE ANALYTICS
BOOK CITATION INDEX
INDEXED

WEB OF SCIENCE™

Selection of our books indexed in the Book Citation Index
in Web of Science™ Core Collection (BKCI)

Interested in publishing with us?
Contact book.department@intechopen.com

Numbers displayed above are based on latest data collected.
For more information visit www.intechopen.com

Meet the editors

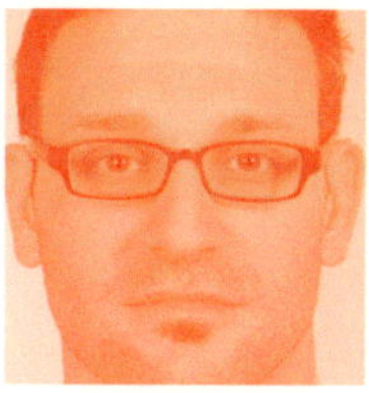

Mike Barbeck has vast experience in regenerative biomedical research working at institutes in Germany. He has researched the principles of biomaterial-mediated tissue regeneration (bone substitute materials and collagen materials) resulting in many papers in peer-reviewed journals. His research has led to further elucidation of cellular fundamentals of the foreign body response to different biomaterials.

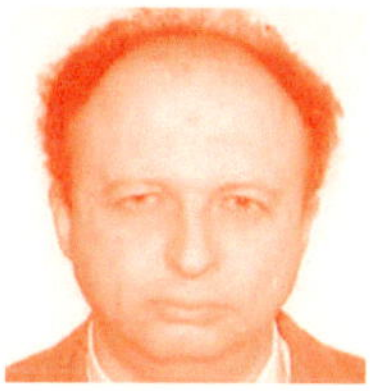

Nahum Rosenberg MD, MOrthop (magna cum laude), FRCS (England), MBA is an orthopedic surgeon with an MD degree from Technion – ITT in 1990. He completed his residency in Orthopedic Surgery at the Rambam Medical Center, Haifa between 1990-97. He received his MOrthop with honors from the Tel Aviv University in 1996 and was a Nuffield Fellow (Orthopedic Surgery) in Oxford University in 1998-9. Dr. Nahum was a Fellow in Orthopedic Surgery at the University of Nottingham in 2002. He completed his MBA from the College of Management Academic Studies, Israel in 2018. Dr. Nahum is a senior orthopedic surgeon at the Rambam Health Care Campus since 2003. He has been an Assistant Clinical Professor in the Faculty of Medicine, Technion -ITT, Haifa since 2007. He is also a Professor in the Department of Traumatology, Orthopedic Surgery and Disaster Medicine in IM Sechenov First Moscow State Medical University 2018-19. Dr. Nahum is a member of the editorial boards in 8 scientific journals, as well as a member of the Shoulder Committee of ISAKOS (International Society of Arthroscopy, Knee Surgery and Orthopedic Sports Medicine). He is the author of 80 peer review scientific publications, and the editor of 7 books. His research interests include: shoulder surgery, the outcome of orthopedic procedures, bone biology, bone regeneration, human biomechanics.

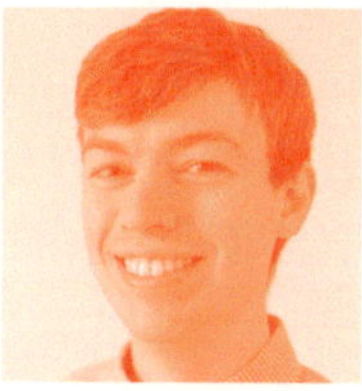

Dr. Patrick Rider is a researcher of biomaterials specializing in dental applications. He received his undergraduate degree in biomaterials science and tissue engineering from the University of Sheffield, and later obtained his Ph.D. from the same university for his research involving the reactive inkjet printing of regenerated silk fibroin to produce dental barrier membranes. After finishing his studies in England, he took up his current position as a member of the Botiss Biomaterials GmbH research and development team in Berlin, Germany.

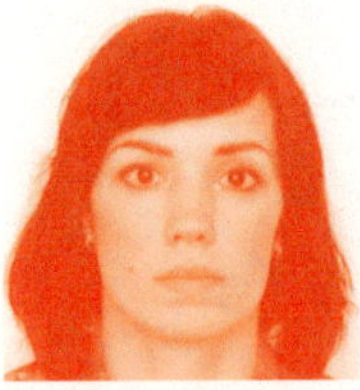

Željka Perić Kačarević was born in Osijek, 1986, where she completed elementary and high school. She received her molecular science degree from the Biology Department in 2010. She completed her postgraduate study in Biomedicine and Health at the Faculty of Medicine Osijek in 2017. Since 2011, she has been employed by the Department of Anatomy and Neuroscience. After 2018 she transferred to the Department of Anatomy Histology, Embryology, Pathology, Histology, Faculty of Dental Medicine and Health, Osijek, Croatia. In scientific research, her experience lies in functional anatomy, fat tissue structure, and its impact on other organic systems.

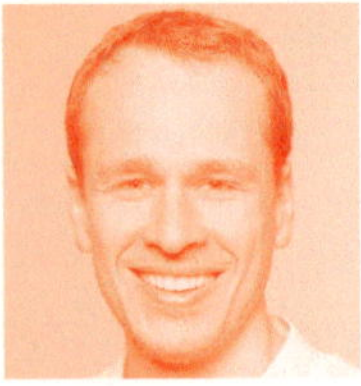

Dr. Ole Jung studied medicine from 2014-2015 at the Universities of Hamburg and Witten/Herdecke with stays in the USA, Switzerland, England, and Poland. From 2015 to 2019, he worked as a group leader and assistant doctor in oral and maxillofacial surgery at the University Medical Center Hamburg-Eppendorf. Since 2019 he has been working in dermatology at the Rostock University Medical Center.

Contents

Preface XI

Section 1
Bone Grafts in Dentistry 1

Chapter 1 3
Marginal Bone Changes around Dental Implants after LIPUS Application: CBCT Study
by Elaf Akram Abdulhameed, Marzuki Omar and A.R. Samsudin

Chapter 2 33
Cell Attachment and Osteoinductive Properties of Tissue Engineered, Demineralized Bone Fibers for Bone Void Filling Applications
by Julie B. McLean, Nigeste Carter, Payal Sohoni and Mark A. Moore

Section 2
Bone Grafts in Orthopaedics 47

Chapter 3 49
Class III Spine Grafts
by Jeffrey G. Marx and Morgan P. Lorio

Chapter 4 63
Allograft Structural Interbody Spacers Compared to PEEK Cages in Cervical Fusion: Benchtop and Clinical Evidence
by Nigeste Carter, Elena C. Gianulis and Mark A. Moore

Chapter 5 83
Bone Graft in the Treatment of the Non-Consolidation of the Scaphoid with Necrosis of the Proximal Pole – A Systematic Review
by Antônio Lourenço Severo, Osvandre Lech, Paulo Cesar Faiad Piluski, Marcelo Barreto Lemos, Carlos Castillo, Danilo Barreto Filho, Daniel Paulo Strack and Ivânio Tagliari

Chapter 6 93
Distraction Osteogenesis: Biological Principles and Its Application in Companion Animals
by Guilherme Domingos, Henrique Armés, Isabel Dias, Carlos Viegas and João Requicha

Section 3
Bone-Related Diseases **111**

Chapter 7 **113**
Thyroid Disorders and Osteoporosis
by Ayotunde Oladunni Ale

Chapter 8 **125**
Relation between Vitamin K and Osteoporosis
by Sawsan Jaghsi

Chapter 9 **137**
Metabolic Disorders in Patients with Chronic Osteomyelitis: Etiology and Pathogenesis
by Archil Tsiskarashvili, Nikolay Zagorodny, Svetlana Rodionova and Dmitry Gorbatyuk

Chapter 10 **155**
Immunological Monitoring of Osteogenesis Disorder
by Olga Viktorovna Berdyugina and Kirill Alexandrovich Berdyugin

Section 4
Biologicals for Bone Tissue Regeneration **177**

Chapter 11 **179**
Application of Adipose-Derived Stem Cells in Treatment of Bone Tissue Defects
by Stevo Najman, Jelena Najdanović and Vladimir Cvetković

Chapter 12 **209**
MicroRNAs as Next Generation Therapeutics in Osteoporosis
by Taruneet Kaur, Rajeev Kapila and Suman Kapila

Preface

"Experimentation and clinical tests have shown that for the graft to take root, not only should it be as viable as possible, but from the very beginning it should have a strong relationship with the host" Vittorio Putti 1912 [1].

Bone has an efficient ability to regenerate. But the critically large defects in bone, either postsurgical or after trauma, progress to nonunion and instability in 10% of patients and therefore require implantation of a bone graft [2]. In the USA alone about half a million bone grafting surgeries are done annually [3]. Furthermore, the rate of bone grafting procedures is expected to rise due to the constantly advancing techniques of bone grafting.

Autologous bone grafting is the gold standard for the reconstruction of critical bone defects. However, autologous grafts have several significant disadvantages, such as donor site morbidity and limited availability. The alternative use of allografts or xenografts is limited due to the risks of rejection, infection, and high nonunion rates. Progress in bone tissue engineering is essential to provide an unlimited source for autologous-like bone grafting source. There is an indication that the method to generate autologous bone-like material, as live autologous bone tissue, originating from patient-specific osteoblast-like cells, grown from bone marrow on β-tricalcium phosphate supporting three-dimensional matrix under optimal biomechanical conditions, is possible (**Figure 1**) [4, 5].

But meanwhile other methods for effective bone grafting are under ongoing development aiming to achieve optimal osteoconductivity and osteoinductivity similar to the autologous bone graft material. Thus, the potential of the newly developed tissue engineering methods for bone grafting is discussed in this book. According to the ongoing research, progress of the methods to create readily available autologous-like bone grafting material that doesn't cause additional surgical morbidity, is anticipated to evolve. Naturally, these methods are expected to fulfill the regulatory requirements, including clinical studies, that will allow the start of widespread clinical use. For this purpose, a thorough understanding of bone regeneration control in vivo by systemic humoral and local factors is essential. In this book, several such factors are presented and discussed.

The classic method of local bone regeneration by means of distraction osteogenesis, which is based on mechanical stimulation at the bone deficient site is presented by Domingos et al. This widespread effective clinical method requires a good understanding of the optimal mechanical and humoral factors – those are presented in the chapter.

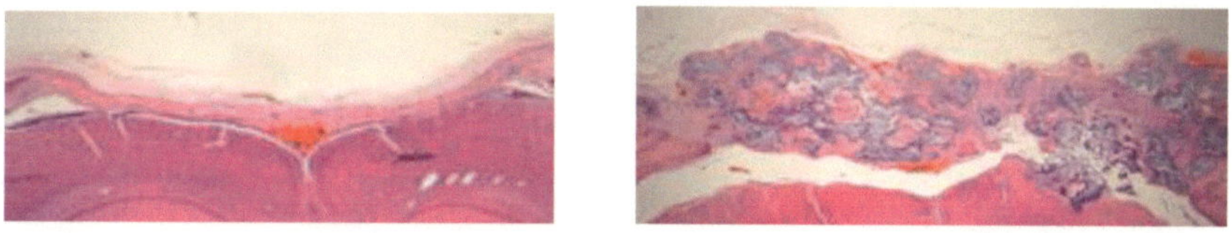

A B

Figure 1.
A- micrograph (HE staining) of a critical bone gap in rat calvarium, 6 weeks after the creation of the gap. No evidence of bone bridging. B- micrograph (HE staining) of bridging of the critical bone gap by young woven bone, 6 weeks after implantation with in vitro generated bone-like tissue.

Berdyugina OV and Berdyugin KA present the immunological aspects related to bone regeneration. Those are not always apparent to the clinicians who are involved in the treatment of bone deficiencies.

The microRNAs control the proliferation and differentiation of osteoblasts and osteoclasts, which influences bone formation, and this is described in the chapter by Kaur T et al. This rarely addressed subject might become an important therapeutic tool in the treatment of bone related disabilities.

The additional important issue of systemic effect of bone damage due to osteomyelitis is reviewed by Tsiskarashvili A et al. The systemic metabolic changes that occur in that situation are crucial for understanding the treatment of bone deficiencies due to osteomyelitis.

The maintenance of bone remodeling is governed by the thyroid hormone. The relationship between thyroid impairment, and bone mass, especially in the aged population, is discussed in the chapter by Ayotunde Oladunni Ale.

The biological effect of vitamin K and bone maintenance is not widely apparent but in the dedicated chapter by Sawsan Jaghsi, this subject is discussed aiming to open an additional niche for possible pharmacological intervention in bone metabolism.

These chapters address the less discussed aspects of bone regeneration and maintenance, therefore the reader may find new areas of interest when approaching the deep understanding of the fascinating area of bone regeneration control.

Mike Barbeck
University Hospital Hamburg-Eppendorf,
Germany

Nahum Rosenberg
Ruth and Bruce Rappaport Faculty of Medicine,
Technion – Israel Institute of Technology,
Haifa, Israel

Patrick Michael Rider
Botiss Biomaterials GmbH,
Germany

Željka Perić Kačarević
University of Osijek,
Croatia

Ole Jung
Department of Dermatology and Venereology,
University Medical Center Rostock,
Germany

References

[1] Donati D, Zolezzi C, Tomba P, Vigano A. Bone grafting: historical and conceptual review, starting with old an old manuscript by Vittorio Putti. Acta Ortop 2007;**78**(1):19-25

[2] Alexander PG, Hofer HR, Clark KL, Tuan RS: Mesenchymal Stem Cells in Musculoskeletal Tissue Engineering. In Principles of Tissue Engineering. 4th edition. Edited by Lanza R, Langer R, Vacanti J. Waltham, MA, USA: Elsevier; 2014:1171-1200

[3] Mauffrey C, Madsen M, Bowles RJ, Seligson D: Bone graft harvest site options in orthopaedic trauma: a prospective in vivo quantification study. Injury 2012,**43**:323-326. 4

[4] Rosenberg N, Rosenberg O. Extracorporeal human bone-like tissue generation. Bone and Joint Research (BJR) 2012;**1**:1-7

[5] Rosenberg N, Rosenberg O. Safety and efficacy of in vitro generated bone-like material for in vivo bone regeneration – a feasibility study. Heliyon (CellPress) 2020;**6**:1-7

Section 1

Bone Grafts in Dentistry

Chapter 1

Marginal Bone Changes around Dental Implants after LIPUS Application: CBCT Study

Elaf Akram Abdulhameed, Marzuki Omar and A.R. Samsudin

Abstract

To assess the effect of LIPUS on marginal bone regeneration during insertion and following loading using CBCT scan imaging, a trial of RCT of 22 subjects needing dental implant was conducted. The participants were randomly allocated into 2 groups; both groups underwent similar two-stage implant surgery of one maxillary dental implant. The control group (n = 11) of the implant site was allowed to heal in a conventional way, while the intervention group (n = 11) was subjected to LIPUS therapy at the implant site (twice a week, 20-minute duration, from week 2 after stage I implant surgery and continued for 10 weeks). Similar ultrasound protocol was repeated 2 weeks after crown installation and again continued for another 10 weeks. The assessment of marginal bone loss around dental implants was carried out at three different views (coronal, sagittal, and axial) of the implant site immediately after surgery, 3 and 6 months later. Statistical analysis of ANOVA within and between two-group analysis that was applied followed by pairwise comparison with confidence interval adjustment showed that there is a significant difference among the groups ($p < 0.05$). The CBCT imaging (coronal view) values suggested that bucccal bone regeneration around the dental implant has significantly increased during the early osseointegration period in the LIPUS-treated subjects than in the control group. LIPUS enhances bone formation in particular buccal bone plate around the dental implant as confirmed by the coronal view.

Keywords: LIPUS, coronal, sagittal, axial, osseointegration

1. Introduction

The introduction of osseointegration, in 1969, by Professor Per-Ingvar Brånemark, at the Institute of Applied Biotechnology, University of Goteborg, [1] opened new avenues in the dental implant treatment for the partially or fully edentulous patients [2]. Titanium endosseous implants are widely used successfully in association with this treatment modality. Various investigations proved this method to be superior for long-term prognosis for dental implant treatment [3, 4].

Osseointegration is a process of connecting structurally and functionally an ordered living bone with load-carrying implant [5]. When histologic features of the osseointegration were observed, functional ankylosis was found without any intrusion of connective or fibrous tissues between the implant surface and bone [6]. However, in some situations, osseointegration does not take place adequately and

IntechOpen

at times leads to implant failure. Continuous investigations looking into implant's chemical and physical characteristics, structures, and the biological responses from the surrounding bone are being conducted to identify its cause.

Implant success depends upon successful osseointegration. Evaluation of the bone surrounding the implant is a common method for observing the implant prognosis [7–9]. Care of the bone that supports the implant is vital for the beneficial results of the implant treatment [10].

Various studies have shown that there were changes in the marginal bone level and loss of different amount of bone that occur mostly during the first year of dental implant placement [11–13]. Assessment of changes in marginal bone height is considered an important parameter in evaluating implant success [14, 15]. Excessive marginal bone loss after implant or following prosthesis may be seen in the first year. However, in the early phase of osseointegration, the process of bone healing is not well understood [16].

One of the etiological factors of marginal bone loss is the disruption of the periosteum and blood supply during flap elevation and placement of implant [17]. Some studies showed that less marginal bone loss was noticed when flapless technique is used as compared with full-thickness flap technique that showed more marginal bone loss during healing period [18–21].

Other studies showed that periosteum disruption not only affects marginal bone level but also has other effects on bone formation around the implant during the healing period that compromise the stability of the implant and delay healing [21, 22].

Previous studies [19, 23] reported that the decreased blood supply to the bone after periosteum elevation has the same effect of flapless technique on the level of marginal bone and bone formation rhythm.

Continuous bone resorption affects function and esthetic. There are several ways to restore and regenerate bone such as advocating bone grafting procedures, usage of growth factors, laser therapy in low levels, and therapeutic ultrasound.

Low-intensity pulsed ultrasound (LIPUS) stimulation is a classical therapeutic modality for bone regeneration. Its efficiency has been widely reported over the years. LIPUS stimulation can be used as a tool to enhance tooth and periodontal regeneration [24].

Della Rocca [25] in her study on the effect of LIPUS on bone regeneration on Wistar rats confirmed that LIPUS can consolidate fractures and reduce bone healing time. It is also shown that LIPUS enhances bone regeneration based on its angiogenic and osteogenic values both before and after dental implant placement [26, 27].

1.1 Ultrasound

1.1.1 History and development of ultrasound

Ultrasound has been discovered 50 years ago for therapeutic and diagnostic uses in the medical field. Ultrasound refers to the sound with frequency greater than that audible by the human ear. It is a mechanical compression-rarefaction wave that travels through the tissue, producing both thermal and nonthermal effects [28].

The thermal effects of ultrasound can increase the temperature of deep tissue with high collagen content to increase the extensibility of the tissue or to control pain. The nonthermal effects of ultrasound can alter cell membrane permeability, thus facilitating tissue healing and transdermal drug penetration. Therapeutic ultrasound may also facilitate calcium resorption. To achieve these treatment outcomes, appropriate frequency, intensity, duty cycle, and duration of ultrasound must be selected and applied.

In evaluating an ultrasound device for the clinical application, one should consider the appropriateness of the available heads and BNRs for the types of problems expected to be treated with the device [28].

1.1.2 Diagnostic uses of ultrasound

Transthoracic ultrasound (US) examination can be used for (1) chest wall lesions; (2) pleural lesions such as pleural effusion, pleural thickening, or pleural tumors; (3) peridiaphragmatic lesions; (4) peripheral pulmonary lesions which abut the pleura; (5) pulmonary lesions with an accessible US window; and (6) mediastinal tumors in contact with the chest wall [29–31].

On US, pleural effusion is characterized by an echo-free or hypo echoic space between the visceral and parietal pleurae that can change shape with respiration. On US, peripheral lung tumors appear as well-defined, homogeneous, hypo echoic, or echogenic nodules with posterior acoustic enhancement.

Diagnostic US is efficiently used for the visceral examinations, e.g., the liver, pancreas, kidneys, etc., at 3 MHz frequency. The neck, breast, and children are examined using a frequency of 5–7 MHz. The increase in the frequency in the ultrasound examination increases the visibility and discrimination of details of the image.

Diagnosis of benign or malignant growth in the uterus, fallopian tubes, and ovary is routinely made in the obstetrics using ultrasound. It is also used for the progressive assessment of pregnancy.

1.1.3 Therapeutic uses of ultrasound

1.1.3.1 Osteoradionecrosis

Harris [32] claimed that therapeutic ultrasound increases the blood supply and the deposition of new healthy callus replacing the necrotic bone. Therefore, therapeutic ultrasound can be used as conservative method of management of osteoradionecrosis of the mandible.

1.1.3.2 In vitro and in vivo bone regeneration

Ultrasound and some other physical factors stimulate the bone healing process by increasing the intracellular calcium levels. Deposition of intracellular calcium enhances the formation of bone [33]. In vivo and in vitro studies have shown that ultrasound treatment increases the activity of alkaline phosphatase in spontaneous and experimental fractures in rats and rabbits as compared with untreated animals [34–36].

Animal and clinical studies conducted in two phases by John et al. [37] reported that ultrasound-treated groups have increased formation of callus. Increased activity of the osteoblasts was observed cytologically in the ultrasound-treated group.

1.1.4 Ultrasound treatment setting parameters

General guidelines of parameters for ultrasound therapy are given for different clinical applications as follow [28]:

- Duty cycle: The proportion of the total treatment time that the ultrasound is on. This can be expressed as a percentage or a ratio: 20 or 1:5 duty cycle, that is, 20% of the time on and 80% of the time off.

- Effective radiating area (ERA): The area of the transducer that radiates ultrasound energy is known as ERA. ERA is smaller in comparison with the area of the treatment head.
- Frequency: Frequency is the measure of compression-refraction cycles per unit of time. It can be expressed in Hertz (Hz) or cycle per second. Frequency used for therapeutic purposes ranges from 1 to 3 MHz. Increment in the frequency decreases the concentration and depth of penetration of the ultrasound energy in the tissues.
- Intensity: Intensity demonstrates power per unit area of the sound head. It is expressed in watts per centimeter squared (W/cm^2). The recommended limit of the intensity for therapeutic purposes is 3 W/cm^2 by the World Health Organization.
- Power: It is the amount of aural energy per unit time. It is expressed in watts (W).
- Pulsed ultrasound: During the treatment, periodic or sporadic supply of ultrasound is known as pulsed ultrasound.
- Spatial average intensity: The average intensity of the ultrasound output over the area of the transducer.
- Spatial average temporal average (SATA) intensity: The spatial average intensity of the ultrasound averaged over the on time and the off time of the pulse.
- Spatial average temporal peak (SATP) intensity: The spatial average intensity of the ultrasound during the on time of the pulse. This is a measure of the amount of energy delivered to the tissue.

1.1.5 Mechanism of action of ultrasound therapy

Although the exact mechanism of LIPUS interaction with the viable tissues and stimulation of bone healing is still unclear, there are several studies that showed that LIPUS stimulates regeneration of the bone and decreases the osseointegration time and promotion of the quality of osseointegration [38].

The mechanism behind the effect of LIPUS on bone regeneration might start from the mechanotransduction pathways of LIPUS on bone wound healing which is considered a complex process as numerous cell types respond to this stimulus involving several pathways. Mechanotransduction refers to the processes through which cells sense and respond to mechanical stimuli by converting them to biochemical signals that elicit specific cellular responses [39]. Typically the mechanical stimulus gets filtered in the conveying medium before reaching the site of mechanotransduction. Cellular responses to mechanotransduction are variable and give rise to a variety of changes and sensations. From definition of mechanotransduction, LIPUS promotes activation of osteoblast and other necessary cells' function which are considered decisive elements in bone healing by increasing proliferation, migration, and differentiation of these cells and changing it from inactive phase to active cells. The cellular responses underlying this mechanism are termed mechanotransduction [40].

Ingber [41] demonstrated in his work that the integrins are the most important key in the transduction of the ultrasound signals with evolutionary conserved mechanoreceptors, are expressed by various cell types, and convert mechanical signal into biochemical response. This form of sensory transduction is responsible for a number of senses and physiological processes in the body, including proprioception, touch, balance, and hearing. Mechanotransduction involves various signal transduction pathways, including the activation of ion channels and other mechanoreceptors in the membrane of the bone cell, resulting in gene regulation in the nucleus [42]. Identification and functional characterization of the mechanotransduction components may improve bone tissue engineering. In this process, a mechanically gated ion channel makes it possible for sound, pressure, or movement to cause a change in the excitability of specialized sensory cells and sensory neurons [43]. The stimulation of a mechanoreceptor causes mechanically sensitive ion channels to open and produce a transduction current that changes the membrane potential of the cell.

Padilla et al. [44] and Sato et al. [45] updated the information in this area of interest that the mechanotransduction pathways involved in cell responses include integrin/mitogen-activated protein kinase (MAPK) and other kinase signaling pathways, gap-junctional intercellular communication, upregulation and clustering of integrins, involvement of the COX-2/PGE2 and iNOS/NO pathways, and activation of mechanoreceptor. Along with the direct effect of ultrasound, sensitizing mechanosensitive receptors, channels of the cell and the indirect effect of acoustic streaming-governed-shear stress on the cell surface (**Figure 1**). Acoustic streaming, giving rise to a unidirectional bulk fluid movement, can improve the circulation of molecules within the extracellular matrix in the culture wall, or trigger fluid flow in vivo, and thereby increase the delivery of cytokines secreted by other cell participants or other essential nutrients, and remove cellular waste products [46]. Tang et al. [47] stressed with his co-worker that the transmembrane mechanoreceptors increased surface expression in rat primary osteoblasts (in vitro study) of a2, a5, b1, and b3 integrins and clustering of b1 and b3 integrins have been shown to be upregulated within 24 hours after 20-minute treatment with LIPUS. In the same cell type, but using continuous ultrasound exposure, enhanced expression of a2, a5, and b1 integrins has also been reported and also showed upregulated expression [36]. After ultrasound exposure in mouse, osteoblasts isolated from long bones, gene expression was also significantly upregulated of a2, a5, and b1 integrins, whereas Watabe et al. [48] revealed in his vitro study that only expression of a5 was enhanced in mouse mandibular and calvaria-derived osteoblasts stimulated with LIPUS. Zhou et al. [49] explained in his amazing work that inhibiting b1 integrin by blocking antibody or RGD peptide in human primary skin fibroblasts led to restoring basal levels of DNA synthesis, which had been upregulated in response to ultrasound before.

Ren et al. [50] has reported that p38 MAPK kinase is crucial for LIPUS to induce and enhance differentiation of human periodontal ligament cells (HPDLC) which are similar to mesenchymal stem cells and can undergo osteogenic differentiation. Treatment of cells with the p38 inhibitor significantly reduced ALP activity, osteocalcin concentration, and matrix mineralization in response to LIPUS, compared to the control group, where no inhibitor was added [44]. Whitney et al. [51] also explained in his study that the LIPUS in continuous mode caused more intense phosphorylation of FAK, Src, p130Cas, CrkII, and Erk1/Erk2 in primary human chondrocyte culture, suggesting that this pathway is involved in US-induced mechanotransduction mechanism. However, several studies in mechanotransduction suggested that voltage-sensitive calcium channels (VSCCs) have been reported to be the key regulators of intracellular calcium signaling in osteoblasts for bone formation [40].

Most recently, Kang et al. [52] studied the effects of 20 minutes a day stimulation by a low-intensity ultrasound (1 MHz, 30 mW/cm^2 continuous sine wave) in combination with cyclic vibratory strain (1 Hz, 10% strain) on MC3T3-E1 cells in a 3D scaffold. The stimulation did not change the cell proliferation over a period of 10 days, but significantly upregulated several gene expressions—COL-I, OC, RUNX2, and OSX—indicating accelerated differentiation.

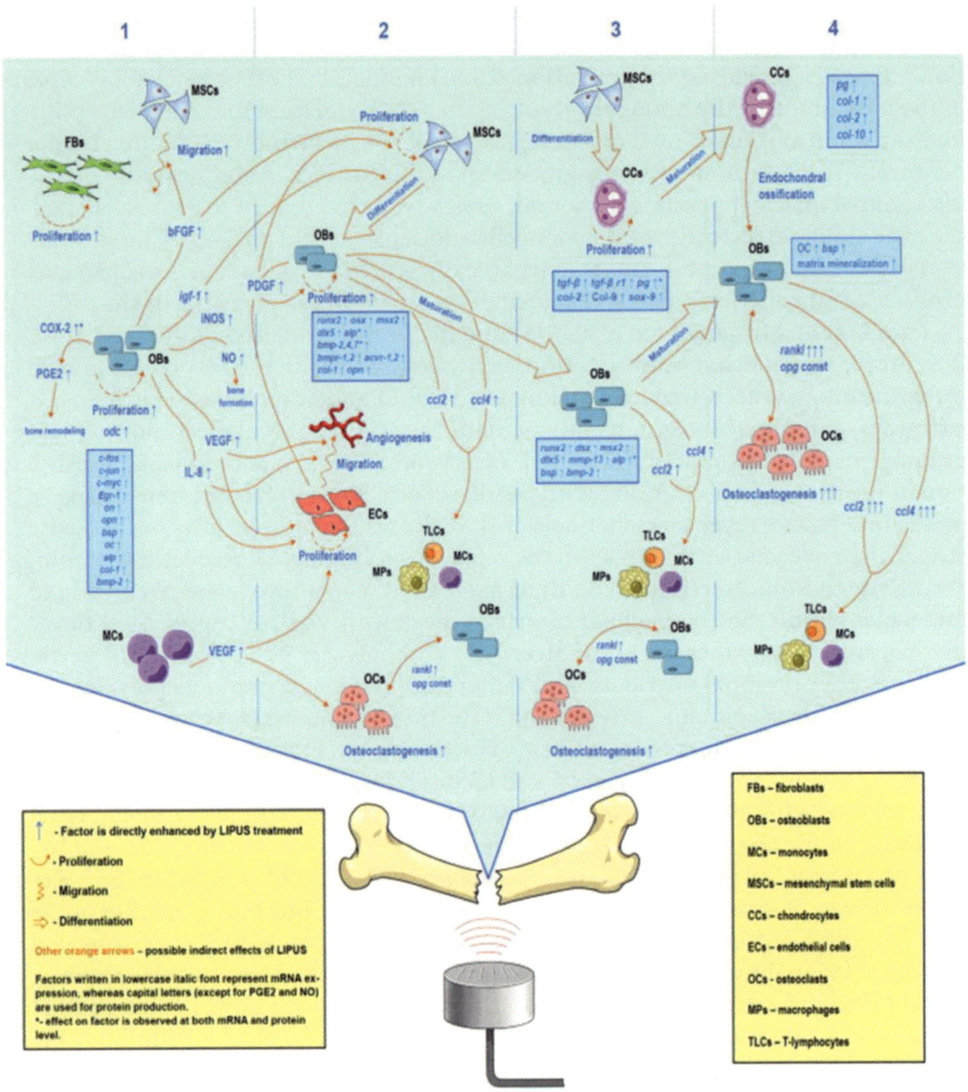

Figure 1.

Summary of hypothetical LIPUS effects on bone cellular events in vitro data. The columns represent the four phases during in vivo endochondral bone fracture healing: phase 1, early events soon after the bone injury: hematoma formation, inflammation, and migration of osteogenic precursors; phase 2, angiogenesis, proliferation of mesenchymal stem cells (MSCs), and osteoblasts and osteogenic differentiation; phase 3, chondrogenesis and maturation of osteoblast; and phase 4, maturation of chondrocytes, woven bone formation, and remodeling [44].

The accessibility of the crucial factors to the compromised cells supports their viability and maintains the indispensable microenvironment in the healing fracture through the regulation of pH and oxygenation, which may be enhanced by the ultrasound treatment. A mechanism of improved oxygen and nutrient transport in response to ultrasound has been suggested by Pitt and Ross [53].

These studies suggest that LIPUS are able to enhance osteogenesis and angiogenesis in vivo and in vitro as was well documented by literature review that angiogenesis precedes osteogenesis process [54]. Angiogenesis is closely associated with osteogenesis where reciprocal interactions between endothelial and osteoblast cells play an important role in bone regeneration [55].

Angiogenesis has a key role in bone repair by not only facilitating the supply of oxygen and nutrients required for bone repair and the removal of waste products but also by providing conduits for the invasion of osteoblast and osteoclast progenitors into the healing site [56]. Vascular endothelial growth factor (VEGF) is a potent and vital angiogenic cytokine. It is a specific mitogen for vascular endothelial cells (ECs) [57]. Shiraishi et al. [58] demonstrated in his vitro study that the application of LIPUS led to the upregulation of interleukin-8, basic fibroblast growth factor, vascular endothelial growth factor, and non-collagenous bone proteins, and the downregulation of osteoclasts resulted in bone regeneration. El-Bialy et al.'s [59] study in vivo has demonstrated that therapeutic LIPUS can promote bone repair and regeneration, accelerate bone fracture healing, and enhance osteogenesis at the distraction site on rabbits ultimately offering long-term benefits to patients.

1.1.6 Ultrasound in dentistry

Low-intensity pulsed ultrasound technique is used for the evaluation of bone growth in the permeable implant surface [60]. Pulsed ultrasound produces a pressure wave which serves as a noninvasive mechanical stimulus and promotes the growth at the site of injury. Amplitude of the pulse is kept as low as 0.3 mm showing no ill effects on the process of recovery. However, mechanism of cellular response produced by ultrasound is not well defined [61, 62]. Low-intensity pulsed ultrasound, which is used for only few minutes in routine, has shown beneficial role in the healing evidenced by experimental and clinical trials [62, 63].

The intensity of ultrasound used for soft tissue application ranges from 500 to 3000 mW/cm^2. Much of the clinical benefits from the ultrasound in physical therapy have been attributed to the controlled heating of the tissue. Because heating bone may also have significant deleterious effects, intensity used for bone application is much lower, in the range 30 mW/cm^2, which does not induce applicable heating of treated hard and soft tissues [64].

1.1.6.1 Applications of ultrasound in dentistry

1. Ultrasound is widely used for fracture detection in dentistry. Fractures of the nasal bone, orbital rim, maxilla, and mandible zygomatic arch are commonly detected by ultrasound. The position of the mandibular condyles is also located by ultrasound. To observe the healing fractures after surgery can be easily performed by ultrasound [66].

2. Focal disease or parotid lesions can be observed easily using an ultrasound.

2. Materials and methods

2.1 Study design

This study was a randomized controlled clinical trial (RCT) in which patients who visited the University Dental Hospital Sharjah (UDHS) for dental treatment and requested for oral rehabilitation of their missing teeth were selected for dental implant therapy. Those patients were examined in the oral surgery implant clinic and provided with new registration serial number. All the odd number patients were in the trial (ultrasound) group, and the even numbers were in the control group.

The aims and objectives of this study were to evaluate the effect of ultrasound therapy on osseointegration using clinical assessments, measurements of RFA values, and radiological assessments using linear measurement of marginal bone loss around the dental implant-supported prostheses using CBCT. The selected age groups were between 20 and 40 years old. All patients were recruited following specific criteria of inclusion and exclusion. Patients of this study were divided into two groups, namely, ultrasound and control; each patient received one dental implant to replace single missing maxillary first or second premolar teeth. In the first trial group (ultrasound), the ultrasound therapy was applied twice a week for 20 minutes that commenced 2 weeks after stage I implant surgery and continued for 10 weeks. At 2 months, uncovery and placement of gingival former for 10 days were carried on for all patients in both groups (ultrasound and control), then the impression taking was done for all patients, and installation of screw-retained porcelain to fused crown was performed 2 weeks later after the impression was taken. The same ultrasound therapy protocol was repeated 2 weeks after the crown installation for another 10 weeks. In the control group, patients were not subjected to application of ultrasound therapy. Clinical data collections composed of measurements of resonance frequency analysis (RFA) values using Osstell ISQ device and linear measurements of different variables using CBCT images taken immediately after the placement of the implant and during follow-up clinical examinations at 3 and 6 months postoperatively.

2.2 Flowchart

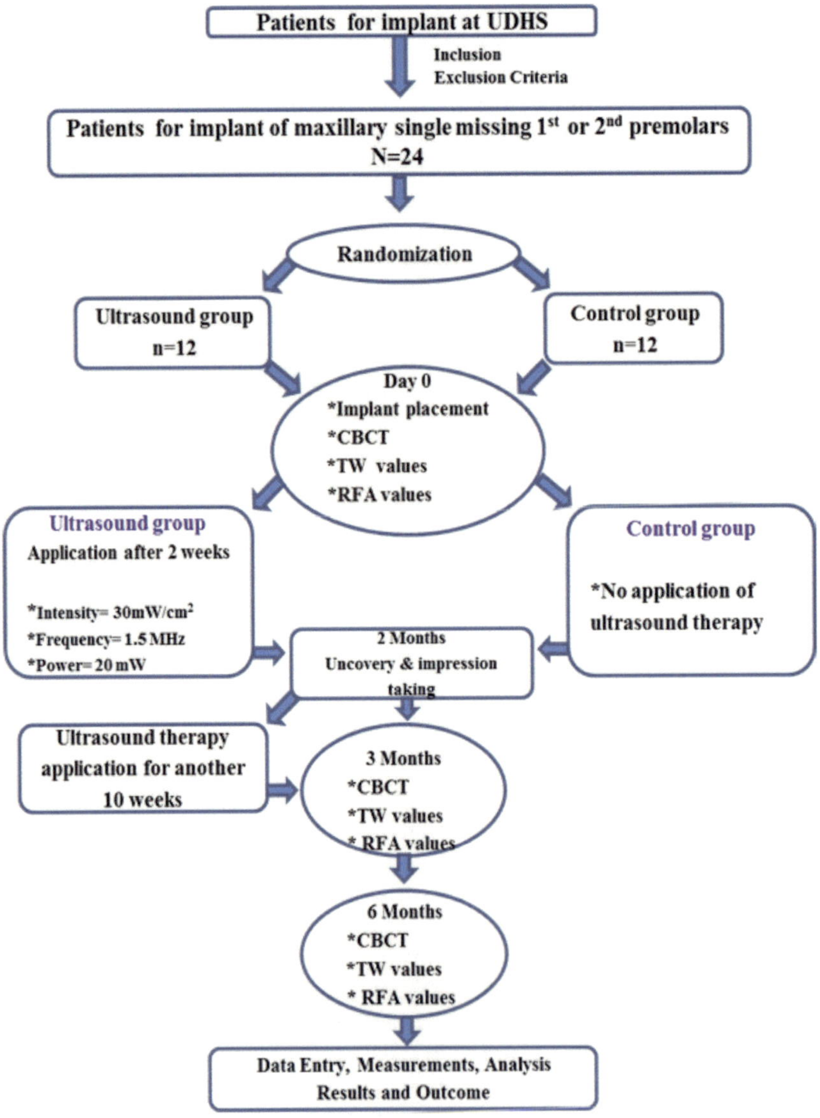

2.3 Clinical methods

2.3.1 Clinical assessment

Thorough medical and dental histories were taken from all patients presented in the study project. General clinical assessment of oral hygiene and gingival and periodontal health in terms of gingival color, contour, size, and consistency was documented. The height and width of the available bone around the potential site of the dental implant were assessed using a bone caliper.

2.3.2 Preoperative radiological screening assessment

An orthopantomogram (OPG) and intraoral periapical radiograph (IOPA) were taken preoperatively during patient selection and were kept in the patient's record; they gave an indication about the location and proximity of the vital structures and anatomical landmarks, bone quality, quantity and the presence of sufficient bone height and width in terms of mesiodistal dimension around the dental implant, absence of pathological lesions that may affect the outcome of dental implant success (periapical cysts, granulomas, osteomyelitis), and the angulation and position of the potential dental implant in relation to the adjacent teeth.

2.3.3 Operative techniques

All patients underwent two stages of implant surgeries. Stage I implant surgery was performed in which one SPI dental implant (THOMMEN Medical SPI ELEMENT MC INICELL) bone level type with a length of 9.5 mm and a diameter of 4 mm was positioned in the maxillary edentulous premolar area in each patient of the 22 sample size. A stage II implant surgery was carried on after 2 months of implant placement in which the dental implant had to be uncovered and impression was taken for crown installation.

2.3.3.1 Group I (ultrasound) group

1. The ultrasound group patients (n = 11) were then subjected to the application of low-intensity pulsed ultrasound 2 weeks following stage I implant surgery placement. The machine employed was Gymna Pulson® 330 Belgium (**Figure 2**). The intensity of ultrasound therapy used was 30 mW/cm^2 with a frequency of 1.5 MHz and temporal average power of 20 mW (**Table 1**). The therapy was delivered intraorally on the buccal part of the implant site for duration of 20 minutes twice a week starting 2 weeks after dental implant placement for the subsequent 10 weeks (**Figure 3**). At 2 months, uncovery and placement of gingival former for 10 days were carried on, then the impression taking was done for all patients, and installation of screw-retained porcelain to fused crown was performed 2 weeks later after the impression was taken. The same ultrasound therapy protocol was repeated 2 weeks after the crown installation for another 10 weeks.

2. Clinical data collections composed of resonance frequency analysis (RFA) value measurements using Osstell ISQ device (**Figure 4**) and linear measurements of CBCT images at three different views were taken immediately after the placement of the implant and in the follow-up clinical examinations at 3 and 6 months postoperatively.

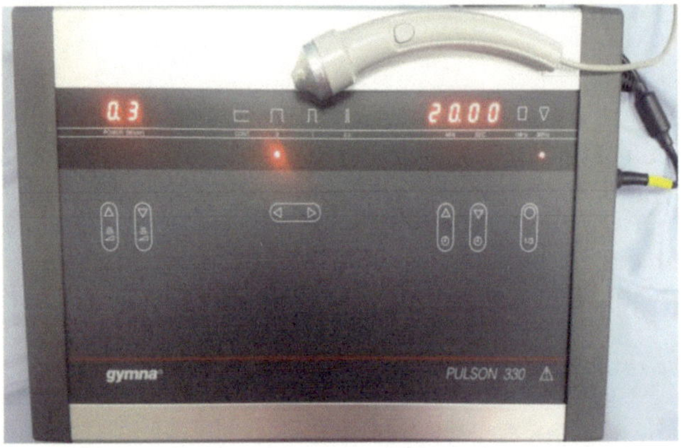

Figure 2.
The therapeutic ultrasound machine Gymna Pulson® 330 with intraoral probe and actual setting parameters on display.

Ultrasound frequency	1.5 MHz
Intensity (SATA)	30 mW/cm^2
Temporal average power	20 W
**Kerr et al. [65].*	

Table 1.
Intraoral ultrasound device: technical specifications of the ultrasound signal.

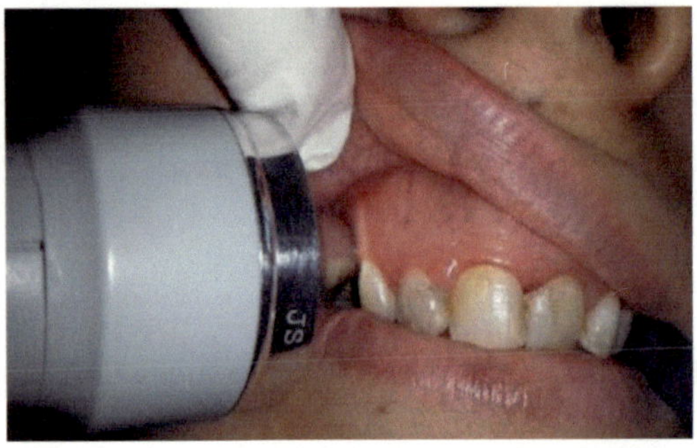

Figure 3.
Ultrasound therapy delivered using probe on the buccal aspect of the implant site.

2.3.3.2 Group II (control)

The control group patients (n = 11) were not subjected to the application of ultrasound therapy. Those patients went through two stages of implant placement surgery. At stage I implant surgery, the dental implant was placed to replace a single missing maxillary premolar tooth. Uncovery and impression were taken for the dental implant at stage II implant surgery, and supra-structure prosthetic construction comprising of screw-retained porcelain fused to metal crown was inserted at 2 months postoperatively. Clinical data collections composed of resonance frequency analysis (RFA) value measurements using Osstell ISQ device and linear measurements of CBCT images at three different views were taken immediately after the placement of the implant and in the follow-up clinical examinations at 3 and 6 months postoperatively.

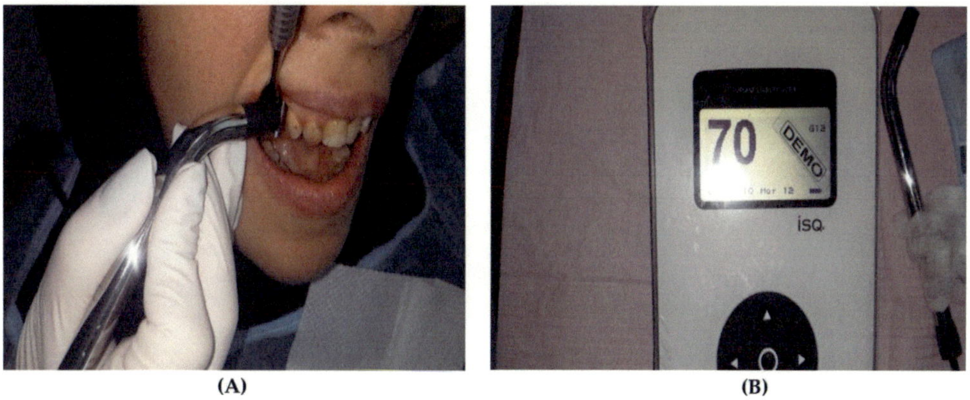

Figure 4.
RFA measurement procedure, the probe close to the SmartPeg™. (A) At bucco-palatal and mesio-distal directions, a value of 70 reveals as primary stability on the day of implant placement surgery (B).

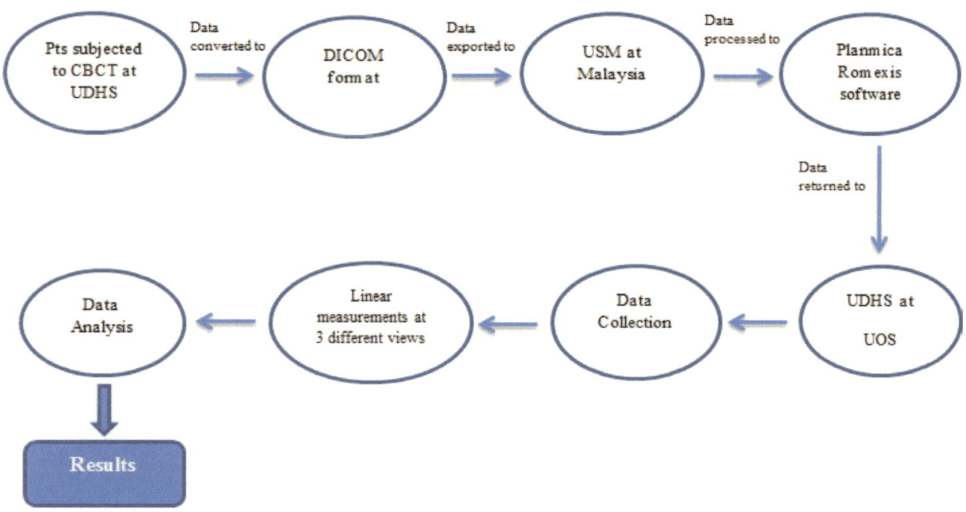

Figure 5.
Flowchart of steps for data transformation from UDHS to USM.

2.4 Data collection

The CBCT scan of each patient was carried out at the Radiographic Department, University Dental Hospital Sharjah, Sharjah, United Arab Emirates. All patients underwent computed tomography scans using GALILEOS; then, the data are converted to DICOM format in which they get exported to USM to be processed using Planmeca Promexis 3D software, and then the data returned to UDHS where data collection started (**Figure 5**).

The machine used produces X-rays in cone shape that centers on the X area of the detector. Its tube detector system can be rotated at 360° around the patient's head which exposes the patient for a series of images to be taken by GALILEOS/ Sirona Dental Systems Scan specifications summarized in **Table 2**.

The cone beam volumetric tomography (CBVT) X-ray unit used in this study was Planmeca ProMax 3D Max. It records the finest details of the patient's oral anatomy. It offers a maximum field view (Ø23 × 26 cm) which explores new possibilities in diagnostic radiology. It has an advanced imaging software system that increases its benefits.

Scanner name	GALILEOS Comfort^{PLUS}
Manufacturer	Sirona Dental Systems GmbH, Bensheim, Germany
Detector type	Image intensifier (I.I.), Thales or Siemens
Focal spot size	0.5
Voltage kV	85
Current mA	10
Exposure time	14 seconds
Number of single exposures 200	200

Table 2.
Specifications of CBCT machine used in Dental clinic, UDHS.

CBVT technology is utilized in Planmeca ProMax 3D Max. It is an advanced, multipurpose, and active imaging machine. It can be utilized in various fields of dentistry that include maxillofacial surgery, implantology, endodontic, orthodontics, periodontics, and for the analysis of TMJ. The newly designed advanced ProMax has evolved into a classical 3D platform with CBVT.

Instead of a continuous beam, each volume is produced by throbbing the X-ray tube during the scanning. It reduces the dose as well as the rotational distortions during the scanning procedure. The total time required for scanning may be from 18 to 26 seconds. However, the exact exposure time may be only 3 seconds. Accurate and distortion-free image for 3D construction is produced by the ScI semiconductor flat panel. Correction for geometric magnification is not required for the images produced by Planmeca ProMax 3D Max.

To ensure immobilization of the patient during exposure, standard methods have been taken as follow:

1. Frankfort plane of the patient parallel to the floor.

2. Midsagittal plane perpendicular to the floor.

3. The patient was asked to bite on the bite block of the machine using the upper and lower incisors to standardize patient's position according to X-ray tube head rotation.

Lead apron was placed on each patient prior to exposure. All metallic objects (e.g., hairpins and earrings) and any intraoral removable prosthesis were removed.

3. Results

3.1 Radiological results using CBCT images

The orthopantomogram (OPG) was shown to be a useful tool for radiological screening of the patient during selection stage. Complex cases such as proximity to vital structures and inadequate bone height and width were excluded from the study. In the CBCT images obtained at day 0, there was adequate availability of bone height and width at the platform of dental implant for both groups. At 3 months, there was an increase of buccal plate thickness of 0.3–0.6 mm in the ultrasound group compared to the control group. At 6 months, there was marginal bone loss around dental implant in the control group and marginal bone increase in height and width in the ultrasound group (**Figure 6A–E**).

3.2 Evaluation of marginal bone changes for both groups at different time intervals

CBCT images were obtained at day 0, 3, and 6 months follow-up. The marginal bone level was assessed and measured at three different views (coronal, sagittal, and axial) at time-point interval.

In the coronal view, there was an overgrowth of the bone width at corono-buccal and corono-palatal and less reduction of the bone height at apico-buccal and apico-palatal in the ultrasound group, but the bony tissue overgrowth was more pronounced at the buccal bone plate at 3 and 6 months rather than at the palatal bone plate. In the control group, the marginal bone loss was more in height and width than the in the ultrasound group (**Table 3**).

In the sagittal view, there was an overgrowth of the bone width at sagitto-mesial and sagitto-distal aspects of dental implants and less reduction of the bone height at apico-mesial and apico-distal in the ultrasound group, but the bony tissue overgrowth was more pronounced at the mesial bone plate at 3 and 6 months. In the control group, there was a reduction in the bone width and height from day 0 to 6 months (**Table 4**).

In the axial view, the bony tissue overgrowth was revealed more at the axio-buccal than axio-palatal at 3 and 6 months in the ultrasound group, while in the control group, there was marginal bone loss in all aspects of dental implant (**Table 5**).

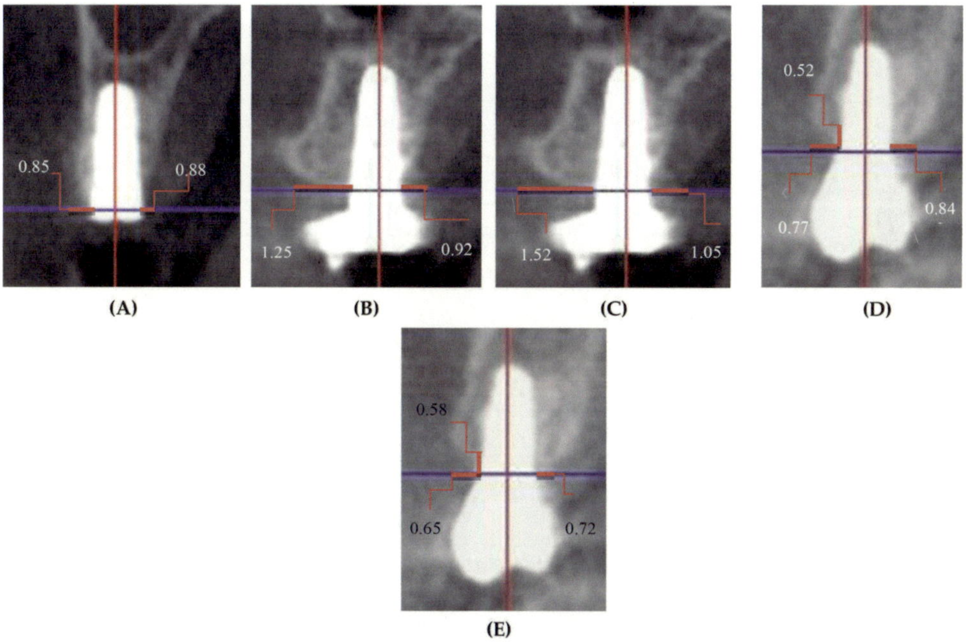

Figure 6.
Representative CBCT images of marginal bone level in the coronal view. Both groups showed an adequate availability of bone height and width at day 0 (A). An overgrowth of buccal bone plate thickness observed in the ultrasound group at 3 and 6 months (B, C). Marginal bone loss around dental implant observed in the control group at 3 and 6 months (D, E).

Time		Ultrasound (n = 11)	Control (n = 11)
		Mean(SD)	Mean(SD)
Day 0	CB**	1.43 (0.24)	1.43 (0.50)
	CP#	1.44 (0.37)	1.42 (0.36)
3 months	CB	1.62 (0.36)	0.92 (0.25)
	CP	1.55 (0.34)	1.37 (0.26)
	AB†	1.20 (0.73)	1.20 (0.39)
	AP‡	0.89 (0.83)	0.87 (0.74)
6 months	CB	1.81 (0.41)	0.85 (0.30)
	CP	1.62 (0.22)	1.02 (0.34)
	AB	1.65 (0.73)	0.88 (0.29)
	AP	1.02 (0.62)	0.76 (0.53)

Day 0 readings for AB and AP are not shown since there are no parameters given.
***CB = corono-buccal*
#CP = corono-palatal
†AB = apico-buccal
‡AP = apico-palatal

Table 3.
Descriptive statistics of linear measurements (mean, SD) of marginal bone changes between ultrasound and control groups in coronal view (values in millimeters).

Time		Ultrasound (n = 11)	Control (n = 11)
		Mean(SD)	Mean(SD)
Day 0	SM**	1.40 (0.30)	1.39 (0.41)
	SD#	1.41 (0.35)	1.38 (0.34)
3 months	SM	1.47 (0.39)	0.88 (0.26)
	SD	1.46 (0.20)	0.92 (0.25)
	AM†	0.89 (0.72)	0.83 (0.74)
	AD‡	0.87 (0.83)	0.84 (0.45)
6 months	SM	1.66 (0.57)	0.65 (0.29)
	SD	1.62 (0.23)	0.78 (0.30)
	AM	1.18 (0.73)	0.75 (0.32)
	AD	1.12 (0.60)	0.71 (0.40)

Day 0 readings for AM and AD are not shown since there are no parameters given.
***SM = sagitto-mesial*
#SD = sagitto-distal
†AM = apico-mesial
‡AD = apico-distal.

Table 4.
Descriptive statistics of linear measurements (mean, SD) of marginal bone changes between ultrasound and control groups in sagittal view (values in millimeters).

Time		Ultrasound (n = 11)	Control (n = 11)
		Mean(SD)	Mean(SD)
Day 0	AM**	1.41 (0.31)	1.40 (0.44)
	AD#	1.42 (0.37)	1.40 (0.33)
	AB†	1.44 (0.37)	1.42 (0.52)
	AP‡	1.45 (0.47)	1.43 (0.36)
3 months	AM	1.52 (0.39)	0.87 (0.25)
	AD	1.48 (0.19)	0.89 (0.27)
	AB	1.60 (0.37)	0.90 (0.30)
	AP	1.53 (0.35)	1.35 (0.18)
6 months	AM	1.66 (0.57)	0.63 (0.30)
	AD	1.63 (0.21)	0.72 (0.30)
	AB	1.82 (0.41)	0.84 (0.22)
	AP	1.63 (0.21)	0.98 (0.34)

**AM = axio-mesial*
#*AD = axio-distal*
†*AB = axio-buccal*
‡*AP = axio-palatal*

Table 5.
Descriptive statistics of linear measurements (mean, SD) of marginal bone changes between ultrasound and control groups in axial view (values in millimeters).

3.3 Comparison of marginal bone changes within each group at three different views

In the coronal view, within the ultrasound group, there was statistically significant increase in the buccal and palatal bones' thickness (height and width) from day 0 to 3 months, day 0 and 6 months, and from 3 to 6 months as p value was less than 0.05, but it was more pronounced at the buccal bone plate, while in the control group, there was no statistically significant increase in bone thickness, and there was marginal bone loss at all aspects of 9*dental implant.

In the sagittal view, within the ultrasound group, there was statistically significant increase in the mesial and distal bones' thickness (height and width) from day 0 to month 3, day 0 and month 6, and from month 3 to month 6 as p value was less than 0.05, while in the control group, there was no statistically significant increase in bone thickness, and there was marginal bone loss at all aspects of dental implant.

In the axial view, within the ultrasound group, there was statistically significant increase in the buccal, palatal, mesial, and distal bones' thickness (height and width) from day 0 to 3 months, day 0 and 6 months, and from 3 months to month 6 as p value was less than 0.05, while in the control group, there was no statistically significant increase in bone thickness.

3.4 Comparison of marginal bone changes between two groups at three different views

In the coronal view, there was statistically significant increase in buccal and palatal bone width between two groups (ultrasound and control) at 3 and 6 months as p value was less than 0.05. Thus, this increase in bone plate width is contributed to ultrasound therapy. There was no statistically significant increase in buccal and palatal bone height at 3 months between ultrasound and control groups, but there was statistically significant increase in buccal and palatal bone height at 6 months. Thus, this increase in bone plate height is contributed by ultrasound therapy.

In the sagittal view, there was statistically significant increase in mesial and distal bone plates' width between two groups (ultrasound and control) at 3 and 6 months as p value was less than 0.05. Thus, this increase in bone plate thickness is contributed by ultrasound therapy. There was no statistically significant increase in mesial and distal bone height at 3 months between ultrasound and control groups, but there was statistically significant increase in mesial and distal bone height at 6 months. Thus, this increase in bone plate height is contributed by ultrasound therapy.

In the axial view, there was statistically significant increase in buccal, palatal, mesial, and distal bone plates' width between two groups (ultrasound and control) at 3 and 6 months as p value was less than 0.05. Thus, this increase in bone plate thickness is contributed by ultrasound therapy.

4. Discussion

4.1 Introduction of marginal bone loss around dental implant

Marginal bone loss is considered to be an inevitable risk factor in implant therapy. The reduction in height and width of marginal bone level affects the success rate of implant treatment in terms of esthetic and function.

The majority of marginal bone loss occurs in the first year after implant placement [67]. Thus, the clinical crown-to-implant ratio rises with time to become more unfavorable as years go by. However, the etiology of long-term marginal bone loss or late implant failure seems to be of different origin and prone to peri-implantitis or occlusal overload [68]. It is important to consider multiple factors together in assessing implant failure rates as interactive effects may be observed in the establishment and maintenance of osseointegration [69, 70]. Thus, in the present study, attempts were made to control the relevant confounding variables (patient gender and age, implant location, implant diameter and neck design, insertion torque, insertion depth, and crown-to-implant ratios).

In this study project, we tried to measure the marginal bone level around the implant and its stability both at the time of implant placement and at the time of loading. For this reason we chose the 3- and 6-month intervals to examine the marginal bone level and implant stability after soft and hard tissue maturation and early bone remodeling [71].

Ultrasound is the generation of sound waves with a frequency above the limit of human audibility of 20 kHz that transfers mechanical energy into the tissues; it is used extensively in sports medicine and physiotherapy. Therapeutic ultrasound can induce angiogenic and bone morphogenetic factors and bone formation in vitro [72].

Dinno et al. [73] demonstrated that intensities of ultrasound of less than 100 mW/cm^2 spatial average and temporal average were nonthermal. Duarte [63] and Pilla et al. [74] reported that low-intensity ultrasound treatment in the range of 30–57 mW/cm^2 yielded minimal temperature changes when applied to the site of a bone fracture. Application of low-intensity pulsed ultrasound (30 mW/cm^2) was considered to have little thermal effect.

4.2 Clinical evaluation of application of ultrasound therapy

All patients in the ultrasound group tolerated the ultrasound therapy very well. The therapy was conducted over 20 minutes comfortably without any rejection from the patients. The results showed that the ultrasound therapy with the intensity set at 30 mW/cm^2 generated minimum heat that did not cause discomfort for the patients. Furthermore, the color of the gingival soft tissue remains pink and did not change to erythematic state at the end of the procedure which further proves there was no inflammation and untoward tissue response following the therapy. Therefore, the pain symptoms from patients were minimal as shown by minimal need for analgesia, and healing of the soft tissue wound in the ultrasound group was excellent. These clinical findings demonstrate wide acceptance of patients toward postoperative ultrasound therapy. Kamath et al. [75] in his study on the effect of LIPUS on healing of femur fracture revealed that there was more significant callous formation at the early stage of femur fracture in the LIPUS group than in the control group. Therefore, even in other parts of the body like femur, there are good results when LIPUS is applied.

In view of the increasing use of high-intensity and low-frequency ultrasonic technology, in medicine and in surgery, better understanding of the benefits or side effects of US application is significant in order to establish appropriate clinical studies. LIPUS has disadvantages besides the advantages as mentioned. Erdogan and Esen [76] showed that the effects of ultrasound therapy on growing bones and brain tissues are unclear. Thus, its use in children and in skull bones should be avoided. Its use in sites with suspected neoplasia and acute infections is contraindicated because of possible accelerated disease progression. Patients should be evaluated for allergic reactions to the coupling gel, and patients with cardiac pacemakers should avoid ultrasound treatment because of possible interaction with the ultrasound signals specially when using US with both high-intensity and high-frequency waves.

Miller et al. [77] mentioned that the induced heat by US is the result of the absorption of US energy in biological tissue and the heat can be concentrated by focused beams until tissue is coagulated for the purpose of tissue ablation. Unlike ultrasound for medical imaging (which transmits ultrasonic waves and processes a returning echo to generate an image), therapeutic ultrasound is a one-way energy delivery that might cause harmful effect in a cumulative way into the tissue, which utilizes a crystal sound head to transmit acoustic waves at 1–3 MHz and at amplitude densities between 0.1 and 3 W/cm^2 [78]. US heating, which can lead to irreversible tissue changes, follows an inverse time-temperature relationship. Depending on the temperature gradients, the effects from ultrasound exposure can include mild heating, coagulative or liquefactive necrosis, tissue vaporization, or all three [77]. Angle et al. [79] demonstrated that the therapeutic ultrasound with frequencies varying between 0.5 and 1.5 MHz and intensities 30–200 mW/cm^2 is known to promote healing, bone deposition, and growth. Nevertheless, therapeutic ultrasound is proposed to deliver energy to deep tissue sites through ultrasonic waves, to produce increases in tissue temperature or nonthermal physiologic changes [78].

Ebadi et al. [80] explained that ultrasonic energy causes soft tissue molecules to vibrate from exposure to the acoustic wave. This increased molecular motion generates frictional heat, thus increasing tissue temperature. The thermal effects of ultrasound are proposed to increase collagen extensibility, increase nerve conduction velocity, alter local vascular perfusion, increase enzymatic activity, alter contractile activity of skeletal muscle, and increase nociceptive threshold [78].

However, in our study, the intensity of LIPUS used was 30 mW/cm^2, and the duration of application was only for 20 minutes, and this treatment was commenced 2 weeks after the acute inflammatory phase has subsided. We feel that this dosage of US therapy is harmless to the active cells in the healing wound which was in the proliferative phase. The dose recommended may be harmful to the cells in the healing wound because they are vulnerable to damage from heat generation or prolonged treatment duration. Therefore, although the mechanotransduction mechanism for cell stimulation following US therapy is an acceptable phenomenon, it may only work favorably within certain limitations of the delivered energy.

4.3 Evaluation of marginal bone level

CBCT images showed adequate availability of bone height and width at the dental implant platform at day 0 for both groups at the time of implant placement. In this study, results obtained using CBCT images were reliable for linear measurements of bone thickness in height and width for both ultrasound-treated group and control group. CBCT enables us to expose the patient to low radiation doses, giving more comfort, and it is an economical procedure [81]. At 3 months, there was an increase of the mean difference of buccal bone plate width of 0.19 mm in the ultrasound group compared to the control group. At 6 months, there was a mean difference marginal bone loss of 0.58 mm in width of the buccal bone plate around the dental implant platform in the control group, while there was 0.38 mm increase in the mean difference of buccal bone width in the ultrasound group. These findings were consistent with the previous study by Chen who investigated the effect of LIPUS on bone regeneration in the rat parietal bone defects [26]. In Chen study, the defects were analyzed with micro-CT (μCT) and then histologically, which demonstrated new bone formation with the newly formed thick and matured bone compared to the one of the control group.

The justification of using LIPUS in this study is to accelerate the bone wound healing processes within the region of interest (ROI) which is the region replacing single missing maxillary premolar following trauma to the bone as implant placement surgery is considered to be a traumatic procedure even though the surgery is minimally invasive to the bone. Our aim in this study is to mimic what happened in natural tissue repair by inducing, triggering, and provocation of the cells related to bone formation by encouragement of mechanotransduction pathways involved in cell responses. These responses include integrin/mitogen-activated protein kinase (MAPK) and other kinase signaling pathways, gap-junctional intercellular communication, upregulation and clustering of integrins, involvement of the COX-2/PGE2 and iNOS/NO pathways, and activation of mechanoreceptor [44]. Mechanotransduction involves various signal transduction pathways, including the activation of ion channels and other mechanoreceptors in the membrane of the bone cell, resulting in gene regulation in the nucleus [42].

Based on time intensity and period of exposure of cells to waves of ultrasound, LIPUS can recruit mesenchymal stem cells from neighboring tissues and other sites in the body in attractive processes (chemotactic) with other biomedical pro-inflammatory mediators (growth factors) that are considered necessary in bone wound healing processes and trigger it from inactive form to active phase when LIPUS is used. This suggests that LIPUS is able to enhance osteogenesis and angiogenesis in vivo and in vitro as was well documented by literature review that angiogenesis precede osteogenesis process [54]. Angiogenesis is closely associated with osteogenesis where reciprocal interactions between endothelial and osteoblast cells play an important role in bone regeneration [55].

In our study, the marginal bone level was assessed and measured at three different views (coronal, sagittal, and axial) in which four points were located and measured per implant site (corono-buccal, corono-palatal, apico-buccal, apico-palatal, sagitto-mesial, sagitto-distal, apico-mesial, apico-distal, axio-buccal, axio-palatal, axio-mesial, and axio-distal), respectively, and at three different time intervals postoperatively at day 0, 3, and 6 months. The results of this study showed an increase in buccal bone width from 1.43 mm at day 0 to 1.81 mm at 6 months which revealed that the mean difference of buccal bone plate width increased by 0.38 mm, while the palatal bone mean difference width was also increased by 0.18 mm at 6 months. In the sagittal view, there was an increase of mean difference of 0.26 mm at the mesial aspect of the dental implant at 6 months in the ultrasound group compared to the control group that had marginal bone loss from 1.43 mm at day 0 to 0.85 mm at 6 months at the buccal bone plate in the coronal view. The reason why the height and width of bone thickness had increased in the ultrasound compared to the control is that LIPUS can promote bone healing and repair by inducing osteogenesis and angiogenesis. Earlier work has shown that the therapeutic range of US stimulates bone formation, osteoblast proliferation, and the synthesis of angiogenic vascular endothelial growth factor (VEGF), basic fibroblast growth factor (FGF), and interleukin 8 [72, 82]. Ramli et al. [83] have proven that ultrasound should be considered to have angiogenic and osteogenic values in their in vivo study looking at ultrasound effects on angiogenesis using the chick chorioallantoic membrane. In vitro ultrasound has also been shown to upregulate the release of the osteogenic cytokine OPG and downregulate RANKL, the ligand of the receptor activator nuclear factor kappa B, which recruits and activates osteoclasts [83].

In this study, the transducer was applied on the buccal aspect of the dental implant very close to the buccal bone plate and showed clinically that at 1.5 MHz frequency, a penetration of up to 2 cm is possible, thus influencing the palatal plate. Ramli et al. [83] demonstrated that the traditional 1- to 3-MHz frequency of ultrasound therapy has a penetration of up to 2 cm. Doan et al. [72] reported that the best effect of therapeutic ultrasound on angiogenesis occurs with intensities between 15 and 30 mW/cm^2 and a frequency of 45 kHz, as the long wave machine has a theoretical advantage of penetrating tissues up to 10 cm.

Results of the control group showed increased loss of bone height from 1.20 mm at 3 months to 0.88 mm at 6 months at the apico-buccal aspect of the dental implant and increased marginal bone loss (MBL) in width from 1.43 mm at day 0 to 0.85 mm at 6 months as compared with LIPUS-treated group. It reveals that LIPUS has a positive effect on the healing of bone, and the loss of marginal bone in the control group was contributed by not using US therapy. This finding is consistent with those of [26, 84–86].

Angle et al. [79] explained in his vitro study, using rat bone marrow stromal cells that the LIPUS intensities below 30 mW/cm^2 are able to provoke phenotypic responses in bone cells. They cultured bone cells under defined conditions with intensities of 2, 15, and 30 mW/cm^2, compared them with the control group (0 mW/cm^2), and then studied them at early (cell activation), middle (differentiation into osteogenic cells), and late (biological mineralization) stages of osteogenic differentiation. They concluded that LIPUS with intensities of 2, 15, and 30 mW/cm^2 showed a positive effect on osteogenic differentiation of rat bone marrow stromal cells in early stage compared with the control group. Monden et al. [87] also suggested that the injured bone may be treated with LIPUS, as LIPUS has the capability to induce the cellular as well as molecular pathways of bone healing. LIPUS treatment matures the newly formed bone in the cortical bone area producing bone differentiation markers, osteocalcin (OCN) and osteopontin (OPN), and reduces the depression by enhancing the periosteal cellular differentiation. In vitro studies have shown that LIPUS leads to the increased expression of genes related to the bone formation. These genes include osteocalcin, aggrecan, bone sialoprotein, insulin-like growth factor-I, collagen types I and X, transforming growth factor beta, alkaline phosphatase, and runt-related gene-2 [88, 89].

Additionally, LIPUS treatment also promotes the synthesis of protein and uptake of calcium by osteoblasts. LIPUS treatment also plays an important role in the remodeling of the bone by stimulating the cyclooxygenase pathway. LIPUS increases the expression of COX-2 gene that promotes the synthesis of prostaglandin E2 (PGE2) in the osteoblasts [88, 89].

Huang et al. [90] concluded in his recent study in vitro that the LIPUS stimulates the expression of BMP-2 which means positive effects of LIPUS on osteogenesis. In vitro study by Sun et al. [91] showed that LIPUS upregulated osteoblasts and downregulated osteoclasts in the rat alveolar mononuclear cells. Lu et al. [92] explained that the mechanical signals from LIPUS could stimulate osteoblasts by means of gene expression and stimulated proteins that were translated by these genes causing activation of apoptotic genes and osteogenesis in acceleration of the tissue remodeling and expedite clinical outcomes as we have seen in our current study.

Iwanabe et al. [93] demonstrated in his recent study in vitro that the number of cells at 5 days after LIPUS exposure was significantly higher than that of the control, while that at 7 days was about 35% higher than that of the control. This means that LIPUS has the potential to be an effective agent in inducing migration, proliferation, and cell differentiation.

In vitro as well as in vivo studies, using animal models showed that LIPUS has stimulatory effect on cellular activity, release of cytokines, and bone healing [94]. Cell physiology is directly affected by LIPUS. It increases the uptake of calcium by the developing cartilage and bone cells in the culture. It also stimulates a large number of genes that help in the process of healing [62]. Barzelai et al. [95] reported that LIPUS not only modulates the expression of genes, but it also enhances the process of angiogenesis and increases the flow of blood at the site of fracture.

4.4 Clinical significance

- LIPUS may be utilized as treatment modality to save dental implant with questionable primary stability during stage I implant placement, with the aim of achieving adequate osseointegration and improving implant success.

- LIPUS can be recruited to promote and accelerate healing time particularly in patients with medical conditions such as diabetes mellitus and other diseases.

- The clinical results shown in this study confirmed that low-intensity pulsed ultrasound (LIPUS) presents low toxicity, noninvasiveness, and repeated applicability. The risk of thermal injury is unfounded.

- Application of LIPUS on dental implant wound at 2 weeks postoperative seems to be a favorable time when the acute inflammatory phase has subsided and the cellular proliferative phase has actively began.

- RFA gives clear image about the stability of the implant and the condition of the bone around implant.

5. Conclusion

5.1 Summary and conclusion

Animal experiments using LIPUS for healing of wounds have shown effective and favorable results with histological evidence. The effects of the ultrasound waves on the cell and molecular biology phenomena of wound healing have further confirmed the fundamental mechanisms underlying this interesting wound healing treatment modality. However, we still lack clinical studies in this field, and our study is one of the few clinical trials of the effect of ultrasound therapy on osseo-integration and marginal bone loss around implant-supported prosthesis, which showed favorable results. We have compared and contrasted two groups of patients receiving implant therapy where the first group was given LIPUS during the early healing period and post loading as an additional treatment modality and the second group was allowed to heal in the conventional way. Comparative bone thickness measurements using CBCT images and implant stability measurements using RFA values showed consistently higher stability with an increase in bone thickness (height and width), and the ultrasound therapy group demonstrated much higher implant stability values than the control group.

The overall clinical results contribute to the following findings:

- LIPUS enhances bone formation around dental implants as confirmed by radiological investigations, RFA values, and pre and post prosthetic loading behaviors.

- LIPUS technique employed in this study promoted increased in buccal bone plate height and width much more than that occurred in the palatal side. This may be attributed to the design of the US delivery probe.

- With an increase in bone height and width, we expect a simultaneous increase in bone-implant contact that leads to higher osseointegration as evidenced by RFA values.

Acknowledgements

This work was supported by Research University Individual (RUI) grant, account no. 1001/PPSG/812207 from Universiti Sains Malaysia (USM).

Abbreviations

μCT	micro-CT
2-D	two dimensional
3-D	three dimensional
AB	apico-buccal
AD	apico-distal
ALP	alkaline phosphatase
AM	apico-mesial
AP	apico-palatal
BMP	bone morphogenetic proteins
CB	corono-buccal

CBCT	cone beam computed tomography
COX-2	cyclooxygenase-2
CP	corono-palatal
DBM	demineralized bone matrix
ECs	endothelia cells
Erk	extracellular signal-regulated kinase
et al.	and another people
FAK	focal adhesion kinase
FGF2	fibroblast growth factor-2
HPDLC	human periodontal ligament cells
iNOS/NO	inducible nitric oxide synthase
ISQ	implant stability quotient
MARK	mitogen-activated protein kinase
MBL	marginal bone loss
MSCs	mesenchymal stem cells
OCN	osteocalcin
OPN	osteopontin
OSX	osteoblast-specific transcription factor Osterix
PGE2	prostaglandin E2
RFA	resonance frequency analysis
ROI	region of interest
SD	sagitto-distal
SM	sagitto-mesial
UDHS	University Dental Hospital Sharjah
US	ultrasound
USM	Universiti Sains Malaysia
VEGF	vascular endothelial growth factor
VSCCs	voltage-sensitive calcium channels
β	beta

Author details

Elaf Akram Abdulhameed[1,2*], Marzuki Omar[2] and A.R. Samsudin[1]

1 Sharjah Institute for Medical Research, University of Sharjah, UAE

2 University Science Malaysia (USM), Malaysia

*Address all correspondence to: elaf.alzubaidi@gmail.com

IntechOpen

© 2019 The Author(s). Licensee IntechOpen. This chapter is distributed under the terms of the Creative Commons Attribution License (http://creativecommons.org/licenses/by/3.0), which permits unrestricted use, distribution, and reproduction in any medium, provided the original work is properly cited. CC BY

References

[1] Jayesh RS, Dhinakarsamy V. Osseointegration. Journal of Pharmacy and Bioallied Sciences. 2015;7(1):226-232

[2] Kishore K, Anne G, Mohan T, Kumar K, Dev J, Rakesh R, et al. Evaluation of crestal bone loss around two different implant systems supporting a mandibular overdenture-a clinical study. Indian Journal of Dental Sciences. 2014;**6**(2):001-004. ISSN: 0976-4003

[3] Eriksson A. The long-term efficacy of currently used dental implants: A review and proposed criteria of success. The International Journal of Oral and Maxillofacial Implants. 1986;**1**:11-25

[4] Jadhav R, Sabane A, Thareja A, Gandhi P. Dental implant in diabetic patients: Statement of facts. Indian Journal of Oral Sciences. 2015;**6**(2):47. DOI: 10.4103/0976-6944.162628

[5] Mavrogenis A, Dimitriou R, Parvizi J, Babis G. Biology of implant osseointegration. Journal of Musculoskeletal and Neuronal Interactions. 2009;**9**(2):61-71

[6] Parithimarkalaignan S, Padmanabhan TV. Osseointegration: An update. Journal of Indian Prosthodontic Society. 2013;**13**(1):2-6. DOI: 10.1007/s13191-013-0252-z

[7] Fyhrie D. Summary—Measuring "bone quality". Journal of Musculoskeletal and Neuronal Interactions. 2004;**5**(4):318-320

[8] Ibrahim N, Parsa A, Hassan B, van der Stelt P, Wismeijer D. Diagnostic imaging of trabecular bone microstructure for oral implants: A literature review. Dento Maxillo Facial Radiology. 2013;**42**(3):20120075. DOI: 10.1259/dmfr.20120075

[9] Sievänen H, Kannus P, Järvinen TL. Bone quality: An empty term. PLoS Medicine. 2007;**4**(3):e27. DOI: 10.1371/journal.pmed.0040027

[10] Marcantonio C, Nicoli LG, Junior E, Zandim-Barcelos DL. Prevalence and possible risk factors of peri-implantitis: A concept review. The Journal of Contemporary Dental Practice. 2015;**16**(9):750-757

[11] Åstrand P, Engquist B, Dahlgren S, Gröndahl K, Engquist E, Feldmann H. Astra Tech and Brånemark system implants: A 5-year prospective study of marginal bone reactions. Clinical Oral Implants Research. 2004;**15**(4):413-420

[12] Enkling N, Johren P, Katsoulis J, Bayer S, Jervoe-Storm PM, Mericske-Stern R, et al. Influence of platform switching on bone-level alterations: A three-year randomized clinical trial. Journal of Dental Research. 2013;**92**(12 Suppl):139S-145S. DOI: 10.1177/0022034513504953

[13] Tadi DP, Pinisetti S, Gujjalapudi M, Kakaraparthi S, Kolasani B, Vadapalli SHB. Evaluation of initial stability and crestal bone loss in immediate implant placement: An in vivo study. Journal of International Society of Preventive and Community Dentistry. 2014;**4**(3):139-144

[14] Nandal S, Ghalaut P, Shekhawat H. A radiological evaluation of marginal bone around dental implants: An in-vivo study. National Journal of Maxillofacial Surgery. 2014;**5**(2):126-137. DOI: 10.4103/0975-5950.154813

[15] Salvi GE, Lang NP. Diagnostic parameters for monitoring peri-implant conditions. The International Journal of Oral and Maxillofacial Implants. 2004;**19**(7):116-127

[16] Hof M, Pommer B, Zukic N, Vasak C, Lorenzoni M, Zechner W. Influence of prosthetic parameters on peri-implant bone resorption in the first year of loading: A multi-factorial analysis. Clinical Implant Dentistry and Related Research. 2015;**17**(1):183-191. DOI: 10.1111/cid.12153

[17] Al-Juboori MJ, Ab Rahman S, Hassan A, Bin Ismail IH, Tawfiq OF. What is the effect of initial implant position on the crestal bone level in flap and flapless technique during healing period? Journal of Periodontal and Implant Science. 2013;**43**(4):153-159. DOI: 10.5051/jpis.2013.43.4.153

[18] Al-Juboori M, Bin AS, Jassan A. Comparison of flapless and conventional flap and the effect on crestal bone resorption during a 12-week healing period. Dental Implantology Update. 2012;**23**(2):9-16

[19] Becker W, Wikesjo UM, Sennerby L, Qahash M, Hujoel P, Goldstein M, et al. Histologic evaluation of implants following flapless and flapped surgery: A study in canines. Journal of Periodontology. 2006;**77**(10):1717-1722. DOI: 10.1902/jop.2006.060090

[20] Gomez-Roman G. Influence of flap design on peri-implant interproximal crestal bone loss around single-tooth implants. The International Journal of Oral and Maxillofacial Implants. 2001;**16**(1):61-67

[21] Jeong SM, Choi BH, Li J, Xuan F. Simultaneous flapless implant placement and peri-implant defect correction: An experimental pilot study in dogs. Journal of Periodontology. 2008;**79**(5):876-880. DOI: 10.1902/jop.2008.070539

[22] Levin MP, Grower MF, Cutright DE, Getter L. The effects of length of surgery on healing of full and partial thickness flaps. Journal of Oral Pathology and Medicine. 1977;**6**(3):152-160

[23] Ozan O, Turkyilmaz I, Yilmaz B. A preliminary report of patients treated with early loaded implants using computerized tomography-guided surgical stents: Flapless versus conventional flapped surgery. Journal of Oral Rehabilitation. 2007;**34**(11):835-840

[24] Rego EB, Takata T, Tanne K, Tanaka E. Current status of low intensity pulsed ultrasound for dental purposes. The Open Dentistry Journal. 2012;**6**(1):220-225

[25] Della Rocca GJ. The science of ultrasound therapy for fracture healing. Indian journal of orthopaedics. 2009;**43**(2):121-126

[26] Chen K, Hao J, Noritake K, Yamashita Y, Kuroda S, Kasugai S. Effects of low intensity pulsed ultrasound stimulation on bone regeneration in rat parietal bone defect model. Journal of Regenerative Medicine. 2013;**2**(1):8-14

[27] Tanzer M, Kantor S, Bobyn J. Enhancement of bone growth into porous intramedullary implants using non-invasive low intensity ultrasound. Journal of Orthopaedic Research. 2001;**19**(2):195-199

[28] Cameron MH. Physical Agents in Rehabilitation: From Research to Practice. Vol. 4. China: Elsevier Health Sciences; 2013

[29] Yang PC. Ultrasound-guided transthoracic biopsy of peripheral lung, pleural, and chest-wall lesions. Journal of Thoracic Imaging. 1997;**12**(4):272-284

[30] Yang PC. Ultrasound-guided transthoracic biopsy of the chest. Radiologic Clinics of North America. 2000;**38**(2):323-343

[31] Yang PC, Lee YC, Yu CJ, Chang DB, Wu HD, Lee LN, et al. Ultrasonographically guided biopsy of thoracic tumors. A comparison of large-bore cutting biopsy with fine-needle aspiration. Cancer. 1992;**69**(10):2553-2560

[32] Harris M. The conservative management of osteoradionecrosis of the mandible with ultrasound therapy. British Journal of Oral and Maxillofacial Surgery. 1992;**30**(5):313-318

[33] Nelson AB, Krispel CM, Sekirnjak C, du Lac S. Long-lasting increases in intrinsic excitability triggered by inhibition. Neuron. 2003;**40**(3):609-620

[34] Leung K, Cheung W, Zhang C, Lee K, Lo H. Low intensity pulsed ultrasound stimulates osteogenic activity of human periosteal cells. Clinical Orthopaedics and Related Research. 2004;**418**:253-259

[35] Yang KH, Parvizi J, Wang SJ, Lewallen DG, Kinnick RR, Greenleaf JF, et al. Exposure to low-intensity ultrasound increases aggrecan gene expression in a rat femur fracture model. Journal of Orthopaedic Research. 1996;**14**(5):802-809

[36] Yang RS, Lin WL, Chen YZ, Tang CH, Huang TH, Lu BY, et al. Regulation by ultrasound treatment on the integrin expression and differentiation of osteoblasts. Bone. 2005;**36**(2):276-283

[37] John P, Poulose C, George B. Therapeutic ultrasound in fracture healing: The mechanism of osteoinduction. Indian Journal of Orthopaedics. 2008;**42**(4):444

[38] Ustun Y, Erdogan O, Kurkcu M, Akova T, Damlar İ. Effects of low-intensity pulsed ultrasound on dental implant osseointegration: A preliminary report. European Journal of Dentistry. 2008;**2**:254-262

[39] Gardinier JD, Majumdar S, Duncan RL, Wang L. Cyclic hydraulic pressure and fluid flow differentially modulate cytoskeleton re-organization in MC3T3 osteoblasts. Cellular and Molecular Bioengineering. 2009;**2**(1):133-143

[40] Katiyar A, Duncan RL, Sarkar K. Ultrasound stimulation increases proliferation of MC3T3-E1 preosteoblast-like cells. Journal of Therapeutic Ultrasound. 2014;**2**(1):1-10. DOI: 10.1186/2050-5736-1182-1181

[41] Ingber D. Integrins as mechanochemical transducers. Current Opinion in Cell Biology. 1991;**3**(5):841-848

[42] Liedert A, Claes L, Ignatius A. Signal transduction pathways involved in mechanotransduction in osteoblastic and mesenchymal stem cells. In: Mechanosensitive Ion Channels. Springer; 2008. pp. 253-265

[43] Gillespie PG, Walker RG. Molecular basis of mechanosensory transduction. Nature. 2001;**413**(6852):194-202

[44] Padilla F, Puts R, Vico L, Raum K. Stimulation of bone repair with ultrasound: A review of the possible mechanic effects. Ultrasonics. 2014;**54**(5):1125-1145

[45] Sato M, Nagata K, Kuroda S, Horiuchi S, Nakamura T, Karima M, et al. Low-intensity pulsed ultrasound activates integrin-mediated mechanotransduction pathway in synovial cells. Annals of Biomedical Engineering. 2014;**42**(10):2156-2163

[46] Argintar E, Edwards S, Delahay J. Bone morphogenetic proteins in orthopaedic trauma surgery. Injury International Journal. 2011;**42**(8):730-734

[47] Tang CH, Yang RS, Huang TH, Lu DY, Chuang WJ, Huang TF, et al.

Ultrasound stimulates cyclooxygenase-2 expression and increases bone formation through integrin, focal adhesion kinase, phosphatidylinositol 3-kinase, and Akt pathway in osteoblasts. Molecular Pharmacology. 2006;**69**(6):2047-2057

[48] Watabe H, Furuhama T, Tani-Ishii N, Mikuni-Takagaki Y. Mechanotransduction activates α 5 β 1 integrin and PI3K/Akt signaling pathways in mandibular osteoblasts. Experimental Cell Research. 2011;**317**(18):2642-2649

[49] Zhou S, Schmelz A, Seufferlein T, Li Y, Zhao J, Bachem MG. Molecular mechanisms of low intensity pulsed ultrasound in human skin fibroblasts. Journal of Biological Chemistry. 2004;**279**(52):54463-54469

[50] Ren L, Yang Z, Song J, Wang Z, Deng F, Li W. Involvement of p38 MAPK pathway in low intensity pulsed ultrasound induced osteogenic differentiation of human periodontal ligament cells. Ultrasonics. 2013;**53**(3):686-690

[51] Whitney NP, Lamb AC, Louw TM, Subramanian A. Integrin-mediated mechanotransduction pathway of low-intensity continuous ultrasound in human chondrocytes. Ultrasound in Medicine and Biology. 2012;**38**(10):1734-1743

[52] Kang KS, Lee SJ, Lee H, Moon W, Cho DW. Effects of combined mechanical stimulation on the proliferation and differentiation of pre-osteoblasts. Experimental and Molecular Medicine. 2011;**43**(6):367-373

[53] Pitt WG, Ross SA. Ultrasound increases the rate of bacterial cell growth. Biotechnology Progress. 2003;**19**(3):1038-1044

[54] Kleinheinz J, Stratmann U, Joos U, Wiesmann H-P. VEGF-activated angiogenesis during bone regeneration. Journal of Oral and Maxillofacial Surgery. 2005;**63**(9):1310-1316

[55] Laranjeira MS, Fernandes MH, Monteiro FJ. Reciprocal induction of human dermal microvascular endothelial cells and human mesenchymal stem cells: Time-dependent profile in a co-culture system. Cell Proliferation. 2012;**45**(4):320-334

[56] Matsumoto T, Goto D, Sato S. Subtraction micro-computed tomography of angiogenesis and osteogenesis during bone repair using synchrotron radiation with a novel contrast agent. Laboratory Investigation. 2013;**93**(9):1054-1063

[57] Chen P, Yin H, Wang Y, Wang Y, Xie L. Inhibition of VEGF expression and corneal neovascularization by shRNA targeting HIF-1α in a mouse model of closed eye contact lens wear. Molecular Vision. 2012;**18**:864-873

[58] Shiraishi R, Masaki C, Toshinaga A, Okinaga T, Nishihara T, Yamanaka N, et al. The effects of low-intensity pulsed ultrasound exposure on gingival cells. Journal of Periodontology. 2011;**82**(10):1498-1503

[59] El-Bialy TH, Royston TJ, Magin RL, Evans CA, Zaki AE-M, Frizzell LA. The effect of pulsed ultrasound on mandibular distraction. Annals of Biomedical Engineering. 2002;**30**(10):1251-1261

[60] De Almeida MS, Maciel CD, Pereira JC. Proposal for an ultrasonic tool to monitor the osseointegration of dental implants. Sensors. 2007;**7**(7):1224-1237

[61] Komatsu DE, Warden SJ. The control of fracture healing and its

therapeutic targeting: Improving upon nature. Journal of Cellular Biochemistry. 2010;**109**(2):302-311

[62] Rubin C, Bolander M, Ryaby JP, Hadjiargyrou M. The use of low-intensity ultrasound to accelerate the healing of fractures. The Journal of Bone and Joint Surgery. American Volume. 2001;**83**(2):259-259

[63] Duarte L. The stimulation of bone growth by ultrasound. Archives of Orthopaedic and Traumatic Surgery. 1983;**101**(3):153-159

[64] Turner-Walker G, Nielsen-Marsh C, Syversen U, Kars H, Collins M. Sub-micron spongiform porosity is the major ultra-structural alteration occurring in archaeological bone. International Journal of Osteoarchaeology. 2002;**12**(6):407-414

[65] Kerr EN, Mealey BL, Noujeim ME, Lasho DJ, Nummikoski PV, Mellonig JT. The effect of ultrasound on bone dimensional changes following extraction: a pilot study. Journal of periodontology. 2008;79(2):283-290

[66] Wilderman MN, Pennel BM, King K, Barron JM. Histogenesis of repair following osseous surgery. Journal of Periodontology. 1970;**41**(10):551-565

[67] Wennström JL, Ekestubbe A, Gröndahl K, Karlsson S, Lindhe J. Implant-supported single-tooth restorations: A 5-year prospective study. Journal of Clinical Periodontology. 2005;**32**(6):567-574

[68] Sakka S, Baroudi K, Nassani MZ. Factors associated with early and late failure of dental implants. Journal of Investigative and Clinical Dentistry. 2012;**3**(4):258-261

[69] Pommer B, Frantal S, Willer J, Posch M, Watzek G, Tepper G. Impact of dental implant length on early failure rates: A meta-analysis of observational studies. Journal of Clinical Periodontology. 2011;**38**(9):856-863

[70] Romeo E, Ghisolfi M, Rozza R, Chiapasco M, Lops D. Short (8-mm) dental implants in the rehabilitation of partial and complete edentulism: A 3-to 14-year longitudinal study. International Journal of Prosthodontics. 2006;**19**(6):586-592

[71] Cardaropoli G, Araújo M, Hayacibara R, Sukekava F, Lindhe J. Healing of extraction sockets and surgically produced–augmented and non-augmented–defects in the alveolar ridge. An experimental study in the dog. Journal of Clinical Periodontology. 2005;**32**(5):435-440

[72] Doan N, Reher P, Meghji S, Harris M. In vitro effects of therapeutic ultrasound on cell proliferation, protein synthesis, and cytokine production by human fibroblasts, osteoblasts, and monocytes. Journal of Oral and Maxillofacial Surgery. 1999;**57**(4):409-419

[73] Dinno M, Dyson M, Young S, Mortimer A, Hart J, Crum L. The significance of membrane changes in the safe and effective use of therapeutic and diagnostic ultrasound. Physics in Medicine and Biology. 1989;**34**(11):1543-1552

[74] Pilla A, Mont M, Nasser P, Khan S, Figueiredo M, Kaufman J, et al. Non-invasive low-intensity pulsed ultrasound accelerates bone healing in the rabbit. Journal of Orthopaedic Trauma. 1990;**4**(3):246-253

[75] Kamath JB, Jayasheelan N, Reddy B, Muhammed S, Savur A. The effect of low-intensity pulsed ultrasound therapy on fracture healing. Muller Journal of Medical Sciences and Research. 2015;**6**(1):49-53

[76] Erdogan Ö, Esen E. Biological aspects and clinical importance of ultrasound therapy in bone healing. Journal of Ultrasound in Medicine. 2009;**28**(6):765-776

[77] Miller DL, Smith NB, Bailey MR, Czarnota GJ, Hynynen K, Makin IRS. Overview of therapeutic ultrasound applications and safety considerations. Journal of Ultrasound in Medicine. 2012;**31**(4):623-634

[78] Allen RJ. Physical agents used in the management of chronic pain by physical therapists. Physical Medicine and Rehabilitation Clinics of North America. 2006;**17**(2):315-345

[79] Angle S, Sena K, Sumner D, Virdi A. Osteogenic differentiation of rat bone marrow stromal cells by various intensities of low-intensity pulsed ultrasound. Ultrasonics. 2011;**51**(3):281-288

[80] Ebadi S, Ansari NN, Henschke N, Naghdi S, van Tulder MW. The effect of continuous ultrasound on chronic low back pain: Protocol of a randomized controlled trial. BMC Musculoskeletal Disorders. 2011;**12**(1):1-6. DOI: 10.1186/1471-2474-1112-1159

[81] Isoda K, Ayukawa Y, Tsukiyama Y, Sogo M, Matsushita Y, Koyano K. Relationship between the bone density estimated by cone-beam computed tomography and the primary stability of dental implants. Clinical Oral Implants Research. 2012;**23**(7):832-836

[82] Reher P, Doan N, Bradnock B, Meghji S, Harris M. Effect of ultrasound on the production of IL-8, basic FGF and VEGF. Cytokine. 1999;**11**(6):416-423

[83] Ramli R, Peter R, Malcolm H, Sajeda M. The effect of ultrasound on angiogenesis: An in vivo study using the chick chorioallantoic membrane. The International Journal of Oral and Maxillofacial Implants. 2009;**24**:591-596

[84] Maddi A, Hai H, Ong S-T, Sharp L, Harris M, Meghji S. Long wave ultrasound may enhance bone regeneration by altering OPG/RANKL ratio in human osteoblast-like cells. Bone. 2006;**39**(2):283-288

[85] Ganzorig K, Kuroda S, Maeda Y, Mansjur K, Sato M, Nagata K, et al. Low-intensity pulsed ultrasound enhances bone formation around miniscrew implants. Archives of Oral Biology. 2015;**60**(6):902-910

[86] Miura K, Motoyoshi M, Inaba M, Iwai H, Karasawa Y, Shimizu N. A preliminary study of the effects of low-intensity pulsed ultrasound exposure on the stability of orthodontic miniscrews in growing rats. The European Journal of Orthodontics. 2014;**36**(4):419-424

[87] Monden K, Sasaki H, Yoshinari M, Yajima Y. Effect of low-intensity pulsed ultrasound (LIPUS) with different frequency on bone defect healing. Journal of Hard Tissue Biology. 2015;**24**(2):189-198

[88] Chen YJ, Wangb CJ, YangL KD, Chang PR, Huango HC, Sunc Y-THYC, et al. Pertussis toxin-sensitive Gai protein and ERK-dependent pathways mediate ultrasound promotion of osteogenic transcription in human osteoblasts1. FEBS Letters. 2003;**554**:154-158

[89] Mukai S, Ito H, Nakagawa Y, Akiyama H, Miyamoto M, Nakamura T. Transforming growth factor-β 1 mediates the effects of low-intensity pulsed ultrasound in chondrocytes. Ultrasound in Medicine & Biology. 2005;**31**(12):1713-1721

[90] Huang W, Hasegawa T, Imai Y, Takeda D, Akashi M, Komori T. Low-intensity pulsed ultrasound enhances

bone morphogenetic protein expression of human mandibular fracture haematoma-derived cells. International Journal of Oral and Maxillofacial Surgery. 2015;**44**(7):929-935

[91] Sun JS, Hong RC, Chang WHS, Chen LT, Lin FH, Liu HC. In vitro effects of low-intensity ultrasound stimulation on the bone cells. Journal of Biomedical Materials Research. 2001;**57**(3):449-456

[92] Lu H, Qin L, Lee K, Cheung W, Chan K, Leung K. Identification of genes responsive to low-intensity pulsed ultrasound stimulations. Biochemical and Biophysical Research Communications. 2009;**378**(3):569-573

[93] Iwanabe Y, Masaki C, Tamura A, Tsuka S, Mukaibo T, Kondo Y, et al. The effect of low-intensity pulsed ultrasound on wound healing using scratch assay in epithelial cells. Journal of Prosthodontic Research. 2016;60(4):308-314. DOI: 10.1016/j.jpor.2016.03.002

[94] Li J, Chang W, Lin J, Ruaan R, Liu H, Sun J. Cytokine release from osteoblasts in response to ultrasound stimulation. Biomaterials. 2003;**24**(13):2379-2385

[95] Barzelai S, Sharabani-Yosef O, Holbova R, Castel D, Walden R, Engelberg S, et al. Low-intensity ultrasound induces angiogenesis in rat hind-limb ischemia. Ultrasound in Medicine and Biology. 2006;**32**(1):139-145

Chapter 2

Cell Attachment and Osteoinductive Properties of Tissue Engineered, Demineralized Bone Fibers for Bone Void Filling Applications

Julie B. McLean, Nigeste Carter, Payal Sohoni and Mark A. Moore

Abstract

Demineralized bone matrices (DBMs) have been used in a wide variety of clinical applications involving bone repair. Ideally, DBMs should provide osteoinductive and osteoconductive properties, while offering versatile handling capabilities. With this, a novel fiber technology, LifeNet Health-Moldable Demineralized Fibers (L-MDF), was recently developed. Human cortical bone was milled and demineralized to produce L-MDF. Subsequently, the fibers were lyophilized and terminally sterilized using low-dose and low-temperature gamma irradiation. Using L929 mouse fibroblasts, L-MDF underwent cytotoxicity testing to confirm lack of a cytotoxic response. An alamarBlue assay and scanning electron microscopy demonstrated L-MDF supported the cellular function and attachment of bone-marrow mesenchymal stem cells (BM-MSCs). Using an enzyme-linked immunosorbent assay, L-MDF demonstrated BMP-2 and 7 levels similar to those reported in the literature. *In vivo* data from an athymic mouse model implanted with L-MDF demonstrated the formation of new bone elements and blood vessels. This study showed that L-MDF have the necessary characteristics of a bone void filler to treat osseous defects.

Keywords: demineralized bone matrix, osteoinductive, osteoconductive, allograft, growth factors, bone formation

1. Introduction

Bone voids may occur due to trauma, surgery, tumor resections, or other factors. For decades, surgeons have used bone grafting to treat a wide variety of bone defects. Bone grafts may contain up to three of the vital properties necessary for bone formation: osteoconductivity, osteoinductivity, and osteogenicity [1]. The property of osteoconductivity describes the way the graft acts as a scaffold on which host cells can attach and proliferate, leading to osseointegration. Osteoinductivity, on the other hand, describes the cellular signaling potential of a graft. Whether endogenous or recombinant, specific growth factors, such as bone morphogenetic protein 2 (BMP-2), attract host cells to a graft and encourage mesenchymal stem cells to differentiate into lineage-committed bone cells. Finally, osteogenicity describes the ability of a bone graft to form bone matrix directly, which can only happen when live cells capable of producing bone matrix are contained within the graft. Bone graft options may contain varying amounts of these properties and are chosen based on the characteristics that the patient needs in order to achieve bone fusion. There are several graft options available, including autograft, synthetic bone substitutes, and allografts.

Autologous bone is harvested from the site of surgery in the patient or a second site, such as the iliac crest. It is still considered the gold standard by many surgeons because it can theoretically provide all three vital properties for bone formation, does not provoke an immune response, and has a long history of use. However, the use of autograft bone is associated with several disadvantages such as donor site morbidity, insufficient supply, and variable quality [2, 3]. Up to 30% of patients experience significant donor site morbidity as well as infection risk, increased operative time, blood loss, and the potential for arterial and nerve injury [4]. Additionally, autograft is limited, and the quality may be poor depending on the patient's health. For example, diabetes, low bone mass, and smoking can all increase the risk of fusion failure as well as intraoperative complications [5].

Synthetic bone substitutes are designed with the goal of mimicking the natural properties of human bone. They can be comprised of a variety of materials including but not limited to, ceramics, cements, and bioactive glass. These grafts are generally biocompatible, osteoconductive, and may be mechanically similar to bone [6, 7]. This category of graft has typically been manufactured to contain porosity similar to bone, but may lack other desirable surface properties, such as hydrophilicity or a rough surface on which cells can attach. Synthetic bone substitutes have gained popularity due to reduced cost and ready availability; however, they may have mismatched resorption rates compared to bone and generally lack osteogenic and osteoinductive properties [8]. Some synthetics, such as recombinant human BMP-2, depend almost solely upon osteoinductivity and often result in rapid bone formation. However, several studies indicate substantial side effects, including osteolysis, heterotopic bone formation, and swelling/edema [9–11]. While synthetics have improved over the last few decades, mimicking natural bone has proven difficult, and allografts, being natural bone, have continued to be a reliable source of grafting material.

Allograft bone is obtained from deceased human donors and has a long history of use. It is readily available in a variety of forms, shapes, and sizes providing surgeons with several graft options suitable for various procedures [12–14]. Allografts can provide up to all three properties necessary for bone formation. For example, mineralized bone allografts have similar osteoconductive properties to autograft while avoiding complications such as donor site morbidity [15]. Some mineralized grafts have been processed to increase desirable characteristics such as increased surface area on which cells can attach as well as increased coefficient of friction to prevent the graft from shifting once implanted. Other allografts, such as demineralized bone matrix (DBM) are both osteoconductive and osteoinductive. To produce DBMs, acid demineralization is used to remove a portion of the mineral component of bone, thus exposing the active signaling proteins necessary to induce new bone formation. The ability of DBMs to facilitate bone healing was demonstrated in clinical applications as early as 1889 when Dr. Nicholas Senn reported using demineralized bone as a vehicle for antiseptics to treat patients with osteomyelitis [16]. However, it was not until 1965, when Dr. Marshall Urist characterized specific proteins trapped within the bone matrix, that it was understood that bone morphogenetic proteins (BMPs) contributed to the osteoinductive property of DBMs [17]. Since the discovery of BMPs, other proteins, such as those associated with angiogenesis, have also been found to contribute to the process of bone healing and regeneration [18]. In addition to containing active signaling proteins, optimal surface characteristics of DBMs are essential for supporting cellular attachment and proliferation. For example, it is crucial to provide enough space for blood vessel formation and for the patient's own cells to migrate into and proliferate on the scaffold [19, 20]. Therefore, some allograft processors work to maintain ideal porosity for cell migration and angiogenesis. Other processes are designed to create a hospitable topography for cell attachment and proliferation as well as to enhance handling characteristics to facilitate implantation and mitigate migration.

DBMs are available in varying forms, including powders, putty, strips, and moldable paste. These grafts often contain carriers such as glycerol, starch, or hyaluronic acid to improve handling. Without a carrier, bone grafts may be difficult to implant in the desired area, or may drift away from the area during surgical irrigation or exposure to blood. However, despite improved handling characteristics, it has been reported that some carriers may inhibit osteoinductive potential [21]. In addition, a carrier dilutes the bone concentration and may easily elute from the surgical site, effectively reducing the implant volume. With these limitations in mind, a novel DBM with unique fiber technology was recently developed as described in Section 2. These fibers (**Figure 1**) are composed solely of demineralized cortical bone and are designed to provide surface features conducive for cellular attachment and easily moldable handling characteristics, all without the addition of a carrier. The purpose of this chapter is to present original research, detailing the composition, osteoinductive nature, cell attachment properties and endogenous bone growth factor content of these bone fibers through *in vivo* and *in vitro* test methods.

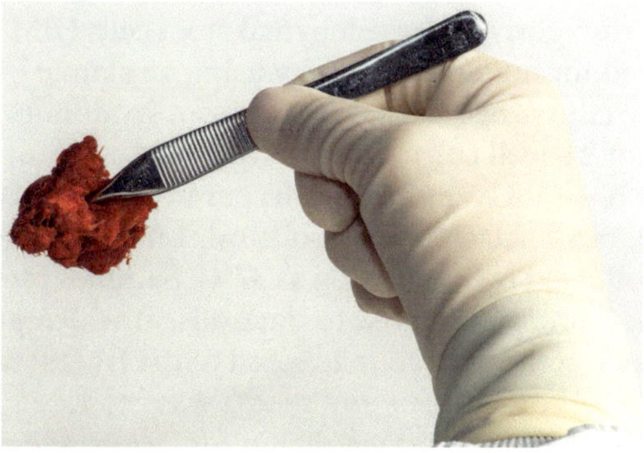

Figure 1.
Rehydrated moldable demineralized fibers.

2. Methodology

2.1 Fiber generation

The fibers described here are referred to as L-MDF (LifeNet Health-Moldable Demineralized Fibers, LifeNet Health, Virginia Beach, VA and clinically available as part of PliaFX® and OraGRAFT® Prime brands). The particular fibers studied below were prepared from human cortical long bones that were aseptically recovered from donors, debrided, and disassociated from marrow and trabecular bone. The resulting tissue was processed by a proprietary computer numerical controlled-milling method (CNC-milled) into long fibers and disinfected using a proprietary process. The fibers were then demineralized using proprietary procedures. Following demineralization, fiber samples were taken to quantify residual calcium levels (average 1.7%) using a calcium reagent kit (Eagle Diagnostics, Cedar Hill, TX).

The demineralized fibers were then freeze-dried, placed in final packaging, and treated via low-dose, low-temperature gamma irradiation, at a level necessary to achieve a sterility assurance level (SAL) of 10^{-6}.

2.2 Cytotoxicity testing of L-MDF using L929 mouse fibroblasts

The cytotoxic potential of L-MDF were quantitatively evaluated by the MTT (3-(4,5-dimethylthiazol-2-yl)-2,5-diphenyltetrazolium bromide) assay using L929 mouse fibroblasts. Three samples of 2.5 cc from each of the six donors (n = 18) were rehydrated with 5 mL sterile saline (0.99% w/v sodium chloride in water). Sample extracts were prepared by incubating 0.2 g of each sample with 1 mL of extraction medium (Minimum Essential Medium supplemented with 10% v/v fetal bovine serum, 100 U mL^{-1} penicillin, 100 μg mL^{-1} streptomycin, and 2 mM L-glutamine) for 24 ± 2 h at 37 ± 1°C. Negative and positive controls were prepared similarly. Extraction medium alone was used as an untreated control "extract" for quantitative comparison of results. L929 mouse fibroblasts were cultured in 96-well microplates to half-confluency and subsequently exposed to 100 μL of sample or control extracts for 24–26 h at 37 ± 1°C. Following extract exposure, cell viability of each well was measured using a MTT assay. The average results for each group were normalized to the untreated control to determine a percent viability. Per ISO 10993-5:2009, percent viability less than 70% indicates a cytotoxic effect.

2.3 *In vitro* metabolic activity of seeded bone marrow-mesenchymal stem cells

Human bone marrow-derived mesenchymal stem cells (BM-MSCs) seeded on L-MDF were measured for metabolic activity using an alamarBlue® assay (Bio-Rad, Raleigh, NC) over the course of 7 days. L-MDF from six donors were placed in triplicate in low-attachment 24-well cell culture plates at a density of 13.1 mg of fiber per cm^2 and seeded with BM-MSCs at 62,500 cells per well on day 0. BM-MSCs without fibers served as the control. After 2–4 h in culture, 1 mL of complete media was added to each well, followed by incubation at 37°C. Samples remained in the incubator until specific time points designated for analysis, at which point media was replaced. The metabolic activity of cells adhered to the fibers was measured after 1, 4 and 7 days in culture. At each time point media was aspirated and replaced with 1 mL of 10% alamarBlue reagent and incubated for an average of 2 h at 37°C. The solution was collected from each sample, centrifuged to pellet any debris, and measured in a 96-well plate at 544 nm excitation/592 nm emission. Fluorescence was recorded using relative fluorescence units (RFUs), and values were normalized to its time-matched control. A one-way ANOVA in conjunction with a Tukey post-hoc was used to determine differences in metabolic activity over time.

2.4 *In vitro* cellular attachment of seeded bone marrow-mesenchymal cells

Scanning electron microscopy (SEM) was used to qualitatively evaluate the attachment and morphology of cells seeded on four L-MDF samples (25 ± 1 mg) at 0.5–1 h, 1 and 7 days in culture. The fibers were placed in separate glass scintillation vials with 1 mL of complete media and incubated at 37°C. Following incubation, excess media was aspirated and BM-MSCs were seeded at 100,000 per cells per vial. At each time point, corresponding vials were removed from the incubator, excess media was removed, and 3 mL of 2.5% glutaraldehyde in cacodylate buffer was added to fix the samples. Cell-seeded samples were rinsed in 0.1 M cacodylate buffer, incubated in 1% osmium tetroxide for 60 min, and then dehydrated in a series of ethanol solutions increasing in concentration up to 100%. Samples were then dried via evaporation of a chemical drying agent, hexamethyldisilazane (HMDS). Prior to imaging, all samples were sputter coated in gold palladium for 200 s at 60 mA, then secured to a holder that was placed inside a vacuum-sealed imaging chamber. Samples were then imaged at a magnification 3000× using a Zeiss Gemini HD Scanning Electron Microscope.

2.5 *In vitro* growth factor analysis

L-MDF were analyzed for the presence of BMP-2 and BMP-7 using an enzyme-linked immunosorbent assay (ELISA) (R&D Systems, Minneapolis MN). L-MDF from six donors were weighed (30 ± 10 mg per donor) and placed in microcentrifuge tubes. Samples were then rehydrated with 5 μL of Dulbecco's Modified Eagle Medium (DMEM) per milligram of fiber, followed by the addition of purified collagenase (14.47 Units/mg of fiber). The samples were digested at 37°C with constant mixing for 16–18 h. Digestion solutions were centrifuged to remove remaining undigested components and the supernatants were collected for testing. The resulting solutions were analyzed for BMP content in triplicate using an ELISA assay. The measured BMP content was averaged across all six donors and results were reported in ng protein/g of demineralized fibers.

2.6 *In vivo* osteoinductive potential (OI)

The osteoinductive potential of L-MDF was evaluated using an *in vivo* athymic mouse model at NAMSA (Northwood, Ohio) following American Society for Testing and Materials (ASTM) F-2529 guidelines. Four 20–25 mg replicates of L-MDF were rehydrated with 100–150 μL of sterile 0.9% w/v sodium chloride and loaded into 0.3 cc sterile syringes. Samples were then compressed to remove excess solution, and implanted bi-laterally between the biceps femoris and superficial gluteal muscle of athymic mice. All mice were euthanized 5 weeks post-implantation by carbon dioxide inhalation. Explants were fixed with 10% formalin and bisected along the long axis. Bisects of each explant were paraffin embedded, and three slides were generated each with 4–6 μm-thick tissue sections. Once stained with hematoxylin and eosin (H&E), slides were evaluated by a blinded pathologist. The presence of cartilage, chondroblasts, chondrocytes, osteoblasts, osteocytes, osteoid, newly formed lamellar bone, and bone marrow were evaluated as new bone elements as they are indicators of endochondral bone formation process.

3. Results

3.1 Cytotoxicity

Cytotoxicity assay results showed that negative and positive controls behaved as expected (i.e., percent viability ≥70% for the negative control groups and <70% for the positive control groups). The average percent viability for negative and positive controls were 94 and 4%, respectively. The average percent viability of L-MDF (91%) was above the 70% threshold, and thus, based on the criteria of the protocol and ISO 10993-5 guidelines, L-MDF are considered to be non-cytotoxic.

3.2 L-MDF supports attachment and sustained metabolic activity of bone marrow-mesenchymal stem cells

Overall, the cellular activity of the BM-MSCs was shown to significantly increase over the course of the 7 day investigation. The results indicated that cells seeded on L-MDF showed a significant increase in proliferation between days 4 (51.3 ± 1.2 RFU) and 7 (59.5 ± 1.5 RFU) compared to day 1 (21.3 ± 0.8 RFU) (**Figure 2**).

SEM images confirmed BM-MSC attachment to L-MDF within 30 min of seeding. Cells appeared rounded with numerous folds and ridges and minimal surface contact (**Figure 3A**). After 1 h in culture, BM-MSCs became elongated and began spreading and increasing surface contact with the fibers (**Figure 3B**). After 1 day, imaging showed flattened cells with multiple adhesion points and cellular extensions as well as extracellular matrix (ECM) secretion (**Figure 3C**). By day 7 in culture, BM-MSCs infiltrated between fibers and demonstrated cell-to-cell interactions (**Figure 3D**).

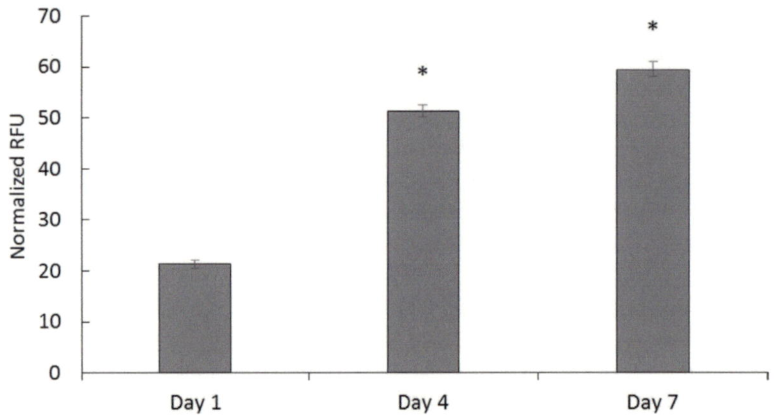

Figure 2.
Proliferation of BM-MSCs attached to L-MDF over 7 days. The average relative fluorescence unit (RFU) values for each set of triplicate test samples were normalized to the average RFU of the corresponding control group (fibers of the respective donor cultured without cells) for all six donors. Asterisks represent statistically significant differences from day 1 proliferation activity.

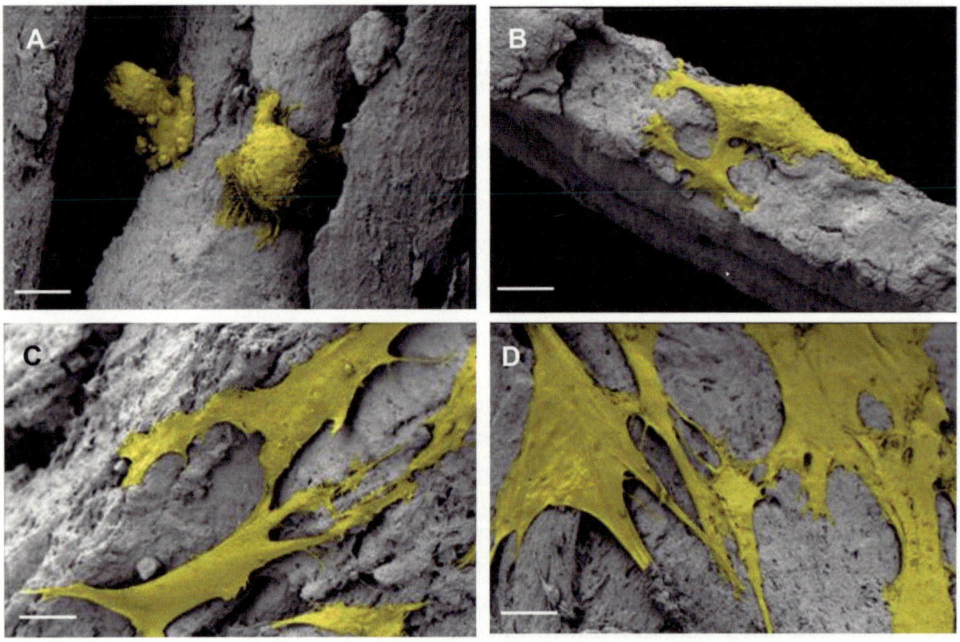

Figure 3.
Representative SEM images illustrating the morphology of cells attached to L-MDF. Following culture for 30 min (A), 1 h (B), 1 day (C) or 7 days (D), respectively, the samples were fixed in 2.5% glutaraldehyde and processed for scanning electron microscopy. Images are representative of all samples evaluated and were taken at 3000× magnification. Scale bar represents 10 μm. Images were pseudo-colored in Adobe Photoshop to distinguish the cells (in yellow) from the fibers.

3.3 L-MDF contains important growth factors and demonstrates new bone formation *in vivo*

The ELISA results indicated the presence of growth factors in L-MDF. The average BMP-2 and 7 concentrations in the samples fibers were 11.24 ± 1.49 and 85.78 ± 6.84 ng/g, respectively (**Figure 4**).

Additionally, in the athymic mouse muscle pouch model, histological analysis revealed new bone elements around and within the implanted scaffold at time of sacrifice (5 weeks; **Figure 5**). Panel A shows a set of merged images that illustrate

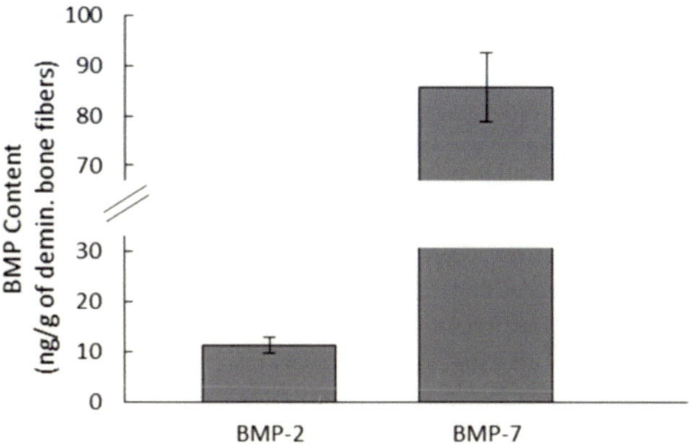

Figure 4.
BMP-2 and BMP-7 content in L-MDF. L-MDF produced from six different donors were digested in collagenase for 16–18 h. Using ELISAs, the resulting digestion solutions were tested for BMP-2 and BMP-7 content in triplicate (mean ∓ SE).

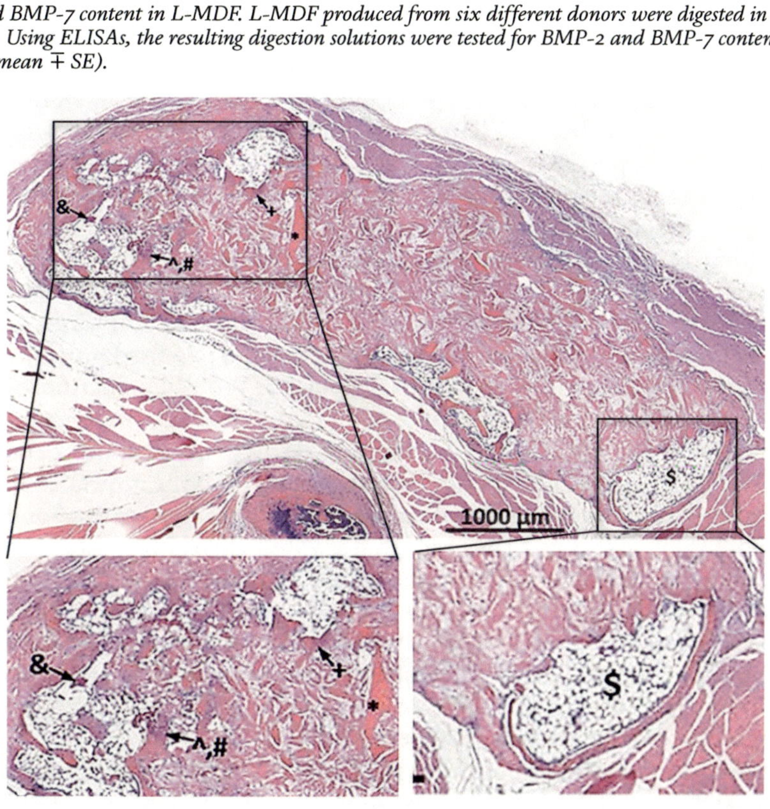

Figure 5.
H&E staining of explants from an athymic nude mouse implanted with L-MDF (*). Merged set of H&E images showing new bone elements present in the entire explant at 35 days post-implantation (4× objective). Expanded areas show the presence of new bone elements such as cartilage (^), chondroblasts/cytes (#), bone marrow ($), new blood vessels (&), and new bone (+) around L-MDF implant (*) at 35 days.

new bone elements present in the explant (4× objective). Panels B and C highlight the presence of new bone elements such as cartilage, chondroblasts/cytes, bone marrow, new blood vessels, and new bone.

4. Discussion

Demineralized bone matrices (DBMs) are widely used in spinal, orthopedic, craniomaxillofacial, and dental procedures to treat bone voids. An ideal DBM provides both osteoinductive and osteoconductive properties to promote new bone formation and provide a scaffold upon which cells can attach and proliferate. Furthermore, DBMs should be malleable and resist graft migration once impacted into a bone defect. To achieve these characteristics important for bone healing, manufacturers use a variety of techniques to process and sterilize DBMs. Despite demineralization being a well-known technique, the proportion of the osteoinductive element—the demineralized bone—of clinically available DBM-based graft materials varies widely by manufacturer. Differences in carrier material and sterilization may also contribute to variability among these grafts. The moldable demineralized fibers described here represent a recently developed allograft configuration that can function as an independent bone void filler without the need of a synthetic carrier. This study was conducted to ensure L-MDF possess the necessary qualities to function in this capacity.

An osteoinductive bone graft has the ability to induce bone growth. Factors such as residual calcium level and growth factor content play important roles in a DBM's ability to grow bone. In particular, residual calcium level can serve as an indicator for the availability of growth factors necessary for bone formation. The literature suggests that DBMs with different degrees of residual calcium show significant differences in osteoinductivity. Zhang et al. evaluated the effects of varying degrees of demineralization, particle size, donor age, and gender on the osteoinductivity of DBM *in vivo* (athymic mouse model) and *in vitro* (alkaline phosphatase assay) [22]. The authors suggested that demineralized bone with a residual calcium level of approximately 2% is "optimally osteoinductive". Similarly, Turonis et al. found that a 2% residual calcium level in human demineralized freeze-dried bone allograft appears to enhance osseous wound healing [23]. The L-MDF samples discussed in this chapter were demineralized using a proprietary and patented process targeted at achieving an optimized level of residual calcium of 1–4%. Furthermore, the presence of specific proteins in DBM is frequently associated with its osteoinductive potential as growth factors can provide signals that direct cellular behavior [18, 22, 24]. In particular, BMP-2 and 7 are important for bone growth as they are known for their "ability to stimulate differentiation of MSCs to osteochondroblastic lineage" [18]. Previous studies have reported a wide span of BMP-2 and BMP-7 levels in demineralized bone, with ranges from 6.5 to 110 and 44 to 125 ng/g demineralized bone, respectively. In this study, ELISA results indicated the presence of BMP-2 and 7 in L-MDF (11.24 ± 1.49 and 85.78 ± 6.84 ng/g) consistent with values reported in the literature. This milieu of growth factors illustrate that L-MDF contain the appropriate trophic factor profile necessary for bone formation and are consistent with expected physiological levels.

The osteoinductive and osteoconductive potential of DBMs are commonly evaluated using an *in vivo* athymic mouse intramuscular pouch model to histologically assess new bone formation [25].

In the study described here, histological analysis revealed the presence of new bone elements demonstrating the osteoinductive potential of L-MDF. In addition, newly formed blood vessels were observed, which can also be indicative of the osteoconductive nature of the bone graft in providing a conducive environment for new bone formation. The surface characteristics of DBMs play an important role in their ability to provide a scaffold for new bone formation [19, 20]. Bone cells need a hospitable environment in which to attach and thrive. In particular, increased surface area, a rough topography, and interconnected networks are known to promote cellular attachment and cell spreading [26]. As demonstrated by the SEM imaging presented here, the long, interconnected L-MDF create a hospitable environment for BM-MSCs to infiltrate and make cell-to-cell connections. The ability of cells not only to quickly attach to the matrix but also maintain a healthy morphology throughout the duration of culture provides evidence of the osteoconductive qualities of L-MDF.

The need for versatile handling has led to the addition of various inert carriers in commercial DBMs. However, studies have shown that carriers may negatively affect the inherent properties of a DBM. In particular, Lee et al. concluded that Poloxamer 407-based hydrogel may inhibit MSC osteoblastic differentiation by filling up spaces between DBM powders, negatively affecting the release of growth factors [21]. In a rat calvarial defect model, investigators found that the two types of DBM had significant differences in bone regeneration, which was attributed to the type of carrier [27]. Furthermore, varying the ratio of carrier to DBM can alter handling characteristics such as malleability and resistance to graft migration. Through *in vivo* and *in vitro* analyses, studies have found that increased bone content in DBMs produces larger amounts of new bone formation [25, 28, 29]. With this is mind, L-MDF were produced by proprietary CNC-milling cortical bone to create specially designed rough surfaces allowing fibers to interlock, allowing this bone void filler to be carrier-free. The roughness also provides numerous attachment points for the cells and their lamellipodia, encouraging a flattened morphology. These interlocking fibers thereby encourage malleability, graft placement in the implant site, and resistance to irrigation, all of which represent ideal handling characteristics.

Finally, terminal sterilization is a processing measure used to ensure the safety of DBMs by reducing the risk of disease transmission. This is in contrast to aseptic processing alone, which introduces no additional bioburden from the environment but alone does not guarantee sterile tissue [30, 31]. Unlike aseptic-only processed tissue, terminal sterilization can result in a graft with a defined sterility assurance level (SAL). For example, an SAL of 10^{-6} indicates a 1 out of 1,000,000 chance that a viable organism exists within any single graft [31]. Although gamma irradiation is currently the most common method for terminally sterilizing allografts, some reports suggests that gamma irradiation can negatively impact the inherent properties of DBMs. There are several factors to consider when evaluating the effects of gamma irradiation on DBMs such as dose and temperature. Irradiation performed in a high dose range or at uncontrolled temperatures can result in denaturing of the osteoinductive signaling proteins, rendering them inactive, and/or structural damage to the collagen matrix due to generation of reactive oxygen species. Weintroub and Reddi evaluated DBM samples which were irradiated on ice at varying doses [32]. Histologic analysis showed DBM irradiated at 0.5–2.5 Mrad were similar to the non-irradiated control, indicating no effect on the induction properties of the implant. In another study, investigators found that DBM irradiated on dry ice (−72°C) demonstrated new bone formation comparable to non-irradiated samples [33]. These results demonstrate DBMs irradiated at low dose and low temperatures are expected to retain properties important to clinical performance. Thus, L-MDF are terminally sterilized to an SAL of 10^{-6} using low-dose, ultra-low temperature gamma irradiation to avoid negative impacts to the osteoinductive and osteoconductive potential, as verified by the results presented here.

5. Conclusion

L-MDF were engineered with the ideal characteristics of a DBM in mind. The cortical bone fibers are demineralized to target optimal levels of residual calcium to yield tissue with osteoinductive potential, and also terminally sterilized to minimize the risk of disease transmission. The results presented here demonstrate that L-MDF exhibit the osteoinductive potential and osteoconductive properties desirable to promote bone formation while also being easy to handle for surgical procedures. These characteristics suggest that L-MDF are a suitable option to treat bone defects in a number of orthopedic, spinal, trauma, craniomaxillofacial, and dental applications.

Acknowledgements

We would like to acknowledge Breanne Gjurich PhD, Evans Wralstad, Alana Sampson MS, Yao Akpamagbo MS, and Davorka Softic MS for their contributions to study design, analysis and interpretation of data presented in the chapter.

Conflicts of interest

JBM, NC, PS, and MM are employees of LifeNet Health, a nonprofit organization.

Author details

Julie B. McLean, Nigeste Carter, Payal Sohoni and Mark A. Moore*
LifeNet Health, Virginia Beach, VA, USA

*Address all correspondence to: mark_moore@lifenethealth.org

IntechOpen

© 2019 The Author(s). Licensee IntechOpen. This chapter is distributed under the terms of the Creative Commons Attribution License (http://creativecommons.org/licenses/by/3.0), which permits unrestricted use, distribution, and reproduction in any medium, provided the original work is properly cited. CC BY

References

[1] Khan WS, Rayan F, Dhinsa BS, Marsh D. An osteoconductive, osteoinductive, and osteogenic tissue-engineered product for trauma and orthopaedic surgery: How far are we? Stem Cells International. 2012;**2012**:236231

[2] Wang W, Yeung KWK. Bone grafts and biomaterials substitutes for bone defect repair: A review. Bioactive Materials. 2017;**2**(4):224-247

[3] Oommen AT, Krishnamoorthy VP, Poonnoose PM, Korula RJ. Fate of bone grafting for acetabular defects in total hip replacement. Indian Journal of Orthopaedics. 2015;**49**(2):181-186

[4] Younger EM, Chapman MW. Morbidity at bone graft donor sites. Journal of Orthopaedic Trauma. 1989;**3**(3):192-195

[5] Park SB, Chung CK. Strategies of spinal fusion on osteoporotic spine. Journal of Korean Neurosurgical Association. 2011;**49**(6):317-322

[6] Lobb DC, DeGeorge BR Jr, Chhabra AB. Bone graft substitutes: Current concepts and future expectations. The Journal of Hand Surgery. 2019;**44**(6):497-505.e2

[7] Klifto CS, Gandi SD, Sapienza A. Bone graft options in upper-extremity surgery. The Journal of Hand Surgery. 2018;**43**(8):755-761.e2

[8] Fernandez de Grado G, Keller L, Idoux-Gillet Y, Wagner Q, Musset A-M, Benkirane-Jessel N, et al. Bone substitutes: A review of their characteristics, clinical use, and perspectives for large bone defects management. Journal of Tissue Engineering. 2018;**9**:1-18

[9] Burkus JK, Sandhu HS, Gornet MF. Influence of rhBMP-2 on the healing patterns associated with allograft interbody constructs in comparison with autograft. Spine (Phila Pa 1976). 2006;**31**(7):775-781

[10] McClellan JW, Mulconrey DS, Forbes RJ, Fullmer N. Vertebral bone resorption after transforaminal lumbar interbody fusion with bone morphogenetic protein (rhBMP-2). Journal of Spinal Disorders and Techniques. 2006;**19**(7):483-486

[11] Lewandrowski KU, Nanson C, Calderon R. Vertebral osteolysis after posterior interbody lumbar fusion with recombinant human bone morphogenetic protein 2: A report of five cases. The Spine Journal. 2007;**7**(5):609-614

[12] James CDT. Sir William Macewen. Proceedings of the Royal Society of Medicine. 1974;**67**(4):237-242

[13] de Boer HH. The history of bone grafts. Clinical Orthopaedics and Related Research. 1988;**226**:292-298

[14] Zimmermann G, Moghaddam A. Allograft bone matrix versus synthetic bone graft substitutes. Injury. 2011;**42**:S16-S21

[15] Miller LE, Block JE. Safety and effectiveness of bone allografts in anterior cervical discectomy and fusion surgery. Spine (Phila Pa 1976). 2011;**36**(24):2045-2050

[16] Senn N. On the healing of aseptic bone cavities by implantation of antiseptic decalcified bone. The American Journal of the Medical Sciences. 1889;**98**:219-243

[17] Urist MR, Strates BS. The classic: Bone morphogenetic protein. Clinical Orthopaedics and Related Research. 2009;**467**(12):3051-3062

[18] Lieberman JR, Daluiski A, Einhorn TA. The role of growth factors

in the repair of bone. Biology and clinical applications. The Journal of Bone and Joint Surgery. American Volume. 2002;**84**(6):1032-1044

[19] Karageorgiou V, Kaplan D. Porosity of 3D biomaterial scaffolds and osteogenesis. Biomaterials. 2005;**26**(27):5474-5491

[20] Rodriguez RU, Kemper N, Breathwaite E, Dutta SM, Hsu EL, Hsu WK, et al. Demineralized bone matrix fibers formable as general and custom 3D printed mold-based implants for promoting bone regeneration. Biofabrication. 2016;**8**(3):035007

[21] Lee JH, Baek HR, Lee KM, Lee HK, Im SB, Kim YS, et al. The effect of poloxamer 407-based hydrogel on the osteoinductivity of demineralized bone matrix. Clinics in Orthopedic Surgery. 2014;**6**(4):455-461

[22] Zhang M, Powers RM Jr, Wolfinbarger L Jr. Effect(s) of the demineralization process on the osteoinductivity of demineralized bone matrix. Journal of Periodontology. 1997;**68**(11):1085-1092

[23] Turonis JW, McPherson JC 3rd, Cuenin MF, Hokett SD, Peacock ME, Sharawy M. The effect of residual calcium in decalcified freeze-dried bone allograft in a critical-sized defect in the Rattus norvegicus calvarium. The Journal of Oral Implantology. 2006;**32**(2):55-62

[24] Wolfinbarger L, Eisenlohr LM, Ruth K. Demineralized bone matrix: Maximizing new bone formation for successful bone implantation. In: Pietrzak WS, editor. Musculoskeletal Tissue Regeneration: Biological Materials and Methods. Totowa, NJ: Humana Press; 2008. pp. 93-117

[25] Boyan BD, Ranly DM, McMillan J, Sunwoo M, Roche K, Schwartz Z. Osteoinductive ability of human allograft formulations. Journal of Periodontology. 2006;**77**(9):1555-1563

[26] Murphy MB, Suzuki RK, Sand TT, Chaput CD, Gregory CA. Short term culture of human mesenchymal stem cells with commercial osteoconductive carriers provides unique insights into biocompatibility. Journal of Clinical Medicine. 2013;**2**(3):49-66

[27] Tavakol S, Khoshzaban A, Azami M, Kashani IR, Tavakol H, Yazdanifar M, et al. The effect of carrier type on bone regeneration of demineralized bone matrix in vivo. The Journal of Craniofacial Surgery. 2013;**24**(6):2135-2140

[28] Han B, Tang B, Nimni ME. Quantitative and sensitive in vitro assay for osteoinductive activity of demineralized bone matrix. Journal of Orthopaedic Research. 2003;**21**(4):648-654

[29] Atti E, Abjornson C, Diegmann M, Zhang K, Cammisa FP, Myers ER. High resolution X-ray computed tomography as a technique to study osteoinductivity of demineralized bone matrix. The Spine Journal. 2003;**3**(5):120

[30] Vangsness CT Jr, Wagner PP, Moore TM, Roberts MR. Overview of safety issues concerning the preparation and processing of soft-tissue allografts. Arthroscopy: The Journal of Arthroscopic and Related Surgery: Official Publication of the Arthroscopy Association of North America and the International Arthroscopy Association. 2006;**22**(12):1351-1358

[31] Vangsness CT Jr, Garcia IA, Mills CR, Kainer MA, Roberts MR, Moore TM. Allograft transplantation in the knee: Tissue regulation, procurement, processing, and sterilization. The American Journal of Sports Medicine. 2003;**31**(3):474-481

[32] Wientroub S, Reddi AH. Influence of irradiation on the osteoinductive potential of demineralized bone matrix. Calcified Tissue International. 1988;**42**(4):255-260

[33] Dziedzic-Goclawska A, Ostrowski K, Stachowicz W, Michalik J, Grzesik W. Effect of radiation sterilization on the osteoinductive properties and the rate of remodeling of bone implants preserved by lyophilization and deep-freezing. Clinical Orthopaedics and Related Research. 1991;**272**:30-37

Section 2

Bone Grafts in Orthopaedics

Chapter 3

Class III Spine Grafts

Jeffrey G. Marx and Morgan P. Lorio

Abstract

This chapter is focused on the USFDA regulation and the related efficacy evidence of bone graft materials, especially Class III drug-device combination products for use in the spine. Nonstructural allograft and cellular allograft products that do not rely on the metabolic activity of living cells are HCT/P products, which require no premarket review for safety and efficacy. Synthetic bone grafts and demineralized bone matrices (DBMs) fall under Class II and require a 510(k) for market clearance, generally on the basis of an animal study. Drug-device combination bone grafts are Class III and require an investigational device exemption (IDE) clinical trial followed by a premarket approval (PMA) application with the FDA to review safety and effectiveness. Currently, there are only two PMA-supported Class III drug-device bone graft substitutes with Level I data that demonstrate equivalence to autograft for safety and effectiveness in spine: Infuse® (rhBMP-2) and i-FACTOR (P-15 peptide). Both of these products have been shown to be effective autograft replacement options, vs. the other technologies, which are autograft extenders. The OP-1 Implant (rhBMP-7) was marketed for a period of time, but it has been removed from the market. This chapter will discuss these products along with their supporting clinical data.

Keywords: spine, bone graft, regulatory approval, clinical evidence, BMP, P-15, infuse

1. Introduction

The ideal bone graft substitute for spinal fusion would have the safety and effectiveness of autograft when used by itself, be supported by quality published clinical evidence, and be available at a reasonable cost. Most of the options available today fall short of these goals. The number and variety of bone grafting products available to choose from is extensive, totaling more than 400 at the current time. The claims about the function and value of these products are confusing, even to those with the time and expertise to evaluate them in-depth. The preclinical and clinical evidence available for making a clinical use decision is also enormously varied and subject to misinterpretation. A large reason for these challenges is that the regulatory pathways and required evidence leading to FDA approval for spinal bone graft substitutes vary widely.

Nonstructural allograft and cellular allograft products, which do not rely on the metabolic activity of living cells, are considered to be HCT/P products under the United States Code of Federal Regulations Title 21—part 1271 (HUMAN CELLS, TISSUES, AND CELLULAR AND TISSUE-BASED PRODUCTS). Section 361 describes products that are minimally manipulated, are for homologous use only, do not have a systemic effect, and are not dependent on the metabolic activity of living cells for their primary function, in addition to other qualifications. Once a manufacturer determines a product meets all of these requirements and follows the appropriate regulations, the manufacturer can place the product on the market by simply notifying the FDA of the intent to do so. There is no premarket review by FDA for safety or effectiveness of such products. Therefore, there are no requirements for preclinical or clinical data. Since most HCT/P products have little to no peer-reviewed human clinical data, the surgeons must extrapolate the likely benefits in their clinical use.

Synthetic bone grafts and demineralized bone matrices (DBMs) fall under Class II under Section 510(k) of the Federal Food, Drug and Cosmetic Act. Section 510(k) describes a regulatory process for the clearance of products that have been demonstrated to the FDA's satisfaction to be "substantially equivalent" in safety and effectiveness to another lawfully marketed device when used for the same purpose. Market clearance requires the filing and review of a 510(k) application and a subsequent FDA review. This review is generally based on a single animal study and bench-top testing comparing the subject device with a predicate. Once again, since most 510(k) cleared products have little to no peer-reviewed human clinical data, surgeons must extrapolate the likely benefits in their clinical use.

Drug-device combination bone grafts are Class III and require an investigational device exemption (IDE) clinical trial followed by a premarket approval (PMA) application. The IDE study requirements include strict oversight from the FDA from statistical and protocol design through clinical follow-up, data integrity and analysis. These IDE studies must be prospective, controlled, blinded and statistically-powered prior to the onset. Moreover, the FDA-required outcomes for approval must be stipulated in the clinical design protocol. The review of both the IDE and PMA filings for drug-device combination products involve both the device (CDRH) and drug (CDER) branches of the FDA. The result of this rigorous process is the highest quality Level I human clinical data available. Surgeons may rely upon this data to make clinical use decisions.

2. Infuse bone graft: bone morphogenetic protein (BMP)

2.1 Bone morphogenetic protein: BMP

In 1965, Dr. Marshall R. Urist showed that demineralized bone matrix (DBM) could induce bone formation when implanted under the skin or intramuscular [1]. Urist pioneered the theory that a substance naturally present in bone was responsible for the osteoinductive bone healing activity of DBM (now Class II). He named this substance, the bone inductive principle, bone morphogenetic protein (BMP) and initiated an extensive and difficult search for these active protein molecules [2]. More than two decades later, advances in molecular biology by Dr. John Wozney's research team at the Genetic Institute described the first isolated extraction and recombinant form of BMP-2 in 1988 [3, 4]. BMP-2 and BMP-7 have been shown to have the most bone forming potential out of the 15 BMPs identified and studied to date [5]. The recombinant protein available commercially today is a synthetic, genetically engineered version of the natural protein.

BMPs are potent bone forming agents in bone regeneration and bone repair activity and are members of the TGF-Beta superfamily of cytokines. BMPs drive mesenchymal stem cells (MSCs) into osteoblastic lineage. These active protein dimeric molecules are osteoinductive and generally require a collagen sponge or ceramic carrier to enhance their handling characteristics. BMPs initiate endochondral bone formation, presumably by stimulating local MSCs and augmenting bone collagen synthesis. The BMP-2 ligand acts as a rigid clamp connecting type I and type II BMP receptor chains (BMPRs) together for transactivation. This activation causes intracellular signaling by phosphorylation of downstream signaling molecules (Smads). Smads ultimately mediate and regulate the transcription of target genes by binding to specific DNA sequences (BMP-responsive elements) [6].

2.1.1 rhBMP-2 pre-clinical

The next direction of rhBMP-2 research was to attempt to define proper dosing of the potent protein and to determine if this dosage would be specific to site or to carrier/scaffold. Formative work in this inquiry was performed in two different models by Sandhu et al. [7, 8].

The investigators first attempted to characterize the dose-response relationship of rhBMP-2 in a canine intertransverse spine fusion model. They compared increasing logarithmic rhBMP-2 doses (58, 115, 230, 460, and 920 mg) on a porous polylactic acid polymer carrier. Successful fusions postoperatively at 3 months were shown throughout this dosing range. A prior study done by this same research team demonstrated superiority of a 2300 mg rhBMP-2 dose to autologous iliac crest bone graft (ICBG) using this same technique. Quality differences above a threshold dose were not reflected in the mechanical, radiographic, or histologic features in the canine intertransverse spine fusion model from a 40-fold variation in rhBMP-2 dose [7].

Learning from the canine work, the investigators continued their work in an ovine lumbar interbody fusion model in conjunction with a cylindrical fenestrated titanium interbody fusion cage (INTER FIX, Medtronic Sofomor Danek, Inc., Memphis, TN). The cage was filled with rhBMP-2-collagen or ICBG (control). The sheep all appeared radiographically fused at 6 months. However, the histologic evaluation revealed that 33% (2/6) of the control group were fused as compared with 100% (6/6) of the rhBMP-2 group ($P < 0.001$). The scar involving the control group was 16-fold more than that seen with the rhBMP-2 group ($P < 0.01$) [8].

A rhesus monkey nonhuman primate model with rhBMP-2 on a collagen carrier within a titanium cage (Sofomor Danek, Memphis, TN) was the subsequent evolutionary step from the ovine model [9]. As optimal dosing for rhesus monkeys had not been previously established, three concentrations of rhBMP-2 [0.00 mg/mL sham (buffer only), 0.75 mg/mL low dose, or 1.50 mg/mL high dose) were tested. The results demonstrated that both the investigational rhBMP-2 groups achieved arthrodesis at 6 months histologically as compared to the sham group. As before with the ovine model, the blinded nonhuman primate model radiographic assessment was suboptimal but the sagittal CT assessment was consistent with the histology. The higher dose rhBMP-2 (1.5 mg/mL) caused faster and denser bone formation; this study established the dose used in the upcoming US IDE trial.

Fusion environments differ. A cage environment places the contained collagen carrier under protected direct compression forces between large vascularized opposing bony vertebral endplate surfaces. Posterolateral fusion presents a difficult environment with limited surface area and an intertransverse process fusion gap under distraction forces. Moreover, the surrounding muscle envelope applies mechanical compression on the graft material and may contribute to a pseudarthrosis or an hourglass configured fusion.

A standard compression resistant carrier with concomitant dosing concentration for rhBMP-2 was deemed necessary. Boden et al. studied a ceramic carrier [60% hydroxyapatite and 40% tricalcium phosphate (TCP)] in a nonhuman primate laminectomy model. Concentrations of rhBMP-2 (0, 6, 9, or 12 mg) were compared to ICBG. Fusion occurred with each rhBMP-2 carrier including the 0 mg/rhBMP-2 ceramic carrier alone group [10]. No significant overgrowth occurred involving the thecal sac, as bone growth induction was confined to ceramic carrier. The ceramic carrier was judged to be satisfactory for posterolateral application.

2.1.2 rhBMP-2 clinical trials

The "elimination" of the gold standard, autologous iliac crest bone graft (ICBG) harvest, in lumbar fusion was scientifically proposed by Burkus et al. in 2002 [11]. Anterior lumbar interbody fusion (ALIF) utilizing a combination of rhBMP-2 (1.50 mg/mL concentration) on an absorbable collagen sponge (ACS) carrier-filled tapered titanium fusion cage was shown to have an equivalent (~90%) radiographic (X-ray and CT) fusion rate to that of ICBG. This 2 year, multicenter, prospective, randomized, nonblinded human trial design compared an investigational Class III drug/device combination product (Infuse®, Medtronic Sofamor Danek, Memphis, Tennessee) on a Type-1 ACS (143 patients) to a control ICBG (136 patients); all 273 patients received the same tapered titanium fusion cage (LT-cage, Medtronic Sofomor Danek, Memphis, Tennessee). Osseous fusion rate was confirmed in 94.5% of the investigational group versus 88.7% of the control group at the two-year follow up. Outcomes of particular surgical interest including operative time (1.6 h), estimated blood loss (109.8 mL), adverse events from iliac crest harvest (0%), reported bone graft site discomfort (0%), and bone graft site appearance complaint (0%) were all less in the investigational group as compared to the control group at 2.0 h, 153.1 mL, 5.9, 32, and 16%, respectively. FDA approval was granted on July 2, 2002 for the rhBMP-2/ACS combination product in conjunction with the tapered titanium fusion cage (Infuse®/LT-Cage or Medtronic Sofamor Danek, Memphis, Tennessee) in the treatment of lumbar degenerative disc disease.

A traditional posterolateral spine fusion application (PLF) was the next step in the evaluation of rhBMP-2 on a ceramic granule carrier (60% hydroxyapatite and 40% TCP) in humans as a forged extrapolation of the seminal nonhuman primate work by Boden et al. [12]. Randomization of 25 patients (whose spondylolisthesis was ≤ Grade 1) into one of three groups was performed; five patients (control group) received autograft PLF with pedicle screw instrumentation, 11 patients received rhBMP-2 PLF with pedicle screw instrumentation, and 9 patients received rhBMP-2 PLF in situ only. A 20 mg rhBMP-2 dose was evenly divided in a bilateral, posterolateral application in those patients receiving rhBMP-2 on a ceramic granule carrier. Load bearing through the hardware until osseous fusion ensued was revelatory in the Oswestry scores. Oswestry scores demonstrated significant improvement in the rhBMP-2 PLF in situ only group at 6 weeks, rhBMP-2 PLF with pedicle screw instrumentation group at 3 months, and control, autograft PLF with pedicle screw instrumentation group, at 6 months. The fusion rate with the combined rhBMP-2 PLF groups (in situ only or with pedicle screw instrumentation) was 100% (20/20) and with the control, autograft PLF with pedicle screw instrumentation, however, was 40% (2/5). The radiographic fusion rate for the combined rhBMP-2 PLF groups was statistically significantly higher than for the control ($P = 0.004$).

A trauma application was then explored in a prospective, controlled, randomized multicenter clinical trial evaluation of patients with open tibial fractures. All 450 patients received intermedullary nail stabilization. Patients were randomized equally ($n = 150$), dividing them among one of three treatments: a standard of care (control group) or alternatively two different concentrations of rh-BMP [(0.75 mg/mL, total dose 6 mg) or (1.5 mg/mL, total dose 12 mg) respectively)] on ACS carrier. The control group standard of care was defined, for purposes of this study, as routine soft tissue management. The specific key measure outcome in the study was defined by the proportion of patients for whom secondary intervention was required due to delayed union or nonunion within the index postoperative year.

The 1.50 mg/mL group demonstrated a 44% reduction in the risk of failure requiring secondary intervention because of delayed union. The 1.50 mg/mL rhBMP-2 group had both significantly accelerated fracture healing and wound healing, higher osseous union rates, significantly fewer secondary interventions, less hardware failure, and less infections (Gustilo-Anderson type III associated injuries). Govender et al. further concluded that the 1.50 mg/mL rhBMP-2 concentration treatment was significantly superior care to the control, standard of care [13]. FDA approval for Infuse® (rhBMP-2 and ACS) in conjunction with an intermedullary nail for acute, open tibial fracture treatment was issued on April 30, 2004.

Between 2005 and 2009, three journal articles were published on the results of the FDA approval studies on 2-stage maxillary sinus floor augmentation [14–16]. Boyne et al. evaluated two concentrations of rhBMP-2/ACS at 0.75 and 1.50 mg/mL versus bone graft control; this pilot study was the first randomized controlled trial (RCT) demonstrating safe de novo bone induction by a recombinant human protein, rhBMP-2. Core biopsies retrieved after subsequent dental implant restoration confirmed normal bone formation in all groups; the proportion of dental implants that remained functionally loaded at 36 months was 62, 67, and 76% in the control group, 0.75 mg/mL rhBMP-2/ACS group, and 1.5 mg/mL rhBMP-2/ACS group, respectively. Triplett et al. performed a pivotal, multicenter, prospective, randomized, parallel evaluation of two treatments for a 2-stage maxillary sinus floor augmentation comparing a 1.50 mg/mL rhBMP-2/ACS group with an autograft control group; this study demonstrated no rhBMP-2 related adverse events at 6 months after dental restoration and similarly effective functional loading performance in both groups. Fiorellini et al. performed a randomized, masked, placebo-controlled, multicenter clinical trial evaluating de novo bone formation for dental implant restoration following tooth extraction using 0.75 mg/mL rhBMP-2/ACS, 1.5 mg/mL rhBMP-2/ACS, placebo control (ACS alone), or no treatment control. The 1.50 mg/mL rhBMP-2/ACS group demonstrated significantly greater (twice as great) bone augmentation compared to both controls ($P \leq 0.05$). Furthermore, bone density and histology disclosed no difference between newly induced and native bone.

A compression resistant matrix consisting of bovine collagen and Beta-tricalcium phosphate-hydroxyapatite in conjunction with rhBMP-2 was next compared to ICBG (control). A prospective, randomized, multi-center trial comparing the clinical and radiographic outcomes of an investigational optimized rhBMP-2 formulation to ICBG in one level instrumented traditional PLF in 463 patients with symptomatic degenerative disc disease (DDD) with spondylolisthesis ≤ Grade 1 [17]. Osseous fusion rate was radiographically (X-ray and CT) confirmed in 96% of the investigational group versus 89% of the control group at a 2 year follow up ($p = 0.014$). Outcomes of particular surgical interest including operative time (2.5 h), estimated blood loss (343.1 mL), reported donor site morbidity (0%), failures because of nonunion (six patients), and number requiring secondary surgeries (20 patients) were all significantly less in the investigational group as compared to the control group at 2.9 h, 448.6 mL, 60%, 18 patients ($p = 0.011$), and 36 patients ($p = 0.015$), respectively. The investigators concluded that clinical outcomes were similar between groups; they further concluded that morbidity was eliminated with the use of the optimized 2 mg/mL rhBMP-2 concentration in the compression resistant matrix. Eight patients (3.3%) with cancer (basal cell carcinoma, lung, lymphoma, ovarian, pancreatic, prostate, squamous cell carcinoma, and vocal cord) were reported in the optimized rhBMP-2 matrix group as compared to two patients (0.9%) with cancer (colon and lymphoma) in the control group. The fourfold increase in cancer in the optimized rhBMP-2 matrix group was not reported as possible device-related adverse events, as the cancer types were heterogeneous and statistically nonsignificant ($p = 0.107$). A nonapproval letter was received by

Medtronic on March 9, 2011 regarding the optimized AMPLIFY rhBMP-2 Matrix. The FDA nonapproval stemmed from the fourfold increased cancer risks in the investigational group and was linked to the high dose rhBMP-2 form of AMPLIFY versus the prior approved low dose forms.

Amidst the high-profile controversy, Yale University Open Data Access (YODA) retrieved Medtronic's safety and efficacy data on file in toto. Contract funding support of both the research and preparation of the work was provided by Medtronic to Yale. The Centre for Reviews and Dissemination (CRD) was then commissioned by the YODA initiative in an unprecedented effort by industry to facilitate unbiased review of the relevant benefits and harms of rhBMP-2 as used specifically in spinal fusion surgery; CRD has no direct financial conflict with Medtronic. Two successive publications in the Annals of Internal Medicine were issued in 2013 regarding the findings of the YODA initiative; the dissimilitude between the two publications were the extraction methods and the different studies included [18, 19]. Simmons et al. found rhBMP-2 had increased fusion rates versus ICBG, 12% higher (CI, 2–23%); Fu et al. found similar overall lumbar fusion rates between rhBMP-2 and ICBG Simmons et al. found nonsignificant increased cancer risk after rhBMP-2 (relative risk, 1.98 [CI 0.86–4.54]); Fu et al. found rhBMP-2 at 24 months had increased cancer risk (risk ratio, 3.45 [95% CI, 1.98–6.00]). Fu et al. also found rhBMP-2 to have associated increased risk for wound complications and dysphagia in off-label use in anterior cervical spine surgery, and nonsignificant increased risk for retrograde ejaculation and urogenital problems after on-label ALIF.

The data synthesis from the YODA initiative and more recent publications report mixed findings with regards to rhBMP-2 usage complications and cancer incidences after rhBMP-2 [20–23]. This same data synthesis suggests that an informed public might have benefited from earlier disclosure and blinded outcome assessment in retrospect.

3. i-FACTOR™: P-15 peptide

In the interest of developing products with greater biological specificity and a potentially better safety profile, a number of peptides (rather than proteins like BMPs) have been evaluated for their role and value in bone formation [24]. Peptides differ from proteins in size and structure, typically being much smaller molecules of between 2 and 50 amino acids compared to proteins (e.g., BMPs), which are much larger (>50 amino acids). Many of these peptide sequences are known for having numerous biochemical cellular signaling roles, especially during de novo tissue formation and in remodeling and injury response. Among the more promising peptides are those found in the cell interaction domain of the master control region of Type I collagen [25]. Type I collagen is comprised of two α1 and one β2 polypeptide chains that wrap around each other to form a right-handed triple helix, a collagen monomer. Numerous monomers polymerize to form the massive, rope-like collagen fibrils found in tissues. Type I collagen not only provides a supportive physical scaffold for cells and confers form and strength to tissues including skin, tendons and, in combination with rigid crystalline hydroxyapatite, bones, it also assumes dynamic, biological functions by regulating tissue assembly, cell differentiation, growth, regeneration, and biomineralization. Numerous functional domains and bioactive peptide sequences on a single collagen molecule are present at regular intervals across the width, and along the length of the polymeric collagen fibril. The high density of bioactive sites on collagen makes it the ideal polyvalent substrate for cells and bioactive factors.

The importance of these peptides and their functions is highlighted by the fact that they have been conserved over 65 M years of evolution as the cell interaction domain remains the same as that found in dinosaur Type I collagen [26]. This segment of the collagen molecule tends to become exposed and more bioavailable during chemical or traumatic cleavage of the collagen molecule. Among the peptides from the cell interaction domain, one referred to as P-15 was found to be 4500 times more potent for cell binding than the others. This peptide is a 15 amino acid sequence that represents a unique “kinked” tertiary protein structure on Type I collagen that facilitates its presentation to mesenchymal stem cells (MSC’s) and their daughter cells along the osteoblastic lineage [27]. P-15 has been found to attract MSC to the implant by providing a favorable environment that facilitates cell attachment. The attraction is followed by a specific receptor-mediated attachment that activates down-stream molecular events via receptor-activated cascade pathways. These events activate and accelerate new bone formation as they attract, attach, and activate bone forming cells. These processes are circular and self-reinforcing once initiated. In addition, P-15 has been shown to benefit biochemical mechanisms such as proliferation, differentiation, migration, cell survival, among others.

In 1996, Qian and Bhatnagar published their first investigations on the P-15 peptide for application in bone tissues. In this paper, they showed that attaching this 15 amino acid peptide (P-15) to a calcium phosphate anorganic bone mineral (ABM) led to dramatic increases in cellular response in culture. Their work suggested that this combination might be a useful addition to the bone grafting armamentarium [28]. The in-vitro model demonstrated the ABM-bound P-15 stimulated human-derived pre-osteoblast resulting in significantly increased number of bound cells and the initiation of down-stream molecular events associated with differentiation and osteoinductive activities. Additionally, it was observed that mechanical forces on the cellular cytoskeleton may be generated by P-15 surface integrin interactions. These forces are believed to contribute to mechanotransduction with profound consequences on cellular differentiation.

Over the subsequent decades, numerous in vitro studies demonstrated that the P-15 peptide would elicit specific biological responses from bone forming lineage cells (pre-osteoblasts as well as MSC.) The stimulation/differentiation of MSC was demonstrated at both the molecular level as seen by upregulation of mRNA production, and the protein level as evidence by the cellular release of bone-regeneration associated proteins and growth factors, including alkaline phosphatase, BMP-2 and Collagen Type I [29]. The mechanism of action that elicits these effects is related to the P-15 peptide “plugging in” to surface receptors on these cells, which turns on the genetically programmed downstream cellular responses.

Qian and Bhatnagar showed that P-15 bound to ABM increases the number of bound human fibroblasts and stimulates cellular activation and spreading [28].

Liu et al. demonstrated that P-15 bound to surface increases the number of bound pre-osteoblastic cells and stimulates cellular activation [30]. The authors also noted a significant increase in specific cell surface integrin activation and focal adhesion kinase activation on surface treated with P-15 compared to control substrates, an indication of the direct biological influence of the P-15 peptide on cells.

Yang et al. demonstrated that P-15 bound to ABM stimulates upregulation of cellular BMP-2 and alkaline phosphatase production and the onset of calcification. Alkaline phosphatase production is an indicator of cellular differentiation to osteoblasts as well as their activity toward bone formation [31].

Yuan et al. found that P-15 bound to ABM stimulates early formation of mineralization nodes [32].

In vivo studies using a rabbit drill hole model demonstrated that ABM-bound P-15 significantly enhances the generation of new bone formation yielding histological evidence of mature bone tissue [33]. The P-15/ABM material yielded statistically more new bone formation at two, four and 8 weeks with over seven-times higher percentage of new bone as compared to ABM alone [33]. A sheep interbody lumbar fusion animal study demonstrated that ABM-bound P-15 yielded fusion rates equivalent to the "gold-standard" of iliac crest bone graft and displayed good trabecular bridging bone structure at 6 months [34]. Finally, rabbit intramuscular implant studies of ABM-bound P-15 established that the P-15 peptide does not support bone formation outside of a bony tissue environment. This can be interpreted as a safety factor, since ectopic bone formation in clinical use is unlikely. These effects translated from tissue culture into animal implantation, showing promise for bone grafting applications with strong bone formation in the absence of ectopic bone formation.

In 1999, the FDA granted the first of two PMA approvals for the use of the P-15 peptide for dental bone grafting to Ceramed on the basis of a prospective, randomized, Level-I IDE study demonstrating safety and effectiveness. This product, Pepgen P-15, has been used in ~500,000 patients to date in the United States.

In 2000, Cerapedics began developing the P-15 peptide technology platform, called i-FACTOR™ bone graft (P-15 Putty), for use in orthopedics and spine surgery indications. i-FACTOR bone graft is a composite bone graft consisting of the synthetic P-15 peptide (biomimetic of the Type I collagen peptide) absorbed onto ABM (naturally-derived calcium phosphate particles) and then suspended in an inert hydrogel carrier. Cerapedics received the first CE mark for i-FACTOR bone graft in 2008 for all orthopedic applications, including spine. Under the CE mark, the product has been used in >50,000 patients to date.

Cerapedics initiated an IDE trial for single level ACDF in an allograft ring in 2006, which culminated in PMA approval in 2015. This FDA-approved trial was prospective, randomized, blinded, controlled and statistically-powered, thus represents Level I study data [35]. In this 319-patient trial, i-FACTOR bone graft successfully met the predefined noninferiority criteria for radiologic fusion (88.9 vs. 85.8% for control), neck disability index (28.8 change vs. 27.4% for control), neurological success (93.7 vs. 93% for control), and safety (97.5 vs. 95.4% for control). More importantly, an FDA-mandated, prospectively designed statistical analysis of the Overall Clinical Success, defined as individual patients who were successful for all four of the primary outcomes, demonstrated statistical superiority to local autograft in overall clinical success (68.8 vs. 56.9%) at 12 months. This statistical superiority was maintained at the 24-month evaluation.

Following the introduction of the i-FACTOR bone graft in the EU, based on a CE-mark, numerous clinical evaluations were performed with i-FACTOR bone graft in the lumbar clinical indication. Mobbs et al. published a prospective ALIF study in which i-FACTOR was used as a stand-alone bone graft inside a PEEK interbody device [36]. In this study, an independent radiological evaluation found a 94% fusion rate by thin cut CT at 24 months, along with a statistical improvement in all clinical evaluations. The authors concluded that, based on their experience, "the study demonstrates a high fusion rate and clinical improvement comparable to the published results for ALIF using autograft or BMP, while avoiding the complications specific to those materials." This study represents an approved use in the EU and Australia, which would be considered off-label in the United States.

Lauweryns et al. published the results from a prospective intra-patient randomized study comparing i-FACTOR bone graft to local autograft in PLIF fusions [37]. In this study, contralateral cages were randomized to be filled with either i-FACTOR bone graft or local autograft, and fusions were assessed by thin cut CT. This study demonstrated faster fusion with i-FACTOR bone graft compared to local autograft. i-FACTOR bone graft was statistically superior with regards to percentage of patients with complete bridging fusion at both 6 months (97.7% for i-FACTOR vs. 59.1% for autograft) and 12 months (97.8% for i-FACTOR vs. 82.2% for autograft). At 24 months, the fusion rates were no longer statistically different. The authors concluded that "i-FACTOR is associated with faster formation of bridging bone when compared to autologous bone in patients undergoing PLIF." This study represents an approved use in the EU and Australia, and would be considered off-label in the United States.

In March 2018, the FDA approved an IDE for Cerapedics to initiate another IDE study. This second prospective IDE study is in single level TLIF procedures. In this study, an advanced formulation of P-15 (P-15 L bone graft) is being randomized against local autograft as the control. This study is expected to enroll 364 patients and has a 2-year endpoint for the PMA filing of Level I data.

Both the well-established mechanism of action regarding the stimulatory effects of P-15 peptide along with the extensive clinical data resulting from an IDE, Level I clinical study, strongly support the safety and effectiveness of P-15 peptide in the form of i-FACTOR bone graft.

4. The OP-1 implant: BMP-7

There is a third drug-device combination spinal bone graft product, which deserves some discussion: the OP-1 implant formerly commercialized by Stryker Biotech under FDA humanitarian device exemptions (HDE) OP-1 was bone morphogenetic protein (BMP)-7 on a collagen delivery carrier. The BMP-7 was bound to the collagen prior to packaging and terminal sterilization. Following study in long bone nonunions, the OP-1 implant was studied as an autograft replacement for primary posterolateral spinal fusion (PLF) under an IDE (IDE G990028).

After failing to meet the primary outcomes of the study to qualify for a PMA approval [rejection at the FDA advisory panel meeting in November, 2007], Stryker Biotech filed an HDE for revision PLF, which was granted in 2004. The Humanitarian Device Exemption (HDE) pathway is a method of gaining very limited FDA approval for a medical device. The device has to be intended to benefit patients in the treatment or diagnosis of a disease or condition that affects or is manifested in not more than 8000 individuals in the United States per year. Although the application is similar to a premarket approval (PMA) application, the product is exempt from effectiveness requirements and, therefore, does not require a well-controlled Level I clinical trial. The application is required to only provide sufficient technical information to demonstrate that the device will not expose patients to an unreasonable or significant risk of illness or injury and the probable benefit to health from the use of the device outweighs the risk of injury or illness from its uses.

The OP-1 device was commercialized by Stryker in the United States until 2010 and then, subsequently sold to Olympus. OP-1 was later removed from the market worldwide.

5. Conclusions

Nonstructural allograft and cellular allograft products marketed as HCT/Ps do not require any FDA review for safety or efficacy. Synthetic bone grafts and DBM's require a 510(k) for clearance on the basis of animal studies, and most of these technologies have little to no meaningful clinical data. Currently, there are only two

PMA-supported Class III drug-device bone graft substitutes available with Level I data that demonstrate equivalence in safety and effectiveness to autograft in the spine: Infuse® (rhBMP-2) and i-FACTOR bone graft (P-15 peptide). Both of these technologies have multiple peer-reviewed clinical studies that can be used to evaluate their effectiveness and make a clinical use decision.

Acknowledgements

The authors would like to thank Celeste Abjornson, PhD; Antonio Brecevich, MD; Tucker Callanan, MS; Christina Dowe, BS; and Frank P. Camissa, JR, MD.

Conflict of interest

Jeffrey G. Marx, PhD, is a full-time employee and an officer of Cerapedics Inc.

Author details

Jeffrey G. Marx[1] and Morgan P. Lorio[2*]

1 Cerapedics Inc., Westminster, CO, USA

2 Advanced Orthopedics and Pain Management, Altamonte Springs, FL, USA

*Address all correspondence to: mloriomd@gmail.com

IntechOpen

© 2019 The Author(s). Licensee IntechOpen. This chapter is distributed under the terms of the Creative Commons Attribution License (http://creativecommons.org/licenses/by/3.0), which permits unrestricted use, distribution, and reproduction in any medium, provided the original work is properly cited. (cc) BY

References

[1] Urist MR. Bone: Formation by autoinduction. Science. 1995;**150**(3698):893-899

[2] Urist MR, Jurist JM Jr, Dubuc FL, Strates BS. Quantitation of new bone formation in intramuscular implants of bone matrix in rabbits. Clinical Orthopaedics and Related Research. 1970;**68**:279-293

[3] Grgurevic L, Pecina M, Vukicevic S. Marshall R. Urist and the discovery of bone morphogenetic proteins. International Orthopaedics (SICOT). 2017;**41**:1065

[4] Wang EA, Rosen V, Cordes P, Hewick RM, Kriz MJ, Luxenberg DP, et al. Purification and characterization of other distinct bone-inducing factors. Proceedings of the National Academy of Sciences of the United States of America. 1988;**85**(24):9484-9488

[5] Sampath TK, Reddi AH. Dissociative extraction and reconstitution of extracellular matrix components involved in local bone differentiation. Proceedings of the National Academy of Sciences of the United States of America. 1981;**78**(12):7599-7603

[6] Simic P, Vukecevic S. Bone morphogenetic proteins: From developmental signals to tissue regeneration. Conference on bone morphogenetic proteins. EMBO Reports. 2008;**8**(4):327-331

[7] Sandu HS, Kanim MA, Kabo JM, Toth JM, Zeegen EN, Liu D, et al. Effective doses of recombinant human bone morphogenetic protein-2 in experimental spinal fusion. Spine. 1996;**21**:2115-2122

[8] Sandhu HS, Toth JM, Diwan AD, Seim HB 3rd, Kanim LE, Kabo JM, et al. Histologic evaluation of the efficacy of rhBMP-2 compared with autograft bone in sheep spinal anterior interbody fusion. Spine (Phila Pa 1976). 2002;**27**(6):567-575

[9] Boden SD, Martin GJ Jr, Horton WC, Truss TL, Sandhu HS. Laparoscopic anterior spina arthrodesis with rhBMP-2 in a titanium interbody threaded cage. Journal of Spinal Disorders. 1998;**11**(2):95-101

[10] Boden SD, Martin GJ Jr, Morone MA, Ugbo JL, Moskovitz PA. Posterolateral lumbar intertransverse process spine arthrodesis with recombinant human bone morphogenetic protein 2/ hydroxyapatite-tricalcium phosphate after laminectomy in the nonhuman primate. Spine (Phila Pa 1976). 1999;**24**(12):1179-1185

[11] Burkus JK et al. Anterior lumbar interbody fusion using rhBMP-2 with tapered interbody cages. Journal of Spinal Disorders. 2002;**15**(5):337-349

[12] Boden SD, Kang J, Sandhu HD, Heller JG. Use of recombinant human bone morphogenetic protein-2 to achieve posterolateral lumbar spine fusion in humans: A prospective, randomized clinical pilot trial 2002 Volvo Award in clinical studies. Spine. 2002;**27**(23):2662-2673

[13] Govender S, Csimma C, Genant HK, Valentin-Opran A, Amit Y, Arbel R, et al. BMP-2 evaluation in surgery for tibial trauma (BESTT) study group. Recombinant human bone morphogenetic protein-2 for treatment of open tibial fractures: A prospective, controlled, randomized study of four hundred and fifty patients. The Journal of Bone and Joint Surgery. American Volume. 2002;**84-A**(12):2123-2134

[14] Boyne PJ, Lilly LC, et al. De novo bone induction by recombinant human morphogenetic protein-2 (rhBMP-2)

in maxillary sinus floor augmentation. Journal of Oral and Maxillofacial Surgery. 2005;**63**:1693-1707

[15] Triplett RG, Nevins M, Marx RE, et al. Pivotal, randomized, parallel evaluation of recombinant human bone morphogenetic protein-2/ absorbable collagen sponge and autogenous bone graft for maxillary sinus floor augmentation. Journal of Oral and Maxillofacial Surgery. 2009;**67**:1947-1960

[16] Fiorellini JP, Howell TH, Cochran D, et al. Randomized study evaluating recombinant human bone morphogenetic protein-2 for extraction socket augmentation. Journal of Periodontal. 2005;**76**(4):605-613

[17] Dimar JR, Glassman SD, Burkus JK, Pryor PW, Hardacker JW, Carreon LY. Clinical and radiographic analysis of an optimized rhBMP-2 formulation as an autograft replacement in posterolateral lumbar spine arthrodesis. Joint Surgery-American Volume. 2009;**91**:1377-1386

[18] Simmonds MC, Brown JV, Heirs MK, Higgins JP, Mannion RJ, Rodgers MA, et al. Safety and effectiveness of recombinant human bone morphogenetic protein-2 for spinal fusion: A meta-analysis of individual-participant data. Annals of Internal Medicine. 2013;**158**(12):877-889

[19] Fu R, Selph S, McDonagh M, Peterson K, Tiwari A, Chou R, et al. Effectiveness and harms of recombinant human bone morphogenetic protein-2 in spine fusion: A systematic review and meta-analysis. Annals of Internal Medicine. 2013;**158**(12):890-902

[20] Carragee EJ, Chu G, Rohatgi R, Hurwitz EL, Weiner BK, Yoon ST, et al. Cancer risk after use of recombinant bone morphogenetic protein-2 for spinal arthrodesis. The Journal of Bone and Joint Surgery. American Volume. 2013;**95**(17):1537-1545

[21] Cooper GS, Kou TD. Risk of cancer after lumbar fusion surgery with recombinant human bone morphogenic protein-2 (rh-BMP-2). Spine (Phila Pa 1976). 2013;**38**(21):1862-1868

[22] Mesfin A, Buchowski JM, Zebala LP, Bakhsh WR, Aronson AB, Fogelson JL, et al. High-dose rhBMP-2 for adults: Major and minor complications: A study of 502 spine cases. The Journal of Bone and Joint Surgery. American Volume. 2013;**95**(17):1546-1553

[23] Carragee EJ, Hurwitz EL, Weiner BK. A critical review of recombinant human bone morphogenetic protein-2 trials in spinal surgery: Emerging safety concerns and lessons learned. The Spine Journal. 2011;**11**:471-491

[24] Visser R, Rico-Llanos GA, Pulkkinen H, Becerra J. Peptides for bone tissue engineering. Journal of Controlled Release. 2016;**244**(Pt A): 122-135

[25] Sweeney SM et al. Candidate cell and matrix interaction domains on the collagen fibril, the predominant protein of vertebrates. The Journal of Biological Chemistry. 2008;**283**(30):21187-21197

[26] Asara JM, Schweitzer MH, Freimark LM, Phillips M, Cantley LC. Protein sequences from mastodon and Tyrannosaurus rex revealed by mass spectrometry. Science. 2007;**316**(5822):280-285

[27] Bhatnagar RS, Qian JJ, Wedrychowska A, Sadeghi M, We YM, Smith N. Design of biomimetic habitats for tissue engineering with P-15, a synthetic peptide analogue of collagen. Tissue Engineering. 1999;**5**(1):53-65

[28] Qian JJ, Bhatnagar RS. Enhanced cell attachment to anorganic bone mineral in the presence of a synthetic peptide related to collagen. Journal of Biomedical Materials Research. 1996;**4**:545-554

[29] Yang XB, Rajendra S, et al. Biomimetic scaffolds for human bone cell growth. Tissue Engineering. 2004;**10**:1148-1158

[30] Liu Q, Limthongkul W, Sidhu G, Shang J, Vaccaro A, Shenck R, et al. Covalent attachment of P15 peptide to titanium surfaces enhances cell attachment, spreading, and osteogenic gene expression. Journal of Orthopaedic Research. 2012;**30**(10):1626-1633

[31] Yang XB, Bhatnagar RS, Li S, Oreffo RO. Biommetic collagen scaffolds for human bone cell growth and differentiation. Tissue Engineering. 2004;**10**(7-8):1148-1159

[32] Yuan L, Huang JS, Hsu CW, Hung IJ. A mineralization-associated membrane protein plays a role in the biological functions of the peptide-coated bovine hydroxyapatite. Journal of Periodontal Research. 2007;**42**:420-428

[33] Lindley EM, Guerra FA, et al. Small peptide bone substitute efficacy in a rabbit cancellous bone model. JBMR. 2010;**94B**:463-468

[34] Shermann BP, Lindley EM, et al. Evaluation of ABM/P-15 versus autograft bone in an ovine lumbar interbody interbody fusion model. European Spine Journal. 2010;**19**:2156-2166

[35] Arnold P et al. Efficacy of i-Factor bone graft versus autograft in anterior cervical discectomy and fusion. Spine. 2017;**41**(13):1075-1083

[36] Mobbs et al. Clinical outcome and fusion rates following ALIF with bone graft substitute i-Factor, an anorganic bone matrix/P-15 composite. Journal of Neurosurgery: Spine. 2014;**21**:867-876

[37] Lauweryns P et al. Prospective analysis of a new bone graft in lumbar interbody fusion: Results of a 2-year prospective clinical and radiological study. International Journal of Spine Surgery. 2015;**9**:2. http://dx.doi.org/10.14444/2002

Chapter 4

Allograft Structural Interbody Spacers Compared to PEEK Cages in Cervical Fusion: Benchtop and Clinical Evidence

Nigeste Carter, Elena C. Gianulis and Mark A. Moore

Abstract

Cervical degenerative disc disease (CDDD) can lead to radiculopathy and myelopathy, resulting in pain, lack of function, and immobility. Anterior cervical discectomy and fusion (ACDF) is a common surgical treatment modality for advanced CDDD. ACDF involves removal of the affected disc(s) followed by replacement with a bone or synthetic graft. Historically, autograft has been considered the gold standard for interbody fusion. However, it is often associated with limitations, including donor site morbidity and limited quality and supply, prompting surgeons to seek alternatives. Two of the most common alternatives are structural bone allografts and polyetheretherketone (PEEK) synthetic cages. Both, advantageously, have similar mechanical properties to autologous bone, with comparable elastic modulus values. However, a lack of osseointegration of PEEK cages has been reported both pre-clinically and clinically. Reported fusion rates assessed radiographically are higher with the use of structural bone allografts compared to PEEK cages, while having a lower incidence of pseudarthrosis. This book chapter will discuss in detail the pre-clinical and clinical performance of structural allografts in comparison to conventional PEEK cages.

Keywords: polyetheretherketone (PEEK), structural bone allograft, anterior cervical discectomy and fusion (ACDF), cervical degenerative disc disease, synthetic cage, allograft, irradiation

1. Introduction

Cervical degenerative disc disease is one of the most common diagnoses for patients suffering from neck and back pain. These symptoms may present with various conditions, such as radiculopathy or myelopathy, involving compression of the nerve root and spinal cord, respectively [1]. Patients may suffer from pain, lack of function, immobility and sensory loss. Initial treatments often include anti-inflammatory medicine, immobilization, and physical therapy [1]. However, when conservative treatment options fail, a surgical approach such as anterior cervical discectomy and fusion (ADCF) may be warranted. This anterior approach involves excising the affected disc(s), removing osteophytes, and decompressing the nerve root or spinal cord. Following disc removal, the residual vertebral space is typically implanted with a bone or synthetic graft, with or without the additional support of plates and screws.

Robinson and Smith described this technique in 1955 [2]. Their approach involved implantation of a horseshoe-shaped bone graft harvested from iliac crest, followed by immobilization. Patients treated with this technique demonstrated promising clinical outcomes [2]. In 1958, Cloward described a similar technique, however, it included decompression of the neural structures and implantation of a bone dowel in the interbody space [3]. Regardless of the approach, a graft was used as a spacer to restore disc height, provide stability, and help promote bone fusion. Autograft, generally taken from the iliac crest, is often considered to be the gold standard for interbody fusion [4]. The use of autograft has led to high fusion rates and clinical success, although there are several disadvantages, such as extended operating time, donor site pain, limited supply, and variable quality depending upon the patient's health [5–8]. In an effort to avoid the complications seen with autografts, there has been a decades-old shift towards the use of alternative interbody spacers for treatment of degenerative disc disease [9, 10]. Two of the most common choices have been structural allograft bone or synthetic cages manufactured using polyetheretherketone (PEEK) [10]. Here, a comparison of the material properties and clinical performance of structural allografts and conventional PEEK cages is provided.

2. Bone graft substitutes as intervertebral spacers in ACDF

Structural bone allografts have been used successfully in a broad range of clinical applications including ACDF procedures [11–13]. Although lacking direct osteogenic potential, structural allografts have similar osteoconductive properties to autograft while avoiding complications such as donor site morbidity [14]. Furthermore, studies have shown similar clinical outcomes when comparing the use of allograft to autograft in ACDF procedures [15, 16]. Other commonly used implants include interbody cages made of various materials, including metals, ceramics, and polymers. Metal implants have been widely used as spinal cages for ACDF procedures. In particular, titanium implants offer mechanical strength, maintenance of vertebral disc height, and are available in various forms including mesh and box implants [4]. However, there are concerns regarding the use of titanium implants due to their mismatched mechanical properties compared to native bone. The difference in elastic modulus between bone and titanium can cause stress shielding, weakening the surrounding bone and increasing risk of peri-prosthetic fractures [17]. Bioactive ceramics serve as an attractive alternative due to their demonstrated biocompatibility, osteoconductive potential, and availability [9]. Despite these advantages, varying porosity of ceramics can lead to brittleness, thus making them less ideal implants for load-bearing applications [18]. Finally, various polymers are used in biomedical applications due to their biocompatibility, chemical and mechanical stability, and wide ranging compositions. However, some polymers are not ideal for orthopedic implants due to their malleable nature and weak mechanical properties [19]. One polymer with desirable mechanical properties is polyetheretherketone (PEEK). Compared to autograft, PEEK cages offer shorter operating time and reduced donor site morbidity [4]. This chapter will focus on the properties of structural allograft bone compared to conventional PEEK implants due to their similar mechanical properties and common use. Pre-clinical studies examining mechanical properties, osteoconduction and osseointegration, and clinical fusion rates in the cervical spine will be presented.

2.1 Structural allograft

Allograft bone, sourced from deceased human donors, is readily available and commonly used [20]. Allogenic bone grafts come in various forms, shapes, and sizes, based on clinical need, and can be either structural or non-structural. The bone is typically processed by physical and chemical means to ensure safety, biocompatibility and clinical suitability. Processing steps can include physical shaping and resizing of the graft for a specific clinical purpose (e.g., an intervertebral body spacer), disinfection and sterilization, and preservation to increase shelf life and simplify storage.

Allograft use in bone grafting procedures dates back many decades, as evidenced by a nineteenth century publication from the Scottish surgeon William Macewen [21, 22]. He successfully reconstructed an infected humerus of a 4 year-old child using allograft tibial segments obtained while treating effects of rickets. Early in the twentieth century, Fred Albee published a book on bone graft applications, laying the foundation for a surge in bone transplantation procedures that is ongoing [23]. Allograft bone is now widely used for spinal, orthopedic, dental, and trauma applications. Notably, allograft usage in the treatment of degenerative cervical disc disease has increased from 14% in 1999 to 59% in 2008 [24]. Of particular interest here, the use of structural allografts in ACDF procedures dates back as early as 1958. Cloward described the use of frozen allograft bone in 46 patients undergoing ACDF [3]. A cylindrical iliac dowel, commonly known as the Cloward dowel, was implanted into the empty interbody space. Forty-four patients demonstrated complete interbody fusion at 3–4 months post-operative. Numerous studies have since been published discussing the use of various structural allografts in ACDF procedures [18]. Structural allografts continue to be used as interbody spacers due to their ability to support mechanical loads and resist failure. Such structural allografts are comprised of either cortical, cancellous or a combination of both cortical and cancellous bone. Cortical bone is more rigid and provides greater structural support, while cancellous bone confers less mechanical strength, but is more porous, providing an osteoconductive scaffold for neovascularization and osseointegration.

Infection due to allograft transplantation remains a risk, albeit rare. A report released by the Centers for Disease Control and Prevention (CDC) in 2005 estimated an overall allograft-associated infection rate of 0.0004%, emphasizing the unlikely event of allograft-associated disease transmission [25]. This number was developed before additional advanced tissue processing methods, including terminal sterilization, were implemented by many tissue providers. Organizations, such as the American Association of Tissue Banks (AATB) and the Food and Drug Administration (FDA), maintain standards for tissue banking, including donor acceptance criteria, tissue procurement and processing methods, and allograft storage [26, 27]. Additionally, FDA published the Current Good Tissue Practice (CGTP) Final Rule, effective in 2005, setting requirements aimed at "preventing the introduction, transmission and spread of communicable diseases" [28]. AATB and FDA guidelines ensure that human allograft tissues are both clinically suitable and safe. Through the combination of rigorous donor screening and tissue processing, risk of disease transmission is virtually eliminated.

2.2 Synthetics: polyetheretherketone (PEEK) cages

Polyetheretherketone (PEEK) is a non-absorbable, semicrystalline polymer processed through a variety of techniques including extrusion, or injection and compression molding [29, 30]. Chemically, PEEK is made up of an aromatic backbone, interconnected by ketone and ether functional groups [30]. The chemical structure of PEEK gives it distinct qualities such as: stability at high temperatures, resistance to chemical and radiation damage, strength and stiffness. PEEK is available in several configurations including neat (unfilled) and carbon-reinforced PEEK (CRPEEK). The addition of composite fillers, such as carbon fiber, provides those forms of PEEK with increased mechanical strength [30].

Developed in 1978, PEEK was initially commercialized for industrial applications such as aircraft and turbine blades due to its high chemical and mechanical resistance [29, 31]. However, in the late 1980s, it emerged as a potential biomaterial for surgical implantation and rapidly gained acceptance as a medical device. In the late 1990s, PEEK was introduced as a spinal cage implant and has also been used for other orthopedic and dental applications [19]. PEEK cages have become a popular choice due to inherent biocompatibility and favorable mechanical properties compared to traditional metal-based cages. PEEK has undergone numerous biocompatibility and cytotoxicity tests in accordance with both FDA and ISO 10993 standards. Morrison et al. evaluated the response from mouse fibroblasts and rat osteoblasts *in vitro* and found PEEK to display excellent biocompatibility [32]. Rivard et al. demonstrated that PEEK particles implanted in New Zealand white rabbits elicited no apparent necrosis or swelling, leading the authors to suggest that it is "harmless" to the spinal cord [33].

Compared to other synthetic implants such as titanium cages, PEEK has an elastic modulus similar to that of native bone, thus reducing the potential impact of stress shielding on the bone healing process [19, 34]. Another advantage of PEEK is radiolucency which allows for radiographic assessment of fusion [35]. Furthermore, due to its ability to resist radiation damage, PEEK is able to be sterilized by electron beam or gamma irradiation. Despite noted advantages, several concerns have been raised due to how PEEK's inert nature and low-surface energy might affect the body's biological response. Adsorption of water at the implant surface plays an important role in protein-surface interactions, and thus cell-surface interactions, which can determine the success of an implant [36]. The hydrophobic nature of PEEK can potentially limit cellular adhesion. This undesirable property has been recently reported in studies finding that conventional smooth PEEK implants have limited osteoconductive properties and limited bone fixation at the implant interface [29, 37]. For example, Phan et al. described a case in which a patient underwent anterior lumbar interbody fusion (ALIF) with a PEEK implant [38]. The authors found evidence of poor integration between the implant and surrounding bone causing the "halo-effect" on CT scans.

These issues have led to several modifications in an attempt to increase PEEK's bioactivity, including surface coating with synthetic osteoconductive material such as titanium, increasing surface roughness and porosity through chemical modifications, and incorporating bioactive particles [34, 39]. Despite these promising modifications, conventional PEEK is still commonly used and is the focus in this chapter.

3. Engineering studies of PEEK and allograft

Interbody spacers require appropriate mechanical properties to be clinically effective. One important property is elastic modulus, the measure of resistance to deformation in response to applied stress. Mismatches in the elastic modulus between the surrounding vertebral bodies and an implant may lead to issues such as subsidence and stress shielding [40]. Clinically, these issues can cause complications such as pseudarthrosis and non-unions. Thus, it is ideal for an implant to have a similar elastic modulus as native bone. Heary et al. measured the elastic modulus and stiffness of various spinal interbody implants including neat and carbon-reinforced PEEK and cancellous and cortical bone [40]. The authors found that the elastic modulus of neat PEEK was similar to cancellous allograft bone, 3.84 and 3.78 GPa, respectively (**Figure 1**). Similarly, carbon-reinforced PEEK demonstrated a comparable elastic modulus to cortical allograft bone, 17.94 and 14.64 GPa, respectively. The study demonstrates the similar elastic modulus of allograft and

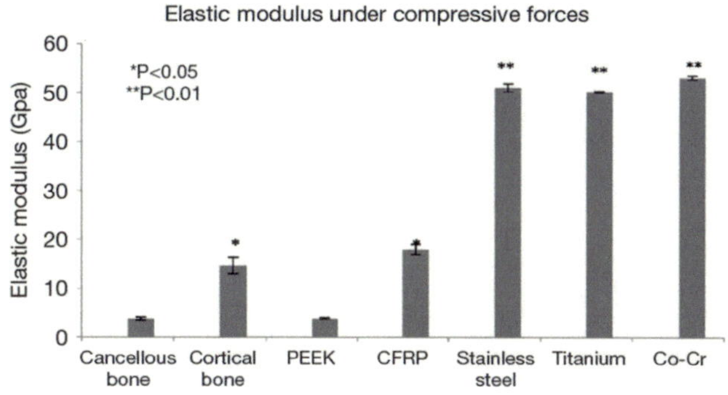

Figure 1.
*Elastic modulus of all materials (*p < 0.05; **p < 0.01). Reprinted with permission from Heary et al. [40].*

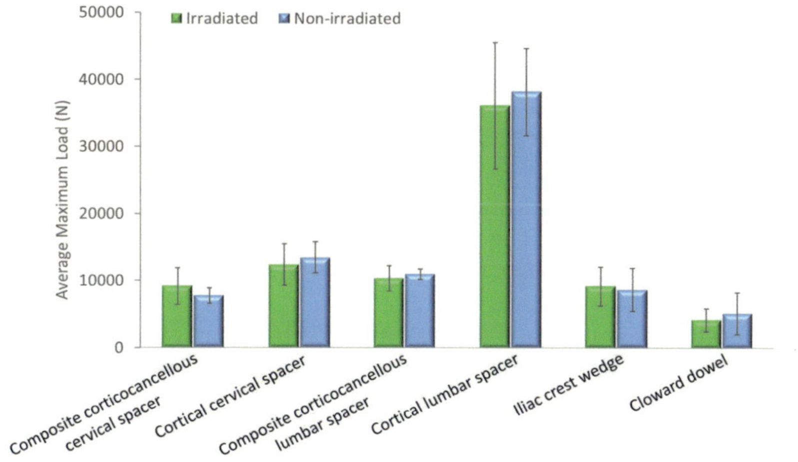

Figure 2.
Compressive strength of disinfected and irradiated vs. disinfected only structural bone allografts used in spinal fusion procedures. Compressive strength was defined as the maximum load that the graft could withstand before graft failure. Disinfected structural allografts were divided into either non-irradiated or irradiated groups, with a targeted absorbed dose of 15 kGy. Irradiation did not significantly alter the compressive strength of any of the structural allografts.

PEEK implants and contrasts with the stiffer stainless steel, titanium, and cobalt-chrome materials.

The success of a spinal fusion procedure depends, in part, on the mechanical strength of the interbody spacer. Failure of the spacer can lead to graft subsidence and non-union. Native vertebral bodies have been reported to withstand average compressive strengths up 2400 N for cervical and 8600 N for lumbar joints [41, 42]. It is desirable for interbody spacers to withstand a compressive strength comparable to that of the relevant autologous bone in that surgical procedure (e.g., cervical vs. lumbar). Since structural allografts are typically processed to disinfect or sterilize, and to preserve for storage before use, these methods have the potential to alter clinically relevant properties. The biomechanical strength of several configurations of structural bone allografts was assessed following disinfection using one such method, the proprietary Allowash® process (United States Patents 5,556,379; 5,820,581; 5,977,034; 6,024,735). In addition, samples were tested with or without a sterilizing dose of gamma irradiation performed at ultra-low temperatures (**Figure 2**). The results indicate that bone grafts can be disinfected and retain a strength greater than that of pertinent vertebral bodies, but can also be sterilized under controlled conditions without negative impact on the clinically relevant

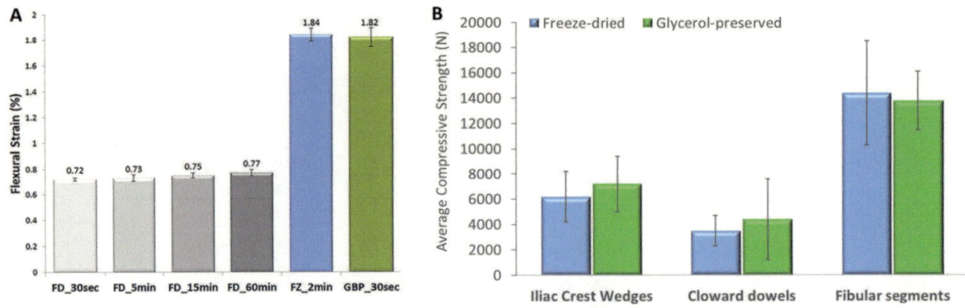

Figure 3.
Biomechanical properties of structural allografts preserved by different methods. Different types of disinfected structural bone allografts were preserved by either freezing, freeze-drying or glycerol preservation, followed by irradiation with a targeted absorbed dose of 15 kGy. Panel (A) shows the average flexural strain of cortical bone allografts preserved by the different approaches. The glycerol-preservation and frozen groups were not significantly different, but both demonstrated significantly greater average maximum flexural strain compared to the freeze-dried group. Modified and reprinted with permission from Samsell et al. [44] according to the Creative Commons Attribution 4.0 International License (https://creativecommons.org/licenses/by/4.0/legalcode). (B) Average compressive strength of structural allografts that were either freeze-dried or preserved using a glycerol-based solution. The compressive strength was not different between the freeze-dried and glycerol-preserved groups for all three graft types.

characteristics of the bone. Additionally, it has been separately demonstrated that moderate doses of irradiation (up to 28.5 kGy) performed at ultra-low temperatures do not alter the compressive strength or elastic modulus of structural allografts compared to non-irradiated controls [43].

Likewise, storage conditions can potentially alter properties of structural bone allografts before use. Traditionally, bone grafts have been provided frozen, with storage at −20°C, or freeze-dried, which allows for storage at room temperature. Frozen grafts require special shipping and storage, and must be thawed prior to use. Freeze-dried allografts can be stored at room temperature, but require rehydration, which may not restore the native biomechanical properties of the graft. More recently, a glycerol-based preservation solution was developed to allow storage of grafts at room temperature [44]. The flexural strain (i.e., elasticity) and compressive strength of various structural bone allografts preserved by either freezing, freeze-drying, or glycerol-based preservation were evaluated. The results demonstrate that the frozen and glycerol-preserved groups were not significantly different, but did display significantly greater flexural strain compared to freeze-dried tissue, even after the freeze-dried bone was rehydrated up to 60 minutes (**Figure 3A**). The compressive strengths of different structural allografts that were either freeze-dried or glycerol-preserved (**Figure 3B**) were found to be unaltered by the preservation method for each type of graft. These results demonstrate that the processing of allograft bone, including disinfection, sterilization by irradiation and varying preservation methods, does not significantly impair clinically relevant characteristics, notwithstanding the increased brittle nature of freeze-dried bone.

4. Pre-clinical literature review: *in vivo* models

In addition to testing mechanical properties, it is also important to evaluate the biocompatibility of bone graft substitutes. Animal models are a common and useful tool to evaluate the *in vivo* response to implantable materials prior to clinical application. Animal studies have demonstrated fibrous tissue growth and lack of osseointegration related to the use of PEEK implants.

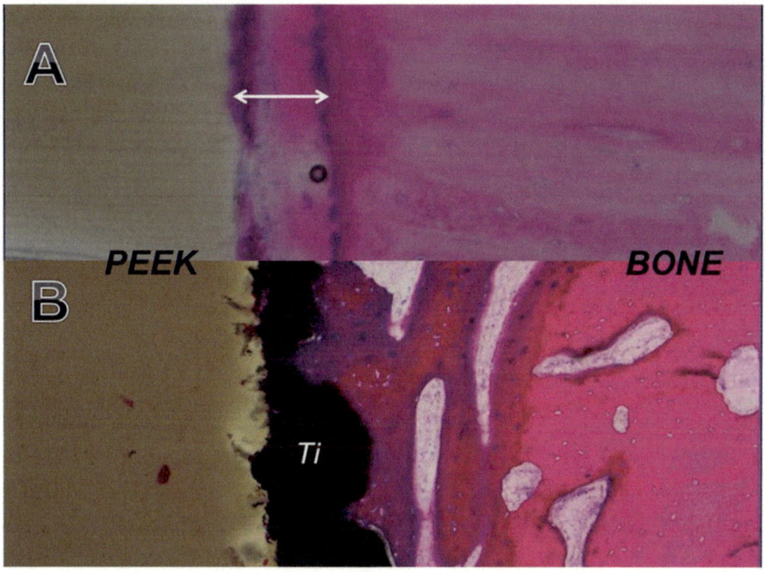

Figure 4.
Histology of PEEK/bone interface at 4 weeks post-implantation into a sheep tibia model. (A) Presence of fibrous tissue (white arrow) between the PEEK implant and adjacent bone—the rim of fibrous tissue results in the halo effect seen on CT imaging. (B) Titanium (Ti)-PEEK/bone interface demonstrating on-growth and ingrowth of bone at the Ti-PEEK/bone interface, with no radiolucent rim evident on CT imaging. Reprinted with permission from Phan et al. [38].

In a technical note, Phan et al. described PEEK's poor integration with the surrounding bone, producing a "PEEK-Halo" effect [38]. This phenomenon is represented by a halo appearance between the implant and bone graft on a CT scan. The authors placed conventional PEEK (c-PEEK) and Ti-sprayed PEEK implants in cortical bone and cancellous bone of adult sheep tibia. Histological analysis of the c-PEEK implant showed a fibrous tissue layer and a gap on the PEEK-bone interface (**Figure 4**). The authors suggest this may be due to inflammatory factors and/or the interaction between PEEK and osteoblastic differentiation. In a cervical interbody fusion model in adult sheep, authors compared the bone-implant interface of conventional PEEK (c-PEEK) and Hydroxyapatite coated PEEK (HA-PEEK) [37]. Micro-CT analysis demonstrated less new bone formation in the c-PEEK group at 6 weeks post-implantation. Furthermore, histological analysis showed a fibrous tissue interface between bone and c-PEEK implants at 6 and 12 weeks post-implantation. Walsh et al. likewise compared the mechanical and histologic properties of conventional PEEK and Ti-PEEK at the bone-implant interface in a sheep model [45]. Sites implanted with c-PEEK appeared static with no bone response. While, encouragingly, Ti-PEEK exhibited in-growth of bone, that is not the focus of this chapter. PEEK-bone implant interface contained a fibrous tissue layer and a gap at 4 and 12 weeks. Direct bone contact for the c-PEEK implants in cancellous bone was minimal at 4 weeks (4.8%) and improved at 12 weeks, but only reached 11.5%. This *in vivo* study is yet another example of fibrous tissue seen at the PEEK interface.

The use of structural allografts in ACDF procedures is well documented, with reported fusion rates similar to that of autologous bone [15, 16]. *In vivo* osseointegration of bone was assessed using a calvarial defect model in athymic rats [44]. A portion of the rat's skull was removed to create a critical size defect, which cannot close on its own. Following creation of the defect site, the investigators implanted human cortical and cancellous bone discs that were preserved by either freezing, freeze-drying, or glycerol-based preservation. At 1 week post-implantation, there

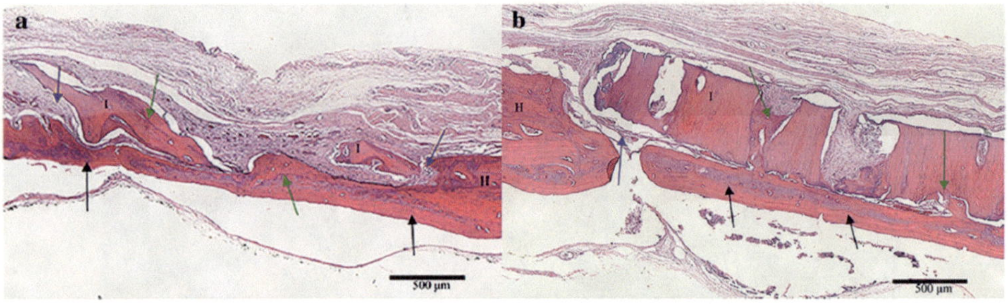

Figure 5.
(a) Glycerol-preserved cancellous bone in a tight-fit rat calvarial defect. The scale is 500 μm. (b) Freeze-dried cortical bone in a tight-fit rat calvarial defect at 6 weeks. The scale is 500 μm. Black arrows mark complete bone bridge formation. Blue arrows indicate soft tissue infiltrate. Green arrows mark osseointegration. H, host bone; I, implant bone. Reprinted with permission from Samsell et al. [44] according to the Creative Commons Attribution 4.0 International License (https://creativecommons.org/licenses/by/4.0/legalcode).

was apparent soft tissue infiltration in all experimental groups, consistent with an early post-operative response. These findings support the biocompatibility of the bone grafts. Additionally, at 6 weeks post-implantation, the authors observed areas of osseointegration similar to autograft (**Figure 5**).

5. Clinical data: fusion, nonunion, and pseudarthrosis rates

Both PEEK and allograft spinal implants have a long history of use in ACDF procedures. While mechanical and pre-clinical results can help predict clinical performance, this is ultimately determined through clinical outcomes. Many studies rely upon radiographic fusion to determine clinical success. According to Zdeblick and Phillips, "most published reports use the 'fusion' criteria required by the FDA, including motion of less than 5° on flexion-extension radiographs and an absence of lucencies around the cages or cage migration" [46]. Some studies also include pseudarthrosis rates. In the following section, we will compare clinical outcomes for allograft and PEEK implants.

Historically, autograft has been considered the gold standard for spinal fusion procedures, and therefore, it is used as the control to which structural allografts or PEEK implants have been compared. In a retrospective review, investigators evaluated radiographic fusion in 66 patients who underwent one-level ACDF with autograft (n = 31) or frozen tricortical iliac crest allograft spacers (n = 35), both with anterior plate fixation [16]. Radiographic outcomes were assessed at an average of 12 months follow-up. One hundred percent of patients in the allograft group demonstrated fusion compared to the 90% of patients in the autograft group, although the difference was not statistically significant. Three patients in the autograft group showed evidence of non-union. The authors suggested that the use of allograft can achieve high fusion rates, while avoiding complications associated with autograft, such as donor site pain. In a similar study, radiographic fusion was assessed in 80 patients who underwent multi-level ACDF procedures using autologous (n = 45) or allogeneic (n = 35) tricortical iliac crest grafts [15]. Radiographic outcomes were assessed in all patients at an average follow-up of 16 months. Successful bone fusion occurred in 100 and 94% of patients in the autograft and allograft group, respectively. Pseudarthrosis occurred in two patients in the allograft group, but was not statistically significant. The authors concluded that allograft can produce solid bone fusion similar to autograft without the associated donor site pain. Finally, in a prospective study, Cho et al. compared the radiographic outcomes of PEEK cages filled with autologous iliac bone marrow vs. autologous iliac crest graft only in 80 patients who underwent ACDF, with the number of levels ranging from 1 to 3 [47]. The study revealed 93% fusion in the autograft only group and 100% fusion rate in autograft filled PEEK cage group at an average follow-up of 10 months. It should be noted that the high fusion rate demonstrated by the PEEK group could potentially be associated with inherent bone healing properties of autograft within the cage.

Structural allografts have been used for decades to treat degenerative cervical disc disease. Numerous studies have evaluated radiographic fusion rates following use of structural bone allografts in ACDF procedures. Abla et al. prospectively evaluated 74 patients who were diagnosed with clinically significant cervical spinal stenosis or spondylosis and required ACDF surgery [48]. The investigators used a corticocancellous composite interbody spacer allograft (**Figure 6**) combined with cervical plate fixation. One-level fusion was performed in 34 patients, two levels in 23 patients, three levels in six patients, and four levels in one patient. Early fusion (at 1–3 months post-operative) was seen in 53% of the patients and by 12 months, 100% of the patients had fusion (**Figure 6**). The authors reported no graft failures, and an overall patient satisfaction of 90% at 12 months follow-up.

Another study, conducted by Graham et al. prospectively compared fusion rates using either freeze-dried or glycerol-preserved Cloward dowel allografts in ACDF procedures [49]. The study evaluated 86 patients with random assignment to either freeze-dried (n = 39) or glycerol-preserved (n = 47) groups (82 and 100 levels, respectively). Radiographic assessment at 6 months follow-up confirmed an overall fusion rate of >95% at all levels. Similarly, Rodway and Gander compared the use of glycerol-preserved vs. frozen interbody corticocancellous composite allografts in 67 patients undergoing ACDF procedures, with the number of levels ranging from 1 to 4 and a 1-year minimum follow-up [50]. Radiographic results demonstrated fusion in 38% of glycerol-preserved and 42% of frozen allografts at 3 months follow-up, and 100% fusion in both groups at 12 months (**Table 1**). Of note, the structural allografts used in each of these studies were sterilized by a low dose of gamma irradiation at ultra-low temperatures. Therefore, the combined results demonstrate the clinical effectiveness of structural allografts in ACDF surgery, regardless of method of preservation or treatment with a sterilizing dose of irradiation.

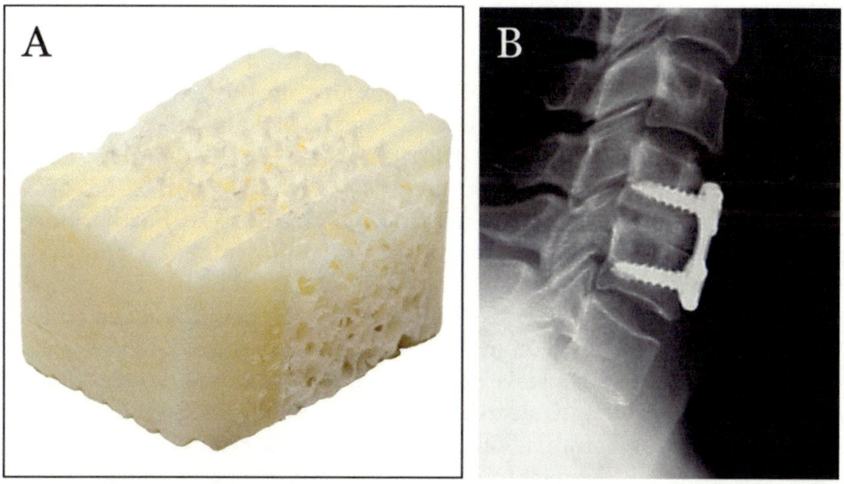

Figure 6.
(A) Structural interbody spacer with cancellous bone sandwiched between two plates of cortical bone. (B) Lateral X-ray 6 months after ACDF was performed in a 47-year old woman from C4-C5 using the structural interbody spacer shown. Complete fusion and good alignment were achieved. Modified and reprinted with permission from Abla et al. [48].

	Frozen				Glycerol-preserved				
	Total patients	Fused grafts	Not fused	% of fused patients	Total patients	Fused grafts	Not fused	% of fused patients	Frozen versus glycerol statistically similar?
Three months	38	16	22	42.1%	29	11	18	37.9%	Yes (P = 0.7343)
12 months	24.5	24.5	0	100%	17.5	17.5	0	100%	Yes (P > 0.999)

*Note that 2 patients had both glycerol-preserved and frozen grafts, 1 level for each type. The results from those patients were counted as 1/2 patients in each group.

Table 1.
Fusion rates by number of patients. Source: "Reprinted with permission from Rodway and Gander [50], according to the Creative Commons Attribution 4.0 International License (https://creativecommons.org/licenses/by/4.0/legalcode)".*

In a separate retrospective study, Muzevic et al. evaluated 154 patients who underwent a first-time ACDF surgery for treatment of cervical degenerative disc disease over a 3-year period [51]. One-level fusion was performed in 48 patients, two-level in 56 patients, three-level in 47 patients, and four-level in three patients using either cortical or corticocancellous structural allografts, along with demineralized bone matrix and cervical plating. Solid fusion was achieved in 98% of patients at a mean follow-up of 6 months, with improved overall treatment outcomes in 82% of patients. Finally, Yue et al. reviewed clinical and radiological outcomes in 71 patients who had ACDF surgery performed using structural freeze-dried fibular allografts an average of 7.2 years prior to the review [52]. The authors found that symptoms remained resolved in more than 82% of patients. They observed fusion in 93% of disc spaces, which was comparable to reported fusion rates for autograft [15, 16, 47, 53, 54]. While approximately 17% of the patients required revision surgery, the authors state that this rate is comparable to that following ACDF performed with autograft. Therefore, they attribute this revision rate to be a reflection of "normal" degeneration with age and not to use of allograft.

Several studies have assessed the clinical outcomes of ACDF procedures with the use of PEEK cages. In a prospective study, investigators assessed bone fusion in 52 patients who underwent anterior cervical discectomy with empty PEEK cages. One-level surgery was performed in 44 patients and 2-level surgery in eight patients [55]. Based on radiographic analyses, the authors confirmed bone fusion at 43 treated levels (72%) at an average of 16 months. The authors note the low fusion rates of empty PEEK cages, but stated that the lack of fusion did not affect clinical outcomes. Similarly, Suess et al. evaluated the clinical and radiographic outcomes of 292 patients who received empty PEEK cages for single-level ACDF procedures [56]. PEEK demonstrated radiographic fusion in 126 patients (43%) at 6 months, 214 patients (73%) at 12 months, and 241 patients (83%) at 18 months. The authors noted that slow and incomplete radiographic fusion could be attributed to the use of empty PEEK cages, and therefore did not recommend their use. Furthermore, they suggest this incomplete fusion may lead to reduced improvement in pain and possible disability. Finally, Kim et al. retrospectively evaluated 68 patients who underwent two and three-level ACDF with PEEK packed with demineralized bone matrix [57]. At an average follow-up of 28 months, PEEK demonstrated 81% overall fusion rate, which is less than reported levels for both autograft and structural allograft.

In a retrospective review, Krause et al. looked at 127 patients who underwent one-level ACDF with structural allograft (composite (61/71), cortical (8/71), or cancellous (2/71)) or PEEK cages to examine the incidence of pseudarthrosis as determined by radiography [58]. Fifty six patients (44%) received PEEK implants while 71 (56%) received structural allografts. All PEEK cages were filled with allogeneic demineralized bone matrix (DBM) or local autograft. The PEEK cohort demonstrated a higher rate of radiographic pseudarthrosis at one or more years after follow-up compared to the allograft cohort, 52 vs. 10% ($p < 0.001$), respectively (**Figure 7**). The investigators concluded that there was a *five-fold higher incidence of pseudarthrosis in patients with PEEK cages*, and almost double the rate of subsequent revision. Furthermore, the investigators suggested PEEK's inability to integrate with organic bone is due to its bio-inertness.

In a similar study, Teton et al. compared pseudarthrosis rates of 62 consecutive patients who underwent multi-level ACDF with structural allograft or PEEK cages, with at least 1 year follow-up [59]. Of 62 patients, 31 received PEEK implants, and 31 received structural allograft. Within the PEEK group, 20 (65%) patients demonstrated radiographic evidence of pseudarthrosis, compared to six (19%) patients implanted with structural allograft ($p < 0.001$), demonstrating *over three-fold higher incidence of pseudarthrosis rates with PEEK*. Furthermore, four patients implanted with PEEK required re-operation due to pseudarthrosis (13%), compared to zero patients with allograft ($p = 0.014$). Additionally, in a retrospective database review, authors analyzed 6130 patients who underwent ACDF with allograft (4063 patients) or intervertebral cages (2067 patients) to compare nonunion rates after

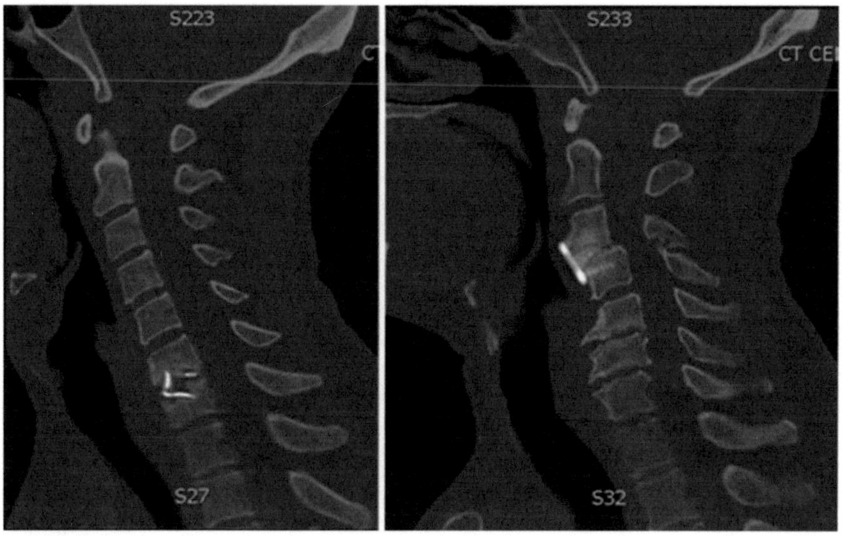

Figure 7.
Sagittal X-ray films obtained in a patient with a PEEK interbody graft and pseudarthrosis (left) and a patient with a structural allograft implant (right) healed 1 year after surgery. Reprinted with permission from Krause et al. [58].

Stratified Analysis; Nonunion Rates Between Allograft and Cage, After Controlling for Number of Levels Treated, Diabetes Status, and Tobacco Use			
	Allograft	Cage	P
One-level ACDF	1.9% (35/1835)	4.2% (35/843)	0.0007
Two-level ACDF	1.7% (28/1641)	6.1% (56/921)	<0.0001
3+ level ACDF	2.9% (17/587)	6.3% (19/303)	0.0155
Diabetes +	2.6% (44/1692)	8.3% (61/738)	<0.0001
Diabetes −	1.5% (36/2371)	3.7% (49/1329)	<0.0001
Tobacco +	2.7% (60/2195)	6.7% (69/1034)	<0.0001
Tobacco −	1.1% (20/1868)	4.0% (41/1033)	<0.0001

ACDF indicates anterior cervical discectomy and fusion.

**PEEK, titanium, mesh, or porous (unstratified due to nature of data base).*

Table 2.
Nonunion Rates Between Structural Allograft and Cages. Source: Reprinted with permission from Pirkle et al. [60].*

Author and year	Number of levels	Graft type	Number of patients	Time of fusion assessment	Fusion rate (%)	Pseudarthrosis rate (%)
Samartzis et al. [16]	2- and 3-level	Autograft	45	16 months	100	N/A
		Structural allograft (tricortical iliac crest)	35		94	
Samartzis et al. [15]	1-level	Autograft	31	12 months	90	N/A
		Structural allograft (tricortical iliac crest)	35		100	
Cho et al. [47]	Multilevel	Autograft	40	Avg. 10 months	93	N/A
		PEEK + autograft	40		100	
Abla et al. [48]	Multilevel	Structural allograft (corticocancellous composite)	74	1–3 months	53	N/A
				12 months	100	
Graham et al. [49]	Multi-level	Allograft (Cloward dowel, freeze-dried)	39	6 months	95	N/A
		Allograft (Cloward dowel, glycerol-preserved)	47		98	
Rodway and Gander [50]	Multi-level	Allograft (corticocancellous composite, glycerol-preserved)	29	3 months	38	N/A
			18	12 months	100	
		Allograft (corticocancellous composite, frozen)	38	3 months	42	
			25	12 months	100	
Muzevic et al. [51]	Multi-level	Allograft (cortical or corticocancellous + DBM)	154	Avg. 6 months	98	N/A
Yue et al. [52]	Multi-level	Allograft (fibular segment, freeze-dried)	71	Avg. 7 years	93	17 ("normal degeneration")
Pechlivanis et al. [55]	1- and 2-level	PEEK	52	Avg. 16 months	72	28 (nonunion)
Suess et al. [56]	1-level	PEEK	292	6 months	43	N/A
				12 months	73	
				18 months	83	

Author and year	Number of levels	Graft type	Number of patients	Time of fusion assessment	Fusion rate (%)	Pseudarthrosis rate (%)
Kim et al. [57]	2- and 3-level	PEEK + DBM	68	Avg. 28 months	81	N/A
Krause et al., [58]	1-level	PEEK + DBM or autograft	56 (47 DBM; 9 autograft)	Avg. 21 months	N/A	52
		Structural allograft (composite, cortical, or cancellous)	71 (61 composite; 8 cortical; 2 cancellous)	Avg. 16 months	N/A	10
Teton et al. [59]	Multi-level	PEEK	31	1 year	N/A	65
		Structural allograft	31		N/A	19
Pirkle et al. [60]	Multi-level	Intervertebral cages	2067	1 year	N/A	5
		Allograft	4063		N/A	2

Table 3.
Clinical fusion and pseudarthrosis rates following ACFD using autograft, structural allograft, or PEEK cages.

1 year post-operative [60]. Cages were unable to be stratified by type and may have been "PEEK, titanium, mesh, or porous." Patients were stratified by the number of levels treated, tobacco use, and diabetic conditions. Overall *nonunion rates were significantly higher in the cage group* (5.32%) than in allograft group (1.97%) ($p < 0.0001$). Notably, patients receiving intervertebral cages showed higher rates of nonunion regardless of other factors such as, levels treated, tobacco use, and diabetes (**Table 2**).

6. Summary

While autograft use is common for bone grafting procedures, it is associated with limitations, including donor site morbidity, limited quantities, and unsatisfactory biological activity. For ACDF, autograft use has steadily declined in favor of alternatives, primarily structural bone allografts and PEEK cages [18, 30]. Favorably, each has mechanical properties similar to autograft, with comparable elastic modulus and sufficient strength for intended applications. However, *in vivo* models demonstrate lack of osseointegration for PEEK, as well as fibrous tissue growth. Poor integration can lead to graft subsidence and pseudarthrosis, and ultimately pain, immobility and sensory loss. In contrast, structural allografts act as an osteoconductive scaffold demonstrating osseointegration in a rat model and have a long history of successful clinical use. These differences are reflected in clinical outcomes, as detailed in this chapter and summarized in **Table 3**. As shown, fusion rates when using PEEK cages were generally lower than when structural allografts were used. Moreover, the use of PEEK cages, and cages in general, in ACDF surgery presented a significantly higher rate of pseudarthrosis vs. structural allografts, leading to a greater rate for the need for subsequent revision surgery.

Due to lack of osseointegration of PEEK reported both pre-clinically and clinically, researchers have modified its surface or sought other materials in attempt to improve clinical outcomes. There are promising advances in porous and titanium coatings and clinical efficacy is being assessed.

In conclusion, although conventional PEEK cages have similar elastic modulus as structural allografts and autografts, they display poorer osseointegration characteristics compared to human bone implants. Comparative clinical analyses indicate that structural allografts yield higher fusion rates and lower incidence of pseudarthrosis than conventional PEEK cages in ACDF procedures.

Acknowledgements

We would like to thank Julie B. McLean, PhD, for editorial assistance.

Conflicts of interest

NC, ECG, and MAM are employees of LifeNet Health, a nonprofit organization.

Author details

Nigeste Carter, Elena C. Gianulis and Mark A. Moore*
LifeNet Health, Virginia Beach, VA, USA

*Address all correspondence to: mark_moore@lifenethealth.org

IntechOpen

© 2019 The Author(s). Licensee IntechOpen. This chapter is distributed under the terms of the Creative Commons Attribution License (http://creativecommons.org/licenses/by/3.0), which permits unrestricted use, distribution, and reproduction in any medium, provided the original work is properly cited.

References

[1] Whitecloud TS 3rd. Modern alternatives and techniques for one-level discectomy and fusion. Clinical Orthopaedics and Related Research. 1999;**359**:67-76

[2] Riley LH Jr, Robinson RA, Johnson KA, Walker AE. The results of anterior interbody fusion of the cervical spine. Review of ninety-three consecutive cases. Journal of Neurosurgery. 1969;**30**(2):127-133

[3] Cloward RB. The anterior approach for removal of ruptured cervical disks. Journal of Neurosurgery. 1958;**15**(6):602-617

[4] Song KJ, Choi BY. Current concepts of anterior cervical discectomy and fusion: A review of literature. Asian Spine Journal. 2014;**8**(4):531-539

[5] Bhadra AK, Raman AS, Casey AT, Crawford RJ. Single-level cervical radiculopathy: Clinical outcome and cost-effectiveness of four techniques of anterior cervical discectomy and fusion and disc arthroplasty. European Spine Journal. 2009;**18**(2):232-237

[6] Shen FH, Samartzis D, Khanna N, Goldberg EJ, An HS. Comparison of clinical and radiographic outcome in instrumented anterior cervical discectomy and fusion with or without direct uncovertebral joint decompression. The Spine Journal. 2004;**4**(6):629-635

[7] Suchomel P, Barsa P, Buchvald P, Svobodnik A, Vanickova E. Autologous versus allogenic bone grafts in instrumented anterior cervical discectomy and fusion: A prospective study with respect to bone union pattern. European Spine Journal: Official Publication of the European Spine Society, the European Spinal Deformity Society, and the European Section of the Cervical Spine Research Society. 2004;**13**(6):510-515

[8] Russell JL, Block JE. Surgical harvesting of bone graft from the ilium: Point of view. Medical Hypotheses. 2000;**55**(6):474-479

[9] Chau AM, Mobbs RJ. Bone graft substitutes in anterior cervical discectomy and fusion. European Spine Journal. 2009;**18**(4):449-464

[10] Chen F, He W, Mahaney K, Noeller J, Mhanna N, Viljoen S, et al. Alternative grafts in anterior cervical fusion. Clinical Neurology and Neurosurgery. 2013;**115**(10):2049-2055

[11] McKoy BE, Wingate JK, Poletti SC, Johnson DR 2nd, Stanley MD, Glaser JA. Fibular allograft after anterior cervical corpectomy: Long term follow-up. The Iowa Orthopaedic Journal. 2002;**22**:42-46

[12] Novell J, Novell-Costa F, Ivorra C, Farinas O, Munilla A, Martinez C. Five-year results of implants inserted into freeze-dried block allografts. Implant Dentistry. 2012;**21**(2):129-135

[13] Richards CJ, Garbuz DS, Pugh L, Masri BA. Revision total knee arthroplasty: Clinical outcome comparison with and without the use of femoral head structural allograft. The Journal of Arthroplasty. 2011;**26**(8):1299-1304

[14] Miller LE, Block JE. Safety and effectiveness of bone allografts in anterior cervical discectomy and fusion surgery. Spine. 2011;**36**(24):2045-2050

[15] Samartzis D, Shen FH, Goldberg EJ, An HS. Is autograft the gold standard in achieving radiographic fusion in one-level anterior cervical discectomy and fusion with rigid anterior plate fixation? Spine. 2005;**30**(15):1756-1761

[16] Samartzis D, Shen FH, Matthews DK, Yoon ST, Goldberg EJ, An HS. Comparison of allograft to autograft in multilevelanterior cervical discectomy and fusion with rigid plate fixation. The Spine Journal. 2003;**3**(6):451-459

[17] Piscitelli P, Iolascon G, Innocenti M, Civinini R, Rubinacci A, Muratore M, et al. Painful prosthesis: Approaching the patient with persistent pain following total hip and knee arthroplasty. Clinical Cases in Mineral and Bone Metabolism. 2013;**10**(2):97-110

[18] Anderson DG, Albert TJ. Bone grafting, implants, and plating options for anterior cervical fusions. The Orthopedic Clinics of North America. 2002;**33**(2):317-328

[19] Ramakrishna S, Mayer J, Wintermantel E, Leong KW. Biomedical applications of polymer-composite materials: A review. Composites Science and Technology. 2001;**61**(9):1189-1224

[20] AAOS Comprehensive Orthopaedic Review 2. 2nd ed. Rosemont, IL: American Academy of Orthopedic Surgeons; 2018

[21] de Boer HH. The history of bone grafts. Clinical Orthopaedics and Related Research;**1988**(226):292-298

[22] James CDT. Sir William Macewen. Proceedings of the Royal Society of Medicine. 1974;**67**(4):237-242

[23] Albee FH. Bone-graft surgery. Clinical Orthopaedics and Related Research. 1996;(324):5-12

[24] McGuire KJ, Harrast J, Herkowitz H, Weinstein JN. Geographic variation in the surgical treatment of degenerative cervical disc disease: American Board of Orthopedic Surgery Quality Improvement Initiative; part II candidates. Spine. 2012;**37**(1):57-66

[25] Center for Disease Control and Prevention (CDC). Allograft-Transmitted Infection: Priorities for Public Health Intervention; 2005

[26] Standards for Tissue Banking. 14th ed. American Association of Tissue Banks; 2016

[27] Regulatory Considerations for Human Cells, Tissues, and Cellular and Tissue-Based Products: Minimal Manipulation and Homologous Use. 2017

[28] US Food and Drug Administration (FDA). Guidance for Industry Current Good Tissue Practice (CGTP) and Additional Requirements for Manufacturers of Human Cells, Tissues, and Cellular and Tissue-Based Products (HCT/Ps); 2011

[29] Toth JM, Wang M, Estes BT, Scifert JL, Seim HB 3rd, Turner AS. Polyetheretherketone as a biomaterial for spinal applications. Biomaterials. 2006;**27**(3):324-334

[30] Kurtz SM, Devine JN. PEEK biomaterials in trauma, orthopedic, and spinal implants. Biomaterials. 2007;**28**(32):4845-4869

[31] Eschbach L. Nonresorbable polymers in bone surgery. Injury. 2000;**31**(Suppl 4):22-27

[32] Morrison C, Macnair R, MacDonald C, Wykman A, Goldie I, Grant MH. In vitro biocompatibility testing of polymers for orthopaedic implants using cultured fibroblasts and osteoblasts. Biomaterials. 1995;**16**(13):987-992

[33] Rivard CH, Rhalmi S, Coillard C. In vivo biocompatibility testing of peek polymer for a spinal implant system: A study in rabbits. Journal of Biomedical Materials Research. 2002;**62**(4):488-498

[34] Ma R, Tang T. Current strategies to improve the

bioactivity of PEEK. International Journal of Molecular Sciences. 2014;**15**(4):5426-5445

[35] Rao PJ, Pelletier MH, Walsh WR, Mobbs RJ. Spine interbody implants: Material selection and modification, functionalization and bioactivation of surfaces to improve osseointegration. Orthopaedic Surgery. 2014;**6**(2):81-89

[36] Kasemo B, Lausmaa J. Material-tissue interfaces: The role of surface properties and processes. Environmental Health Perspectives. 1994;**102**(Suppl 5):41-45

[37] Walsh WR, Pelletier MH, Bertollo N, Christou C, Tan C. Does PEEK/HA enhance bone formation compared with PEEK in a sheep cervical fusion model? Clinical Orthopaedics and Related Research. 2016;**474**(11):2364-2372

[38] Phan K, Hogan JA, Assem Y, Mobbs RJ. PEEK-Halo effect in interbody fusion. Journal of Clinical Neuroscience. 2016;**24**:138-140

[39] Almasi D, Iqbal N, Sadeghi M, Sudin I, Abdul Kadir MR, Kamarul T. Preparation methods for improving PEEK's bioactivity for orthopedic and dental application: A review. International Journal of Biomaterials. 2016;**2016**:8202653

[40] Heary RF, Parvathreddy N, Sampath S, Agarwal N. Elastic modulus in the selection of interbody implants. Journal of Spine Surgery. 2017;**3**(2):163-167

[41] Przybyla AS, Skrzypiec D, Pollintine P, Dolan P, Adams MA. Strength of the cervical spine in compression and bending. Spine. 2007;**32**(15):1612-1620

[42] Mosekilde L, Mosekilde L. Iliac crest trabecular bone volume as predictor for vertebral compressive strength, ash density and trabecular bone volume in normal individuals. Bone. 1988;**9**(4):195-199

[43] Balsly CR, Cotter AT, Williams LA, Gaskins BD, Moore MA, Wolfinbarger L Jr. Effect of low dose and moderate dose gamma irradiation on the mechanical properties of bone and soft tissue allografts. Cell and Tissue Banking. 2008;**9**(4):289-298

[44] Samsell B, Softic D, Qin X, McLean J, Sohoni P, Gonzales K, et al. Preservation of allograft bone using a glycerol solution: A compilation of original preclinical research. Biomaterials Research. 2019;**23**:5

[45] Walsh WR, Bertollo N, Christou C, Schaffner D, Mobbs RJ. Plasma-sprayed titanium coating to polyetheretherketone improves the bone-implant interface. The Spine Journal. 2015;**15**(5):1041-1049

[46] Zdeblick TA, Phillips FM. Interbody cage devices. Spine. 2003; **28**(15 Suppl):S2-S7

[47] Cho DY, Liau WR, Lee WY, Liu JT, Chiu CL, Sheu PC. Preliminary experience using a polyetheretherketone (PEEK) cage in the treatment of cervical disc disease. Neurosurgery. 2002;**51**(6):1343-1349. Discussion 9-50

[48] Abla AA, El Kadi H, Bost J, Maroon JC, Wert M. Allograft composite cortical and cancellous bone graft for anterior cervical fusion. Contemporary Neurosurgery. 2005;**27**(8):1-6

[49] Graham RS, Samsell BJ, Proffer A, Moore MA, Vega RA, Stary JM, et al. Evaluation of glycerol-preserved bone allografts in cervical spine fusion: A prospective, randomized controlled trial. Journal of Neurosurgery. Spine. 2015;**22**(1):1-10

[50] Rodway I, Gander J. Comparison of fusion rates between glycerol-preserved and frozen composite allografts in

cervical fusion. International Scholarly Research Notices. 2014;**2014**:960142

[51] Muzevic D, Splavski B, Boop FA, Arnautovic KI. Anterior cervical discectomy with instrumented allograft fusion: Lordosis restoration and comparison of functional outcomes among patients of different age groups. World Neurosurgery. 2018;**109**:e233-ee43

[52] Yue WM, Brodner W, Highland TR. Long-term results after anterior cervical discectomy and fusion with allograft and plating: A 5- 1-year radiologic and clinical follow-up study. Spine. 2005;**30**(19):2138-2144

[53] Geisler FH, Caspar W, Pitzen T, Johnson TA. Reoperation in patients after anterior cervical plate stabilization in degenerative disease. Spine. 1998;**23**(8):911-920

[54] Schneeberger AG, Boos N, Schwarzenbach O, Aebi M. Anterior cervical interbody fusion with plate fixation for chronic spondylotic radiculopathy: A 2- -year follow-up. Journal of Spinal Disorders. 1999;**12**(3):215-220. Discussion 21

[55] Pechlivanis I, Thuring T, Brenke C, Seiz M, Thome C, Barth M, et al. Non-fusion rates in anterior cervical discectomy and implantation of empty polyetheretherketone cages. Spine. 2011;**36**(1):15-20

[56] Suess O, Schomaker M, Cabraja M, Danne M, Kombos T, Hanna M. Empty polyetheretherketone (PEEK) cages in anterior cervical diskectomy and fusion (ACDF) show slow radiographic fusion that reduces clinical improvement: Results from the prospective multicenter "PIERCE-PEEK" study. Patient Safety in Surgery. 2017;**11**:12

[57] Kim YS, Park JY, Moon BJ, Kim SD, Lee JK. Is stand alone PEEK cage the gold standard in multilevel anterior cervical discectomy and fusion (ACDF)? Results of a minimum 1-year follow up. Journal of Clinical Neuroscience. 2018;**47**:341-346

[58] Krause KL, Obayashi JT, Bridges KJ, Raslan AM, Than KD. Fivefold higher rate of pseudarthrosis with polyetheretherketone interbody device than with structural allograft used for 1-level anterior cervical discectomy and fusion. Journal of Neurosurgery. 2018;**30**(1):46-51

[59] Teton Z, II BC, Ahmed Raslan M, Khoi Than M. Use of Polyetheretherketone Interbody Devices for Multi-Level Anterior Cervical Discectomy and Fusion Results in a Three-Fold Higher Rate of Pseudarthrosis Compared to Structural Allograft. American Association of Neurological Surgeons; 2019

[60] Pirkle S, Kaskovich S, Cook DJ, Ho A, Shi LL, Lee MJ. Cages in ACDF are associated with a higher nonunion rate than allograft: A stratified comparative analysis of 6130 patients. Spine. 2019;**44**(6):384-388

Chapter 5

Bone Graft in the Treatment of the Non-Consolidation of the Scaphoid with Necrosis of the Proximal Pole – A Systematic Review

Antônio Lourenço Severo, Osvandre Lech, Paulo Cesar Faiad Piluski, Marcelo Barreto Lemos, Carlos Castillo, Danilo Barreto Filho, Daniel Paulo Strack and Ivânio Tagliari

Abstract

The scaphoid fractures are the most common of the carpal bones, corresponding to 60; 10% of these progress to nonconsolidation, moreover, 3% can present necrosis of the proximal pole. There are various methods of treatment using vascularized (VBG) and nonvascularised bone grafts (NVBG). To evaluate and compare the rate of scaphoid consolidation with necrosis of the proximal pole using different surgical techniques. The authors conducted a systematic review of the literature using the following databases: PubMed and Bireme/Lilacs, where 13 case series were selected (10 with use of VBG and 3 of NVBG), according to inclusion and exclusion criteria. In most cases the vascularized bone grafts were used, especially those based on intercompartmental supraretinacular artery 1 and 2 due to greater reproducibility in performing the surgical technique.

Keywords: scaphoid, bone graft, scaphoid fractures, carpal bones, vascularized bone grafts, nonvascularised bone grafts

1. Introduction

The scaphoid fractures are the most common of the carpal bones, corresponding to 60% of these fractures. In spite of the existing consolidation without surgical treatment, some series of cases indicate rates of nonconsolidation of up to 10% [1]. Recent data suggest that the major risk factor for the nonconsolidation is the displacement of the fragments, which is associated with nonconsolidation rates of up to 55% [2].

Avascular necrosis has an estimate of occurrence of 3% in all cases of scaphoid fractures and occurs predominantly in the proximal pole, which has been attributed to the peculiarity of vascularization of this bone; studies on this subject describe that the arterial supply of the scaphoid occurs through three vessels (volar side, dorsal and distal) named according to spatial relationship with the scaphoid [3–5].

IntechOpen

More recently some studies showed that there are two arteries: one fully dorsal and another limited to the tubercle [6].

For the diagnosis of avascular necrosis the use of magnetic resonance imaging (MRI) has been recommended, which has an accuracy of up to 68%, increasing to 83% when associated with the use of gadolinium contrast. However, the gold standard is the intraoperative assessment of the absence of bleeding in the proximal fragment [7].

Several treatment techniques have been described using bone grafts, both vascularized (VBG) and nonvascularized bone grafts (NVBG). The use of nonvascularized bone grafts began with Adams and Leonard in 1928, who used cortical graft of the tibia embedded in the proximal and distal fragment through the back access via [8].

In 1934, Murray [9] described the embedded tibial graft usage through the tuberosity of the scaphoid; Bernard and Stubins in 1928 described the withdrawal of this bone pin from styloid process of the radius [10].

Matti in 1936 developed the technique in which an excavation in the proximal and distal scaphoid fragments was performed through the dorsal via, and that was later filled with cancellous bone graft [11]. Russi in 1960 modified Matti's technique using the volar via to preserve the vascularization of the scaphoid, performing niche filling with cancellous bone graft in a single block [12].

In 1970, Fisk observed the intense reabsorption of the volar portion of the fragments and the instability that follows, where distal fragment tends to flexion and the proximal fragment tends to stretch together with the semilunate, and later proposing the use of cortical cancellous graft correcting this deformity [13]. Later, Segmüller in 1973 [14] followed the precepts described by Fisk, but described the association of the use of osteosynthesis material (traction screw). Consequently, Fernandez, in 1984, described this technique in detail [15].

In 1965, Roy-Camille [16] published the technique of the VBG taken from the tuberosity of the scaphoid. Later, in 1986, Kuhlmann described the technique in which VBG removed from the medial portion and the volar portion of the distal radius were used for treatment of failures occurring after use of Matti-Russe technique [17].

In [18], work describing the vascularized graft taken from the distal portion of the radius with the vascularization based of intercompartmental supraretinacular artery 1 and 2 (1,2 ICSRA) was published.

In a recent systematic review [19], it was concluded that the consolidation rate of scaphoid fracture that evolved to a nonconsolidation with use in vascularized bone graft was of 88 versus 47% with use of nonvascularized graft.

In face of these data, this study aimed to carry out an updated literature review about the consolidation rates with use of different types of grafts (vascularized and nonvascularized) used for the treatment of scaphoid nonunion with necrosis of the proximal pole.

2. Methodology

A search was conducted in the current medical literature, by searching in the databases PubMed and Bireme/Lilacs using combinations of keywords below [20] (**Table 1**):

1. Bone graft scaphoid

2. Nonunion scaphoid

3. Vascularized bone graft nonunion scaphoid

4. Cancellous bone graft scaphoid

5. Pseudoarthrosis scaphoid

Term used on the search	Number of articles on PubMed	Articles selected from PubMed	Number of articles on Bireme	Articles selected from Bireme
Bone graft scaphoid	267	22	167	24
Nonunion scaphoid	273	19	182	18
Vascularized bone graft nonunion scaphoid	22	20	34	16
Structural bone graft nonunion scaphoid	10	8	6	5
Pseudoarthrosis scaphoid	66	10	273	13

Table 1.
Search in the current medical literature through the PubMed and Bireme/Lilacs data base.

All articles that made no reference to the use of bone graft to the treatment of nonunion of the scaphoid were excluded, which made reference to the use of graft in skeletally immature individuals, citing the use of bone grafts in other pathologies of the carpus and published articles for more than 20 years.

Thus the following selection was obtained.

Within the selected articles any work that made no reference to the occurrence of avascular necrosis of the proximal pole were excluded.

Therefore, a total of 13 articles were used for the analysis of the results.

3. Analysis of results

After the literature review, it can be seen that in the last two decades there is a tendency to the preference for the use of vascularized bone grafts in cases of non-consolidation of the scaphoid, especially when there are signs of avascular necrosis of the proximal pole, the main indication for the use of these grafts.

A systematic review of the literature highlights the use of various techniques of vascularized bone grafts (VBG), including: VBG based on capsular circulation, VBG based on metaphyseal circulation of the distal radius, VBG based on the volar circulation of the distal radius, based on the VBG supraretinacular artery between the 1st and 2nd extensor compartment (1,2 ICSRA), VBG coming from femoral condyle and coming from the iliac crest; the latter achieved using microanastomosis in the radial artery. All techniques show high consolidation rates, with an average of 89% (**Table 2**).

Steinmann et al. [21] in his work, made use of the distal radius graft with 1,2 ICSRA technique described by Zaindenberg; reached consolidation rates of 100% in 44 cases treated with this technique. Of these, eight had necrosis of the proximal pole. Tsai et al. [22] also by use of the technique 1,2 ICRSA reached consolidation rate of 80% (4 of 5 patients). Liang et al. [23] using the same technique described above had consolidation rates of 100%. However, unlike the previous work, [24] also used the vascularized bone graft technique based on 1,2 ICRSA, reaching consolidation rates of 100% in 10 patients, 5 cases with necrosis of the proximal pole of the scaphoid (**Tables 2** and **4**).

However, the study done by [25] in which vascularized bone graft based on 1,2 ICSRA was also used, shows consolidation rates well below comparing to the studies cited above. This work achieved consolidation rates of only 27% in 22 cases of nonconsolidation of the scaphoid and if only the cases with signs of necrosis of the proximal pole are considered, this percentage decreases to 12.5% (**Tables 2** and **4**).

Steinmann et al. [21] describe high rates of consolidation using distal radio bone graft based on capsular circulation, reaching 80% of consolidation, 10 cases were evaluated

Author	Consolidation rate	Kind of vascularized graft
[21]	100%	VBG based on 1,2 ICSRA
[22]	80%	VBG based on 1,2 ICSRA
[23]	100%	VBG based on 1,2 ICSRA
[24]	100%	VBG based on 1,2 ICSRA
[25]	27%	VBG based on 1,2 ICSRA
[26]	80%	VBG based on capsulate circulation
[27]	87%	VBG based on the first metacarpal artery
[28]	89%	VBG based on 1,2 ICSRA
[29]	73%	VBG based on the anterior transverse carpal artery
[30]	100% 40%	VBG from the femural condyle 1,2 ICRA

Vascularized bone graft (VBG), supraretinacular artery between compartments 1 and 2 [1,2 ICSRA].

Table 2.
Consolidation rates according to the technique used to the use of vascularized bone graft.

where all had necrosis of the proximal pole. The authors highlight the lack of need for dissection of small vessels as a great advantage of this technique (**Tables 2** and **4**).

Using the bone graft taken from the base of the thumb with the vascularization based on the first metacarpal artery, [27] have reached the consolidation rate of 87% in the series of 24 patients. In this work, four cases with necrosis of the proximal pole were included and all obtained radiographic consolidation. Despite the need for dissection of a small vessel, the authors report as an advantage the constancy in all cases of the first metacarpal artery (**Tables 2** and **4**).

In the study of [28] they realized the prospective evaluation of 46 patients who were treated with the use of vascularized bone graft based on 1,2 ICSRSA versus 40 patients treated with the use of nonvascularized bone graft taken from the distal radius and they obtained a statistically significant result in favor of the use of vascularized bone graft with a rate of 89.1 versus 72.5% with use of nonvascularized graft. Within the group of patients who underwent VBG use, 21 presented necrosis of the proximal pole and of these 19 have achieved consolidation (90.5%) (**Tables 2** and **4**).

In the study of [29] using VBG of the volar portion of the distal radius based in the anterior transverse carpal artery, 73% of consolidation rates were obtained in 30 cases. In this series two cases had signs of avascular necrosis of the proximal pole and neither obtained consolidation with the proposed treatment (**Tables 2** and **4**).

In their study, [30] compared consolidation rates into two groups treated with VBG: in a group of 22 patients they used graft taken from the distal radius with circulation based on 1,2 ICSRA and another group with 12 patients they used bone graft free from the femoral condyle. They achieved a statistically superior results using graft derived from the femoral condyle which reached the rate of 100 versus 40% of consolidation with graft originated from the distal radius (**Tables 2** and **4**).

Regarding the techniques that describe the use of NVBG for the treatment of nonunion of the scaphoid with necrosis of the proximal pole, only three series of case were found in this study that did not have the defined exclusion criteria. Matsuki et al. [31] proposed an investigation to assess the rate of consolidation of the proximal pole of the scaphoid fractures using NVBG associated with the fastening with Herbert bone screws; where 11 patients were evaluated and obtained consolidation in all of them (**Tables 3** and **4**). Using the same technique, [32] investigated 17 patients with 1 year follow up and obtained a consolidation rate of 52% (**Tables 3** and **4**). Ribak et al. [28] carried out the research on the consolidation rate

Author	Consolidation rate	Kind of nonvascularized graft
[31]	100%	Corticocancellous bone graft of the iliac crest
[32]	52%	Corticocancellous bone graft of the iliac crest
[28]	72%	Corticocancellous bone graft of the distal radius.

Table 3.
Consolidation rate according to the technique used for use of nonvascularized bone graft.

Author	NPP cases	Consolidation rates	Kind of graft
[21]	8	100% (8/8)	VBG based on 1,2 ICSRA
[22]	5	80% (4/5)	VBG based on 1,2 ICSRA
[23]	11	100% (11/11)	VBG based on 1,2 ICSRA
[24]	5	100% (5/5)	VBG based on 1,2 ICSRA
[25]	16	12,5% (2/16)	VBG based on 1,2 ICSRA
[26]	10	80% (8/10)	VBG based on capsular circulation EOV baseado na circulação capsular
[27]	4	100% (4/4)	VBG based on the first metacarpal artery EOV baseado na 1ª artéria metacarpal
[28]	21	19/21 (90.5%)	1,2 ICRA
[29]	2	0/2 (0%)	VBG based on the anterior transverse carpal artery exclusion of all in Portuguese that are in the table
[30]	10 12	4/10 (40%) 12/12 (100%)	1,2 ICRA VBG from the femural condyle
[31]	11	11/11 (100%)	Corticocancellous bone graft of the iliac crest Enxerto ósseo cortico esponjoso da crista ilíaca
[32]	17	52% (9/17)	Corticocancellous bone graft of the iliac crest Enxerto ósseo cortico esponjoso da crista ilíaca
[28]	16	68% (11/16)	Corticocancellous bone graft of the distal radius Enxerto ósseo cortico esponjoso do rádio distal

Table 4.
Consolidation rates, considering only cases with necrosis of the proximal pole of the scaphoid (NPP), vascularized bone graft (VBG), supraretinacular artery between compartments 1 and 2 [1,2 ICSRA].

with use of NVBG in 40 patients; of these, 16 presented necrosis of the proximal pole and the consolidation was achieved in 11 of them (**Tables 3** and **4**).

4. Discussion

The evidence supports that the arterial supply of the proximal pole is poor in comparison to the two-thirds of the distal scaphoid. The proximal pole for being entirely intraarticular is covered with hyaline cartilage with only one ligament insertion (radio-scaphoid-lunate ligament). So its vascularization is entirely dependent on intraosseous circulation. Thus, when there is loss of continuity solution due to deviation fracture, this circulation is impaired favoring the occurrence of non-consolidation [33, 34].

Tsai et al. [22] cites two basic reasons for the preference for the use of vascularized bone graft (VBG) regarding the use of vascularized bone graft not (NVBG): the shorter consolidation time, which implies a faster functional recovery, and ability to carry blood supply to a nonvascularized bone.

Since the publication of [18], who obtained 100% of consolidation in cases of nonconsolidation of the scaphoid, there is a growing interest in indicating the use of VBG based on the circulation of the dorsal radius, particularly with the use of the extensor intercompartmental supraretinacular artery between 1 and 2 [1,2 ICSRA]. Supporting this data in a recent publication, [19] published a meta-analysis study which showed a consolidation rate of 88 versus 47% using VBG and NVBG, respectively. The 1,2 ICRSA runs superficially on the retinaculum of the extentions and heads distally to the radial metaphyseal bone. According to the studies using this technique, easy identification and dissection of the artery are the major advantages. This came accordingly to the work of [35], which showed a consolidation rate of 93% using the technique described by Zaidenberg.

In [21, 23, 24], the 1,2 ICRSA technique was also used in their work, all reaching a consolidation rate of 100%. The three authors consider this a technically easier procedure, compared with other VBG techniques, also for being limited to only one incision. In addition, the correction DISI (dorsal intercalated segment instability) was obtained, caused by the curvature of the humpback scaphoid, a factor that helps increasing the range of motion postoperatively. Opposed to these studies, [7], the restoration of carpal geometry is essential for the consolidation, however the techniques that use bone graft derived from the distal radius, would provide a too small bone graft for humpback correction, i.e., the DISI. Thus, a means of achieving VBG that met this condition was the use of bone graft originated from the medial femoral condyle. The disadvantage of this technique would be the need of microsurgical technique usage for small vessel anastomosis, on the other hand, a graft with excellent quality would be obtained, that would offer greater rigidity when compared to graft taken from the distal radius. However, it should be noted that the technique that uses graft free from the femoral condyle requires microsurgical technique mastery, requiring specific training and long learning curve [30].

Jones et al. [30] compared two groups: VBG from the femoral condyle based on the VBG versus 1,2 ICSRA with consolidation rates of 100 and 40%, respectively. Ribak et al. [28] obtained consolidation of 89% using VBG based on 1,2 ICSRA versus consolidation of 72% using NVBG obtained from the distal radius. But for [25] using the VBG based on the 1,2 ICSRA concluded that this technique was ineffective in the series, with consolidation rates of 27% and reducing to 12.5% if we consider only cases of necrosis of the proximal pole.

Bertelli et al. [27] observed consolidation rates in 21 of 24 patients using the VBG based on the first metacarpal artery. These authors prefer to use of VBG due to the greater effectiveness in promoting bone consolidation compared to nonvascularized bone grafts, even in difficult situations such as avascular necrosis of the proximal pole.

The use of VBG using the capsular movement of the distal radius was described by [26] in which obtained consolidation rates of 80%. For these authors, this is a relatively simple technique that eliminates the need for dissection of small vessels or microanastomoses, and lead to a lower risk of vascular injury. A limitation of this technique, however, lies in failing to correct the humpback scaphoid deformity.

Jessu et al. [29] used VBG based on the anterior transverse carpal artery, i.e., vascularized bone grafts proposed by [34], obtained consolidation rate of 73% in 30 patients with nonunion of the scaphoid, however the two cases of proximal pole necrosis were not consolidated. The authors considered the consolidation rate disappointing, but still consider this to be an advantageous technique, mainly for its unique volar approach that reduces morbidity, but its realization requires long learning curve.

All the studies that use the 1,2 ICSRA technique highlight the easy viewing and dissection of the pedicle, which make this technique extremely useful for the treatment of nonunion of the scaphoid with necrosis of the proximal pole [21–25, 28].

The studies that use NVBG, basically used cortical cancellous bone grafts, simple techniques that have as an advantage the easy material removal. But there was an important change in consolidation rates, where [31] achieved great overall results, amounting to consolidation of 100% in 11 patients with necrosis of the proximal pole of the scaphoid. [28, 32], on the other hand, reached a much lower rate of 72 and 55%, respectively.

5. Conclusion

There is preference for the use of vascularized bone graft in relation to non-vascularized bone grafts, although the surgical technique is more detailed and demanding specific training, mainly in cases requiring vascular microsurgery, works using the technique for vascularized bone grafts reflect a better reproduction of positive results compared to conventional bone grafts. Therefore, according to this systematic review, there is no consensus in the literature that the use of vascularized bone graft can be effective in all cases for scaphoid consolidation with necrosis of the proximal pole.

Author details

Antônio Lourenço Severo[1]*, Osvandre Lech[2], Paulo Cesar Faiad Piluski[2], Marcelo Barreto Lemos[3], Carlos Castillo[2], Danilo Barreto Filho[4], Daniel Paulo Strack[5,6] and Ivânio Tagliari[7]

1 Hand Surgery and Microsurgery of Univ. Federal Fronteira Sul (UFFS), Hospital São Vicente de Paulo (HSVP), Instituto Ortopedia e Traumatologia (IOT), Passo Fundo, RS, Brazil

2 UFFS, HSVP, IOT Shoulder and Elbow Surgery Department, Passo Fundo, RS, Brazil

3 UFFS, HSVP, IOT Hand Surgery and Microsurgery Department, Passo Fundo, RS, Brazil

4 Hand Surgery Department at MIguel Riet Correa Jr. FURG-EBSERH University Hospital

5 Orthopedics and Traumatology Department Center, IJUÍ, RS, Brazil

6 Unimed Noroeste

7 UPF Graduate Program in Projects and Manufacturing Processes, HSVP Research Center/Unit 02, IOTRS, Passo Fundo, RS, Brazil

*Address all correspondence to: antoniolsevero@gmail.com

IntechOpen

© 2020 The Author(s). Licensee IntechOpen. This chapter is distributed under the terms of the Creative Commons Attribution License (http://creativecommons.org/licenses/by/3.0), which permits unrestricted use, distribution, and reproduction in any medium, provided the original work is properly cited.

References

[1] Geert A, Buijze LO, Ring D. Management of scaphoid nonunion. Journal of Hand Surgery. 2012;**37A**:1095-1100

[2] Talal A-J, Mannan A, Giannoudis P. The use of the free vascularised bone graft for nonunion of the scaphoid: A systematic review. Journal of Orthopaedic Surgery and Research. 2014;**9**:21

[3] Grettve S. Arterial anatomy of the carpal bones. Acta Anatomica. 1955;**25**:331

[4] Minne J, Depreux R, Mestdagh H. Les pédicules artérieles du massif carpien. Lille Médical. 1973;**18**:1174

[5] Taleisnik J, Kelly PJ. The extraosseous and intraosseous blood supply of the scaphoid bone. The Journal of Bone and Joint Surgery. American Volume. 1966;**48**:1125-1137

[6] Gelberman RH, Menon J. The vascularity of the scaphoid bone. Journal of Hand Surgery. 1980;**5**:508-513

[7] Sanjeev K, Bishop AT, Shin A. Role of vascularized bone grafts in the treatment of scaphoid nonunions associated with proximal pole avascular necrosis and carpal collapse. Journal of Hand Surgery. 2011;**36**:722-725

[8] Adams JD, Leonard RD. Fracture of the carpal scaphoid a new method of treatment with a report of one case. NEJM. 1928;**198**(8):401-404

[9] Murray J. Bone graft for non union of the carpal scaphoid. British Journal of Surgery. 1934;**22**:63-68

[10] Bernard L, Leonard RD. Fracture of the carpal scaphoid: A new method of treatment with a report of one case. NEJM. 1928;**198**(8):401-404

[11] Matti H. Technik und resultate meiner pseudarthosenoperation. Zentralblatt für Chirurgie. 1936;**63**:1442-1453

[12] Russe O. Fracture of navicular carpal: Diagnosis, non operative and operative treatment. JBJS. 1960;**42A**(5):759-768

[13] Fisk GR. Carpal instability and the fractured scaphoid. Annals of the Royal College of Surgeons of England. 1970;**46**:63-76

[14] Segmüller G. Navikulare-pseudarthrose. In: Operative Stabilisierung am Handskelet. Bern: Verlag Hans Huber; 1973. pp. 99-104

[15] Fernandez DL. A technique for anterior wedge-sheped grafts for scaphoid non-union with carpal instability. The Journal of Hand Surgery. 1984;**9**:733-737

[16] Roy-Camille R, Fractures ET pseudarthroses D. Scaphoid moyen utilisation d'um gref for pedicule. Actual Chir Orthop Raymond Poincare. 1965;**4**:197-214

[17] Trumble TE, Vo D. Proximal pole scaphoid fractures and nonunion. Journal of the American Society for Surgery of the Hand. 2001;**3**:155-171

[18] Zaidenberg C, Siebert JW, Angrigiani C. A new vascularized boné graft for scaphoid nonunion. The Journal of Hand Surgery. 1991;**16**(A):474-478

[19] Merrel GA, Wolfe S, Slade JF. Treatment of scaphoid nonunions: Quantitative meta-analysis of the literature. Journal of Hand Surgery. 2003;**27**:685-691

[20] Kelly AL, Gerad PS. Understanding systematic reviews and meta-analyses in orthopaedics. Journal of the American Academy of Orthopaedic Surgeons. 2013;**21**:0245-0255

[21] Steinmann SP, Bishop AT, Berger RA. Use of the 1,2 intercompartmental supraretinacular artery as vascularized pedicle bone graft for difficult scaphoid nonunion. The Journal of Hand Surgery. 2002;**27a**:391-401

[22] Tsai TT, Chao EK, Tu YK, Chen AC, Lee MS, Ueng SW. Management of scaphoid nonunion with avascular necrosis using 1,2intercompartmental supraretinacular arterial bone grafts. Chang Gung Medical Journal. 2002;**25**:321-328

[23] Liang K, Ke Z, Chen L, Nie M, Cheng Y, Deng Z. Scaphoid nonunion reconstructed with vascularized bone-grafting pedicled on 1,2 intercompartmental supraretin-aculararter y and external fixation. European Review for Medical and Pharmacological Sciences. 2013;**17**:1447-1454

[24] Uerpairojkit C, Leechavengvongs S, Witoonchart K. Primary vascularized distal radius bone graft for nonunion of the scaphoid. Journal of Hand Surgery. 2000;**25b**(3):266-22470

[25] Straw RG, Davis TRC, Dias JJ. Scaphoid nonunion: Treatment with a pedicledvascularized bone graft based on the 1,2 intercompartmental supraretinacularbranch of the radial artery. Journal of Hand Surgery. 2002;**27b**(5):413-416

[26] Sotereanos DG, Nickolaos AD, Dailiana ZH, Sarris IK, Konstantinos NM. A capsular-based vascularized distal radius graft for proximal pole scaphoid pseudarthrosis. Journal of Hand Surgery. 2006;**31a**:580-587

[27] Bertelli JA, Tacca CP, Rost J. Thumb metacarpal vascularized bone graft in long-standing scaphoid nonunion—A useful graft ,via dorsal or palmar approach: A cohort study of 24 patients. Journal of Hand Surgery. 2004;**29a**:1089-1097

[28] Ribak S, Medina CEG, Mattar R, Ulson HJR, Resende MR, Etchebehere M. Treatment of scaphoid nonunion with vascularised and nonvascularised dorsal bone grafting from the distal radius. International Orthopaedics. 2010;**34**:683-688

[29] Jessu MA, Wavreille GB, Strouk C, Fontaine BC. Chantelot b.scaphoid nonunions treated by kuhlmann's vascularized bone graft: Radiographic outcomes and complications. Chirurgie de la Main. 2008;**27**:87-96

[30] Jones DB Jr, Burger H, Bishop AT, Shin AY. Treatment of scaphoi waist nonunion with na avascular proximal pole and carpal colapse: A comparisson of two vascularized boné grafts. The Journal of Bone and Joint Surgery. American Volume. 2008;**90**:2616-2625

[31] Matsuki H, Junichi I, Iwasaki N, Uchiyama S, Minami A, Kato H. Non-vascularized bone graft with Herbert-type screw fixation for proximal pole scaphoid nonunion. Journal of Orthopaedic Science. 2011;**16**:749-755

[32] Randall RR, Ridge O, Carter PR. Iliac crest bone grafting and Herbert screw fixation of nonunions of the scaphoid with avascular proximal poles. Journal of Hand Surgery. 1995;**20A**:818-831

[33] Geissler WB, Slade JF. Fractures of the carpal bones. In: Green DP. Green's Operative Hand Surgery. 6th ed. Vol. 1. Elsevier Churchill Living Stone; 2010. p. 639-707

[34] Caporrino FA, Faloppa F, Dos Santos JBG, et al. Tratamento Cirurgico da Não consolidação do Escafóide com enxerto vascularizado da extremidade dorsal e distal do radio, baseado na artéria supraretinacular

1,2. Revista Brasileira de Ortopedia. 2003;**38**(9):522-533

[35] Kuhlmann JN, Mimoum M, Boabighi A, Baux S. Vascularized bone graft pedicled on the volar carpal artery for non-union of the scaphoid. Journal of Hand Surgery (British). 1987;**12**(2):203-210

Chapter 6

Distraction Osteogenesis: Biological Principles and Its Application in Companion Animals

Guilherme Domingos, Henrique Armés, Isabel Dias, Carlos Viegas and João Requicha

Abstract

Distraction osteogenesis is a surgical technique widely used in orthopedic surgery for treatment of various pathological skeletal conditions, namely correction of limb-length discrepancies, angular deformity and treatment of distal and severely comminuted fractures, or bone defects through bone transport. The basic principle consists on the gradual distraction of two bone segments, previously submitted to a corticotomy and promptly fixated generally using of circular external skeletal fixation. New bone tissue is generated in the bone gap between the two segments. This review aims to describe the biological fundaments and principles of this technique, the surgical steps performed to attempt distraction osteogenesis, and its possible complications with main focus on its application in companion animals.

Keywords: distraction osteogenesis, principles, bone regeneration, companion animals

1. Introduction

Distraction osteogenesis (DO) can be defined as the mechanical induction of bone tissue produced after the section and slowly separation of two bone segments, stabilized and subjected through a slow, gradual, and stable distraction. This is possible due to the inherent capacity of bone tissue to regenerate and remodel according to the mechanical and tension forces to which it is gradually submitted [1, 2].

The DO is a technique widely used in human and veterinary medicine, both in adult and pediatric orthopedics. It is used in the treatment of various diseases such as limb length discrepancies, bone deformities secondary to trauma, infections or malformations, and even as a compensation after surgical excision of bone tumors [3]. The physiological bone growth is a result of the tension exercised over the bone physis and the soft tissue resistance. This forces act on the same plane but in opposite directions [4].

The basic of the procedure should respect the principles defined by Ilizarov, Bastiani, and other pioneers in orthopedic research: (i) the osteotomy will be of low energy preserving the vascularization and the soft tissue envelope; (ii) the fixation mechanism applied to both segments must be stable; (iii) after the corticotomy a latency period will be applied, and (iv) the distraction rate (DR) must be appropriate for the level and type of bone in which osteogenesis is being performed [5].

After the separation of both segments, three temporal phases of DO can be defined: latency period, distraction period, and consolidation period [3].

2. Osteotomy and corticotomy

The DO procedure begins with the transverse section at a diaphyseal or metaphyseal level of the long bone to be elongated. Ilizarov described three methods to create fractures, including osteotomy, corticotomy, and osteoclasis. The osteogenic potential of the osteotomy or corticotomy depends on three main factors: the localization in bone, the type of technique used, and the latency period subsequently applied [6, 7].

Regarding the localization, some researchers in the past referred that the bone lengthening should be performed in the middle of the diaphysis of the long bone, and when necessary elongation was obtained, a bone graft from the ilium crest could be applied on the distraction focus to promote its consolidation. Later, Ilizarov recognized the metaphysis as the ideal site for the osteotomy, due to its massive trabecular bone area, rich in collateral vascularization, and higher potential for fracture recovery. Other researchers compared the regenerated bone quality at the diaphysis and metaphysis after DO, while using different latency periods. In the metaphysis, latency periods of 0 and 7 days allowed a greater osteogenesis and a faster remodeling and consolidation, when compared to the diaphysis elongation. A latency period of 14–21 days was associated with a premature consolidation in both regions. Bone mineralization of the newly formed tissue was faster at the metaphysis than at the diaphysis. Curiously, when there was no latency period, the distraction was successful and the consolidation faster. The latency of 7 days did not reveal the risk of premature consolidation; however, the consolidation and bone formation were slower than where there was no latency period. *Post mortem* torsion and bending test revealed that the bone tissue elongated on the metaphysis was tougher and more resistant. Histologically, the osteogenesis is observed to be based on intra-membranous ossification and, when a longer latency period is performed, increased proliferation of cartilaginous tissue at the osteotomy focus is detected, resulting in an endochondral ossification which may end up resulting in a slower process. The same study revealed that the metaphysis has more viable characteristics for the DO than the diaphysis [8].

Kojimoto and collaborators showed, in rabbits, the importance of the periosteum, referring that when it is removed, a bone callus is not formed and the bone lengthening can fail [9]. Ilizarov considered the preservation of the periosteum, and the medulla vascularization as mandatory to obtain better results on a DO [7, 10, 11]. Ilizarov developed the subperiostal osteotomy technique in which the anterior, medial, and lateral portions of the cortex are sectioned, and the posterior side is the manually fractured, thus preserving the medullar vasculature. Although Ilizarov defends the importance of the medullar vasculature, other authors question its importance [9, 12, 13].

3. Segment stabilization

The distraction is performed using an external fixation system, and this can be a circular Ilizarov or and longitudinal monoplane unilateral frame [3]. It is imperative to keep an adequate stabilization of the fracture, its alignment, and osteodistraction [11, 14].

The external fixator frame rigidity must prevent unnecessary micro-movements at the osteotomy site, but, at the same time, it should be compliant to allow bone tissue inducting micro-movements along the axial axis [14–16]. A stable external fixator with less stiffness decreases the time to achieve bone consolidation. Moreover, the time of consolidation with low mechanical score (less rigid) is smaller when compared to more rigid fixations [2].

Kusec and colleagues compared the bone tissue formed by DO using a unilateral distractor and an Ilizarov distractor, in a population of 15 German Shepherd dogs. No histological or radiographic differences were found on the newly formed bone tissue. The regeneration progressed in centripetally from the cortex and the intramembranous ossification was predominant at the medullar portion of the distraction focus [17]. The Ilizarov fixator, comparing to Wagner, Orthofix, and Oxford unilateral frames, is also flexible with a consistent stiffness to bending moments in anteroposterior and lateral planes. Moreover, the Ilizarov fixator is more resistant to axial compression with increasing load and is more flexible in the axial direction compared with the other devices [18].

During bone lengthening, the distraction moment where the screws are tightened or loosened in the external device frame may create instability on the distraction focus and therefore adversely affect the procedure. The use of new compounds, such as highly dense plastics, interconnected with metal alloys, helps to prevent instability during the adjustment period [19].

4. Latency period

The latency period begins immediately after the osteotomy and extends to the beginning of the distraction. This may be characterized as a "rest" period after the corticotomy to allow a tissue response to the iatrogenic trauma. This response includes a proliferation of fibroblast and the induction of a state of periosteal reactivity, phenomena which occur at the beginning of a fracture regeneration [3]. The latency period allows an organization of the hematoma and the fibrous tissue matrix, which will serve as a mold to the osteoblast proliferation, that on the first 24 hours produce osteoid at the bone surfaces. This period also allows a periosteal and endosteal revascularization [7, 10, 20].

In rabbits, the importance of the latency period was demonstrated in a tibial DO. A 7-day latency period allowed a greater regeneration at the distraction focus and increased vasculature, in opposition to a DO without latency period characterized by a fibrous tissue formation [21]. Other studies showed that the existence of a latency period allows the formation of cartilaginous tissue which leads to regeneration based on an endochondral ossification, a mechanism that is slower that its intramembranous counterpart [8].

Regarding the duration of this period, there is no consensus and several studies report variable periods from 0 to 21 days [1, 7, 8, 10]. There are several factors that influence the appropriate latency period, such as: age, the osteotomy localization, the soft tissue trauma or the existence of a primary pathology. A longer latency period may allow a premature consolidation, being then necessary to produce another fracture in order to continue the lengthening. And a shorter latency period might predispose to a bone non-union [3]. In Veterinary Orthopedics, the recommended latency period is 2–3 days for immature animal or 5–7 days to mature animal [1], inferior to the usual 5–10 days reported in humans [3].

5. Distraction period

During the distraction period, the bone segments undergo a stable and constant tension force, becoming metabolically active. The formation of bone tissue occurs along the distractive stress line, in the lengthening focus at the extremities of both bone segments. During this regenerative process, the bone tissue formation can reach 200–400 μm/day, which is 4–8 times superior to the physiological bone growth that occurs in the physis of a healthy growing dog [22].

With the distraction onset, tensile forces develop at the fracture focus, while at the same time collagen is deposited by proliferating fibroblast and organized into linear fibrils. This tissue becomes radiographically visible after 7–14 days of distraction, and with the continuous process, a radiolucency zone is formed at the center of the fracture focus, the fibrous interzone (FIZ). This zone divides the regenerated bone in equal parts, and it is rich in chondrocytes, fibroblast, and ovoid cell morphologically intermediate between a fibroblast and osteoblast. The FIZ remains avascular during most part of the distraction, after its completion, it is rapidly vascularized and mineralized during the consolidation period [3]. When the FIZ cells differentiate in osteoblasts, they begin to deposit bone matrix forming the micro-column formation zones (MCFZ). These micro-columns are similar to stalactites and stalagmites and are identified as cones of 150–200 μm. This mineralization proceeds longitudinally along the collagen fibers, parallel to the distraction forces. Between the FIZ and MCFZ, a connective tissue is formed, and this contains highly proliferative cells identical to those that arise in a primary ossification center [3].The fibroblast and osteoblast are arranged along the longitudinal collagen fibers at the distraction site and the later deposit osteoid directly into this fibrils [2] (**Figure 1**).

Although controversial, most histological studies regarding Ilizarov's method confirm that bone formation during a DO is primarily based in intramembranous ossification [8, 23]. In humans and in animal models of osteodistraction on both long bones and mandible, performed in dogs, rabbits, and sheep, intramembranous ossification prevails over its endochondral counterpart [9, 22, 24, 25], mainly on the ending stage [26]; however, three distinct ossification methods have already been identified. Endochondral ossification can be identified in all DO periods [9, 24, 27] and it is usually identified at the FIZ junctions and at new mineralized membranes originated from the corticotomy site [26, 28]. The ossification ratio between an intramembranous and endochondral ossification is 5–1, respectively [18, 26].

A third ossification phenomenon was histologically identified and termed transchondroid ossification, characterized by a bone formed from cells similar to chondrocytes and with a transition from fibrous tissue to chondroid bone tissue, a tissue intermediate between bone and cartilage, which undergoes a gradual transition to bone tissue without a blood capillary invasion [23, 28]. Other authors have

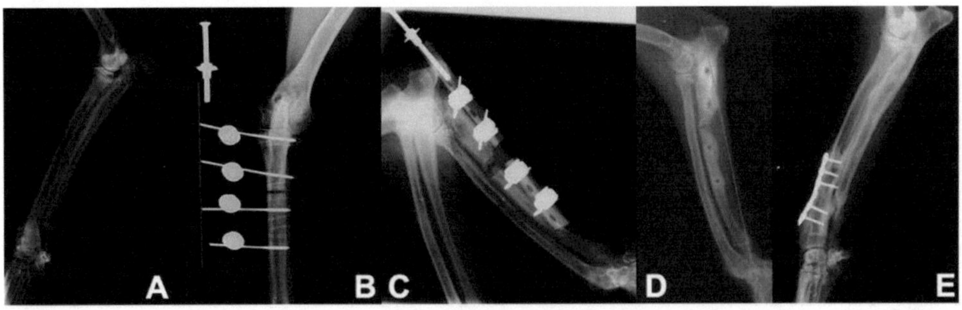

Figure 1.
Representative radiographic images of a distraction osteogenesis procedure performed in a 7-month-old female Greyhound dog due to a premature distal ulnar physis closure with proximal consequences in elbow joint. (A) Lateral view of the lower right thoracic limb. (B) Cranial view of the limb after the application of the distractor in the ulna. (C) Lateral view upon 11 days of distraction. (D) Lateral view at the end of the consolidation period and after the removal of the distractor. (E) After ulnar bone consolidation and lengthening, a realignment of the radius with an osteosynthesis plate was performed to fully rehabilitate the limb.

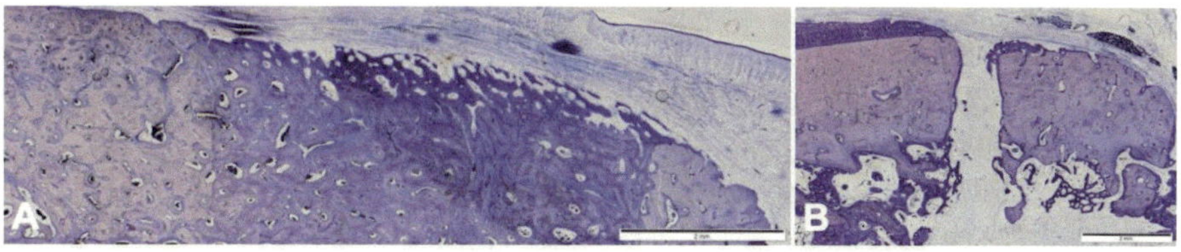

Figure 2.
Representative histologic images of a mandibular bone after distraction osteogenesis. (A) Distraction area successfully filled with new regenerated bone. (B) Bone defect occupied by connective tissue, a failure probably due to mobility of one of the fragments. Magnification ×40, Levai Laczko staining. Courtesy of Prof. Fernando Muñoz, Department of Clinical Veterinarian Sciences, University of Santiago de Compostela.

shown that cells similar to hypertrophied chondrocyte go through an osteogenic differentiation with deposition of type 1 and type 2 collagen fibers [29]. The cartilage that forms during a DO is usually located near the periosteum, but not within the limits of the cortex on the distraction focus [3] (**Figure 2**).

During the distraction period occurs an enormous angiogenic response. At the lengthening site, a peak of blood circulation nine times superior to that of normal bone tissue may occur. This hypervolemia persists for a significant amount of time, as it was shown that 17 weeks after the procedure the local volemia remains twice the normal value [23, 30].

It is believed that bone regeneration occurs in response to a slow and stable mechanical tensile force, applied to the bone callus and under which the living tissues become metabolically active, this phenomenon is called mechano-transduction [7, 10]. Ilizarov's experiments demonstrated that mitochondria of the skeletal muscular tissue hypertrophied and become more active, resulting in increased cellular volume and functional activity of the cell's nucleus [10].

During the distraction period, it is advised to do a radiographic assessment of the patient every 7–10 days, in order to evaluate the regenerated bone tissue, and if necessary, readjust the distraction rate (DR) [1]. Once the idealized bone length is achieved, the distraction ends. Marking the beginning of the consolidation period where the bone and osteoid are mineralized and remodeled [3].

6. Distraction rate and distraction rhythm

The distraction rate (DR), defined as the tension gradually applied to the bone, is measured in millimeters per day, the normal being 1 mm/day. However, this may vary according with the bone or the site of the bone we want to lengthen [3].

The total amount of distraction performed daily, the DR, is based on the same factors that should be considered for the ideal latency period [7, 10]. The typical DR in Veterinary Medicine should range from 0.75 to 2 mm/day, which is similar to what happens in Human Orthopedics [31–33]. Variables like age, osteotomy technique, and localization will influence the choice of a correct DR. We can correlate excessive DRs with muscular contractures and articular subluxations [34, 35]. The choice of an appropriate DR is essential in the prevention of premature consolidation of the regenerated tissue and soft tissue damage, as well as in the maintenance of articular congruity and biomechanical stability [1].

Ilizarov proposed an ideal DR of 1 mm/day for bone regeneration, and he based himself on his study in 120 dogs, using DR of 0.5, 1, and 2 mm/day. When using 0.5 mm/day, he noticed an increase in premature closures. And while using a DR of 2 mm/day Ilizarov reported increased tissue damage due to exceeding the tissues' revascularization capacity [14]. Recent studies suggest that DR between 0.5 and 2 mm/day are appropriate, and that the ideal DR must be based on individual characteristics such as age, osteotomy site, and need for angular correction [12, 35].

The distraction rhythm (DRy), the number of lengthening times made per day, influences the quality and quantity of the regenerated bone tissue and is important in the preservation of the soft tissue integrity during the procedure [7, 10, 34]. Ilizarov observed, using a canine model, that by using an automatic distractor capable of performing a DRy of 60 times per day, would produce a significantly better quality of bone when compared with DRy of 1–4 times per day. A DR of 1 mm a day with a DRy of 4 times a day was determined as ideal [7, 10]. In a goat model of tibia lengthening, DRy of 1, 4, and 720 times per day would not affect the strength, rigidity, and histomorphometric characteristic of the regenerated bone and would not affect the somatosensory potential of the peripheral nerves [34, 36]. Another study using the same animal model concluded that increasing the DRy would result in less muscular degeneration [39]. In Veterinary Medicine, it is recommended DRy of 2–4 times per day [9, 18, 31, 33].

7. Consolidation period

When finished the distraction period, the external fixator is maintained in order to confer stability to the regenerated tissue and allow its mineralization and consolidation [3]. In this period, the FIZ starts to mineralize and the central region becomes radiographically sclerotic. During the following weeks, the columns of regenerated tissue become homogeneous as the primary bone tissue is replaced by Haversian bone. In small animals, it will take around 8–12 weeks to form a new cortex and medullary cavity [7, 10, 36, 37].

Over time, the longitudinally oriented trabeculae are transformed into transverse plaques, incorporating the collagen template [7, 8, 10, 36]. The bone microcolumns are covered with osteoblasts that actively produce osteoid. Each column is accompanied by a large vascular channel that preserves the ideal distance in order to allow a diffusion gradient between cells. The activity of bone cells during a DO is similar to what occurs during a fracture healing [8, 28, 38]. However, what happens at a tissue level, the continuous recruitment and activation of cells capable of producing and reabsorbing bone, significantly exceeds a fracture healing process [39]. Simultaneously during the extensive bone production, a remodeling occurs, producing *porosis* of the bone cortex and margins of the regenerated bone. After 2–3 months in animal and 4–6 months in humans, the Havers channels, through which blood vessels and nerves pass, are formed [11, 12, 38]. The bone marrow components, in the regenerated bone appear after 4 months. Bone remodeling is complete after 5–7 months in small animals and 12–24 months in humans. After this remodeling period, the mechanical integrity of the cortex is restored [1].

The consolidation period after a DO was investigated in a 20-year retrospective study, based on 115 animals submitted to a corticotomy and application of a circular external fixator [2]. The authors concluded that the radius requires less time to consolidate than the tibia and presented the hypothesis that this occurs due to during the march, the radius bears weight in a parallel axis and the tibia carries the weight through an oblique axis [40]. Another hypothesis is based on the fact that dogs bear around 60% of their weight on the thoracic limbs, therefore the weight carried by a radius is superior to what is supported by a tibia [41–43]. In experimental rabbit model, the effects of an angular osteotomy after a DO were studied, revealing that a 30° axis deviation at the distraction focus resulted in a 50% reduction of the regenerated bone [44]. In humans, the femur is referred to consolidate faster than the tibia [45]. Ilizarov's original technique described that the consolidation period before fixator removal should be 1 month/cm of new regenerated bone [46].

The bone formation can be controlled through tomography, scintigraphy, ultrasound, and bone densitometry; however, radiographs continue to be the more practical method to determine the consolidation efficiency and when the bone is ready to remove the external fixation system [1, 38].

Nowadays, numerous studies are focused on the molecular mechanism behind a DO, such as, the genetic expression of the bone morphogenic proteins (BMPs 2 and 4) which is induced by tension and mechanic stress [47, 48]. Other molecular signs, such as the insulin-like growth factor type 1 (IGF-1), transforming growth factor beta (TGFb) and fibroblastic growth factor 1 (FGF-1), associated with osteoblast proliferation and its differentiation from mesenchymal cells were identified at the distraction site [49, 50]. Another study identified that it is possible to accelerate the ossification process during a DO by administrating a recombinant homologous growth hormone [51].

Tissue engineering approaches have already been applied to promote bone regeneration at DO. The use of mesenchymal stem cells (MSCs) from autologous origin, isolated from the bone marrow or adipose tissue, or from human xenogeneic origin has been described in different animal models of DO like rats, rabbits, pigs, dogs, and sheep with promising outcomes; nonetheless many of the mechanism behind the process remain to be investigated, for example, the recruitment and activation of MSCs upon the initial stimulation by surgical trauma. Growth and differentiation factors, hormonal proteins, and pharmacological agents can be added in combination to the distraction site. The number of cells transplanted is measured in cell over DR (number of cells in millions divided by total distractions in millimeters) ranged from 0.03 to 5.00 M/mm. The cells can be injected after the distraction period, loaded into scaffolds and then transplanted to the distraction focus during the osteotomy or during the latency period [52]. Genetically modified MSCs have also been evaluated using growth and differentiation factors including bone morphogenetic protein-7 (BMP-7) [53, 54], BMP-2 [55, 56], basic fibroblast growth factor (bFGF) [57], transforming growth factor-β (TGFβ), and insulin-like growth factor-1 [58], as well as genes encoding transcription factors, such as osterix (Osx) [59, 60] and runt-related transcription factor 2 (Run×2) [61] with distinct effects reported in the improvement of bone regeneration [52].

8. Craniofacial distraction osteogenesis

Djasim and collaborators created guidelines for craniofacial DO. They collected data from dog, rat, sheep, goat, rabbit, pig, and rhesus monkey models based on data from previous craniofacial DO studies. With the premise that intramembranous bones of the skull have a different vascular supply compared to long bones, therefore DO parameters suitable for orthopedic DO might be suboptimal for craniofacial DO. They concluded that a latency period may not be necessary in some animals such as sheep and pigs, and in others it produces far better-quality bone tissue as seen in rats and rabbits. They reaffirmed that the ideal distraction rate should be 1 mm/day, which should be halved when using rats and determined an ideal consolidation period of 6–8 weeks [62]. Another review in mandibular DO showed that the latency period ranged from 2 to 7 days. The distraction rate ranged from 0.4 to 2.4 mm/day. The total distraction gap obtained ranged from 3.2 to 20 mm, and the consolidation period ranged from 4 days to 10 weeks [52].

9. Distraction osteogenesis after oncologic surgery

DO can also provide an option for limb sparing surgery upon resection of primary bone tumors, such as osteosarcomas. The bone transport osteogenesis (BTO), an adaption of the DO technique, is used to preserve limb function after resection of large segmental bone defects. Briefly, after the tumor excision, an osteotomy is performed on the proximal bone segment, creating a distraction focus and resulting on a small portion of healthy bone which will act as the transport segment. Then using an external ring fixator, this segment is slowly distracted in the defect direction, creating regenerated tissue resulting in bone union and a bridged effect. The distraction should continue until 3 days after the segments touch in order to compress the distal healthy bone, turning it metabolically active, this process is called docking. Successful docking is achieved when the transport segment heals with the adjacent bone. It is possible to predict the timing of docking by measuring the distance between the two bones on radiographs and calculating the number of days required to achieve contact based upon the DR. The surgeon should consider grafting when the transport segment is approximately less than 0.5 cm from contact with the docking site. When owners strongly wish to avoid further surgery, autologous bone marrow graft, obtained from the patient, could be mixed with canine demineralized bone matrix (DBM) into the docking site, acting as a vehicle of mesenchymal stem cells and osteoinductive signals [63, 64].

BTO surged as an alternative to cadaveric allograft bone transports, which was seen as the main limb salvage procedure in alternative to amputation; however, complications such as non-union, graft fracture, and infection are referred in the literature. One study reported that nearly one half of the patients develop infection may be associated with the lack of intrinsic blood supply surrounding the allograft and tumor resection area [65]. This high complication rate could lead to soft tissue lost, chronic pain, non-weight-bearing lameness, multiple surgeries, and even amputation [66–68].

The extent of the needed tissue resection can be planned based on detailed radiographs, scintigraphy, or ideally, a preoperative magnetic resonance imaging (MRI) which will be essential to help build the fixator frame, and assess the extent of the tumor involvement within the bone marrow, as it commonly exceeds the extent detected on radiographs. The surgeon should plan to excise at least 2 cm of bone proximal to the most proximal extent of tumor identified [63]. The patients with better outcome in DO upon oncologic surgery are those whose tumors are located in the distal radius or ulna, due to bigger pancarpal arthrodesis success [64]. The best candidates for limb salvage are those whose tumors involve less than 50% of the bone and have minimal soft tissue involvement. In theory, the extension of tumor treatable with this technique is limited to by the ability to achieve appropriate margins. There must be at least enough bone remaining in the proximal radius to create a transport segment and to place three wires above the transport segment. Dogs with infected allografts after prior limb salvage surgery are suitable candidates for bone transport, unless they have had recent radiation therapy. Patients with pathologic fracture, multicentric neoplasia, metastasis or severe intercurrent health conditions should not be considered as favorable candidates [63].

After the tumor resection, BTO is similar to a conventional DO, a latency period of 3 days is sufficient unless the dog is receiving chemotherapy treatment. In those cases, a longer latency period of up to 7 days should be applied. Afterwards, the distraction should consist on a DR of 1 mm/day and DRy of 2–4 times a day. Immediately after a chemotherapy session, distraction should be ceased for 3 days before being restarted. This waiting period can be eliminated if the patient shows signs of premature consolidation. Radiographic reassessment should be made every 10–14 days during bone transport and every 3–4 weeks after docking. Some animals may require higher DR to prevent premature consolidation, while other may require occasional "resting" period of 2–5 days. If the regenerated bone begins to be progressively thinning, ductile, and with "hourglass" shape in radiographs, it is recommended to slow or stop distraction for a few days. Conversely, if the wires in the transport segment begin to bend in the direction of distraction, the DR should increase for 2–3 days (1.5–2 mm/day) to help preventing premature consolidation. The radiographs and fixator should also be regularly evaluated to adjust DR and DRY, document broken wires, evidence of tumor recurrence, progression of mineralization of regenerate bone, and time of docking [63].

Fixators should be removed when peripheral bridging of the central radiolucent zone within the regenerate tissue is evident on radiographs, the columns of new bone are mineralized, and when the docking site union has been achieved. It can be difficult to evaluate the stability of the docking site before removing the fixator frame, due to the concentration of metal hardware. If doubt exists regarding effective union, the fixator removal can be delayed provided the patient is not having substantial soft-tissue problems. Osteosarcoma patients should be restaged every 2–3 months to evaluate for metastasis or local tumor recurrence [63].

Negative effects of systemic chemotherapy and radiotherapy are reported in distraction osteogenesis [69–71]. Chemotherapy likely impedes the osteoblasts to cope with the increased functional demand and compromises bone callus formation during a DO. High dose chemotherapy reduces colony forming unit fibroblast by 50% in the bone marrow, by 10% on cortical bone, and 20% in trabecular bone [72]. However, two studies compared patients who underwent DO with and without chemotherapy and it did not demonstrate any difference in the bone healing process between patient groups [73, 74]. The hypothesis proposed is that DO's effect on osteoblast may counteract the inhibitory effects of chemotherapy [75].

In humans, some bone sarcomas, most commonly Ewing sarcoma, adjuvant radiotherapy is a treatment option, being reported adverse effects of radiation therapy on up to 74% of patients [76–78], namely wound healing problems, infection, muscle and joint contracture, ankylosis, osteitis, non-union, pathological fractures, tendon adhesion, and radiation induced sarcoma [76–79]. In a rabbit tibia model, it was demonstrated that radiation exposure decreases the quantity and quality of regenerate and angiogenesis during a DO [80]. Also, in a rabbit mandible model, it was found that osteogenesis is delayed after a 60-Gy dose of radiation, even though viable osteoblast and osteocytes may still be present [81]. It is therefore likely that distraction osteogenesis is negatively affected by radiation [75].

10. Complications of distraction osteogenesis

The complication associated with a DO include muscular contractures, subluxations, vascular and nerve lesions, premature or delayed consolidation, and even bone non-union. The placement of intramedullary pins near a nerve or large caliber blood vessel can lead to damage on those structures during the lengthening [1].

Neuromuscular lesions are rarely associated with lengthening phases unless they exceed 30% of the limb size [33, 82, 83]. Subluxations are associated with muscular contractures and can occur in substantially excessive lengthening. Premature consolidations can be prevented with an adequate DR and DRy. Delayed consolidations are multifactorial but are more commonly reported cases where an excessive DR was applied. Bone non-union is on its own associated to an infectious process. A strict radiographic protocol allows a control, assessment, and readjustment in order to avoid these complications [1].

One of the limitations of this technique is the long period necessary for the newly formed bone to mature, mineralize, and consolidate. The external fixators must be kept until the end of the consolidation period in order to confer the stability necessary to obtain better quality bone [3].

During a femoral lengthening, the muscles inserted therein are responsible for the majority of the complication that may occur. The quadriceps, glutes, and abductors can influence the lengthening progression, and the tension exercised on the soft tissues causes pain, reduces the articular mobility, and deforms the regenerated bone column. To achieve a successful lengthening, it is imperative that one understands this concept and adjust the surgical technique and patient management to minimize its impact [5].

Stogov and collaborators showed, in dogs, that a high frequency (120 DRy) of 3 mm/day does not only produce viable bone, but also produce compensatory alterations to the muscle tissue that would prevent catabolic alterations on the anterior tibial muscle during a tibia elongation. These authors referred that a high frequency lengthening amount that does not exceed 15% of the initial tibial length, does not result in considerable damage to the anterior tibial muscle. Using a DR of 3 mm/day while increasing the DRy (180 automated distractions per day) can produce a consistent regenerated bone [84].

As mentioned before, the soft tissues are a limitation factor for the procedure [34, 82, 85]. Lengthening exceeding 20% the original bone measure is reported to damage peripheral nerves, muscular, and tendon structures. Thus, physical rehabilitation during the procedures could decrease the severity of the muscular contractures and prevents articular diseases. The double-level or bi-level lengthening, which consist on creating two fracture focus and therefore two focus of bone distraction can reduce by half the distraction period duration, dispersing the distraction forces applied at the soft tissues and reducing the degenerative effects [1]. The correction of biapical radial deformities in dogs has been described with success using bi-level hinged external fixators as posterior distraction [86].

Taking into consideration that the DO can also occur along a transverse axis, perpendicular to the longitudinal bone axis, it is also possible to perform a widening of bone tissue. Some authors have already successfully preformed bone transports, in order to correct a defect on a long bone they perform a DO on the contralateral bone and use the regenerated tissue as graft to the affected limb. It has been performed in the same bone tibia-tibia but also in ipsilateral ulnar and radial bone transports, tibial-humeral and fibular-tibial, and this procedure is also performed in human medicine [87].

It is worth referring a recent study in humans, which applied a multidirectional DO device, a new technique with the goal of correcting cranial deformities in children [88].

Conflict of interest

The authors declare no conflict of interest with any financial organization regarding the material discussed in the chapter.

Author details

Guilherme Domingos[1], Henrique Armés[1,2], Isabel Dias[3], Carlos Viegas[3] and João Requicha[1,3]*

1 Faculty of Veterinary Medicine, University Lusófona, Lisbon, Portugal

2 Hospital Veterinário de São Bento, Lisbon, Portugal

3 Department of Veterinary Sciences, University of Trás-os-Montes e Alto Douro, Vila Real, Portugal

*Address all correspondence to: jfrequicha@gmail.com

IntechOpen

© 2019 The Author(s). Licensee IntechOpen. This chapter is distributed under the terms of the Creative Commons Attribution License (http://creativecommons.org/licenses/by/3.0), which permits unrestricted use, distribution, and reproduction in any medium, provided the original work is properly cited.

References

[1] Welch RD, Lewis DD. Distraction osteogenesis. The Veterinary Clinics of North America. Small Animal Practice. 1999;**29**(5):1187-1205

[2] Tuohy JL, Marcellin-Little DJ, Griffith EH. Durations of bone consolidation and external fixation after distraction osteogenesis in dogs. Veterinary Surgery. 2014;**43**:903-911

[3] Sailhan F. Bone lengthening (distraction osteogenesis): A literature review. Osteoporosis International. 2011;**22**(6):2011-2015

[4] Merloz P. Bone regeneration and limb lengthening. Osteoporosis International. 2011;**22**(6): 2033-2036

[5] Nayagam S. Femoral lengthening with a rail external fixator: Tips and tricks. Strategies in Trauma and Limb Reconstruction. 2010;**5**(3):137-144

[6] Ilizarov GA, Zarubin VI. Method of treatment of long bone defects by lengthening of one of the fragments with Ilizarov technique. In: Transosseous Compression, Distraction and Compression-Distraction Osteosynthesis in Traumatology and Orthopedics. Collection of Scientific Works from Kurgan Research Scientific Institute. Vol. 2. Russia: Kurgan Research Scientific Institute; 1976

[7] Ilizarov GA. The tension-stress effect on the genesis and growth of tissues: Part I. The influence of the rate and frequency of distraction. Clinical Orthopaedics and Related Research. 1989;**239**:249-281

[8] Aronson J, Shen X. Experimental healing of distraction osteogenesis comparing metaphyseal with diaphyseal sites. Clinical Orthopaedics and Related Research. 1994;**301**:25-30

[9] Kojimoto H, Yasui N, Goto T, Matsuda SY. Bone lengthening in rabbits by callus distraction. The role of periosteum and endosteum. Journal of Bone and Joint Surgery. British Volume (London). 1988;**70**(4):543-549

[10] Ilizarov GA. The tension-stress effect on the genesis and growth of tissues: Part II. The influence of the rate and frequency of distraction. Clinical Orthopaedics and Related Research. 1989;**239**:263-285

[11] Ilizarov GA. Transosseous Osteosynthesis: Theoretical and Clinical Aspects of the Regeneration and Growth of Tissue. New York: Springer Verlag; 1992

[12] Frierson M, Ibrahim K, Boles M, et al. Distraction osteogenesis. A comparison of corticotomy techniques. Clinical Orthopaedics. 1994;**301**:19-24

[13] Marcellin-Little DJ, Ferretti A. Improving bone healing with the circular external fixation method. Veterinary Forums. 1997;7:40-47

[14] Ilizarov GA. Clinical application of the tension-stress effect for limb lengthening. Clinical Orthopaedics. 1990;**250**:8-26

[15] Paley D, Fleming B, Catagni M, et al. Mechanical evaluation of external fixators used in limb lengthening. Clinical Orthopaedics and Related Research. 1990;**250**:50-57

[16] Lewis DO, Bronson DG, Welch RD. Effect of individual components on the axial stiffness of single ring IMEX circular external skeletal fixation system constructs. Veterinary and Comparative Orthopaedics and Traumatology. 1997;**10**:80

[17] Kusec V, Jelic M, Borovecki F, Kos J, Vukicevic S, Korzinek K. Distraction osteogenesis by Ilizarov and unilateral external fixators in a canine model. International Orthopaedics. 2003;**27**(1):47-52

[18] Younger AS, Morrison J, MacKenzie WG. Biomechanics of external fixation and limb lengthening. Foot and Ankle Clinics. 2004;**9**(3):433-448

[19] Stallings JT, Lewis DD, Welch RD, et al. An introduction to distraction osteogenesis and the principles of the Ilizarov method. Veterinary and Comparative Orthopaedics and Traumatology. 1998;**11**:59-67

[20] White SH, Kenwright J. The importance of delay in distraction of osteotomies. The Orthopedic Clinics of North America. 1991;**22**:569-579

[21] Fjeld TO, Steen H. Limb lengthening by low rate epiphyseal distraction. An experimental study in the caprine tibia. Journal of Orthopaedic Research. 1988;**6**:360-368

[22] Aronson J, Good B, Stewart C, Harrison B, Harp J. Preliminary studies of mineralization during distraction osteogenesis. Clinical Orthopaedics and Related Research. 1990;**250**:43-49

[23] Choi IH, Chung CY, Cho TJ, Yoo WJ. Angiogenesis and mineralization during distraction osteogenesis. Journal of Korean Medical Science. 2002;**17**(4):435-447

[24] Delloye C, Delefortrie G, Coutelier L, Vincent A. Bone regenerate formation in cortical bone during distraction lengthening. An experimental study. Clinical Orthopaedics. 1990;**250**:34-42

[25] Ali MN, Ejiri S, Kobayashi T, Anwar RB, Oda K, Ohshima H, et al. Histologic study of the cellular events during rat mandibular distraction osteogenesis. Oral Surgery, Oral Medicine, Oral Pathology, Oral Radiology, and Endodontics. 2009;**107**(3):325-335

[26] Fink B, Pollnau C, Vogel M, Skripitz R, Enderle A. Histomorphometry of distraction osteogenesis during experimental tibial lengthening. Journal of Orthopaedic Trauma. 2003;**17**(2):113-118

[27] Jazrawi LM, Majeska RJ, Klein ML, Kagel E, Stromberg L, Einhorn TA. Bone and cartilage formation in an experimental model of distraction osteogenesis. Journal of Orthopaedic Trauma. 1998;**12**(2):111-116

[28] Yasui N, Sato M, Ochi T, et al. Three modes of ossification during distraction osteogenesis in the rat. Journal of Bone and Joint Surgery. British Volume (London). 1997;**79**(5):824-830

[29] Li G, Virdi AS, Ashhurst DE, Simpson AH, Triffitt JT. Tissues formed during distraction osteogenesis in the rabbit are determined by the distraction rate: Localization of the cells that express the mRNAs and the distribution of types I and II collagens. Cell Biology International. 2000;**24**(1):25-33

[30] Choi IH, Ahn JH, Chung CY, Cho TJ. Vascular proliferation and blood supply during distraction osteogenesis: A scanning electron microscopic observation. Journal of Orthopaedic Research. 2000;**18**(5):698-705

[31] Ferretti A. The application of the Ilizarov technique to veterinary medicine. In: Bianchi Maiocchi A, Aronson J, editors. Operative Principles of Ilizarov. Baltimore: Williams & Wilkins; 1991

[32] Latte Y. A specific vet Ilizarov apparatus for the treatment of fractures, delayed union, non-union and mal

union. In: Proceedings of the Veterinary Orthopedic Society; 1991. p. 51

[33] Marcellin-Little DJ, Ferretti A, Roe SC, DeYoung DJ. Hinged Ilizarov external fixation for correction of antebrachial deformities. Veterinary Surgery. 1998;**27**(3):231-245

[34] Birch JG, Samchukov ML, Welch, RD, et al. The effect of rhythm of distraction during limb lengthening: An experimental investigation. In: Proceedings of the Fourth Annual ASAMI Scientific Meeting; New Orleans; 1994. p. 7

[35] Catagni MA, Malzev V, Kirienko A. Correction of angular deformities. In: Bianchi-Maiocchi A, editor. Advances in Ilizarov Apparatus Assembly. Milan: Medicalplastic; 1994

[36] Welch RD, Birch JG, Samchukov ML. Histomorphology of distraction osteogenesis in a caprine tibial lengthening model. Journal of Bone and Mineral Research. 1998;**13**:1-9

[37] Latte Y. Studies of 63 cases treated by Ilizarov apparatus: Indications, results, complications. In: Proceedings of the Veterinary Orthopedic Society; Alberta, Canada; 1993. p. 12

[38] Aronson J. Temporal and spatial increases in blood flow during distraction osteogenesis. Clinical Orthopaedics. 1994;**301**:124-131

[39] Welch RD. Biology of distraction osteogenesis. In: Proceedings of the Annual Meeting of the American College of Veterinary Surgeons; Chicago, USA; 1995. p. 305

[40] Agostinho FS, Rahal SC, Miqueleto NS, Verdugo MR, Inamassu LR, El-Warrak AO. Kinematic analysis of Labrador retrievers and Rottweilers trotting on a treadmill. Veterinary and Comparative Orthopaedics and Traumatology. 2011;**24**:185-191

[41] Levine D, Marcellin-Little DJ, Millis DL, et al. Effects of partial immersion in water on vertical ground reaction forces and weight distribution in dogs. American Journal of Veterinary Research. 2010;**71**:1413-1416

[42] Molsa SH, Hielm-Bjorkman AK, Laitinen-Vapaavuori OM. Force platform analysis in clinically healthy Rottweilers: Comparison with Labrador retrievers. Veterinary Surgery. 2010;**9**:701-707

[43] Brady RB, Sidiropoulos AN, Bennett HJ, et al. Evaluation of gait related variables in lean and obese dogs at a trot. American Journal of Veterinary Research. 2013;**74**:757-762

[44] Richards M, Goulet JA, Weiss JA, Waanders NA, Schaffler MB, Goldstein SA. Bone regeneration and fracture healing. Experience with distraction osteogenesis model. Clinical Orthopaedics and Related Research. 1998;**355**(Suppl):S191-S204

[45] Fischgrund J, Paley D, Suter C. Variables affecting time to bone healing during limb lengthening. Clinical Orthopaedics and Related Research. 1994;**301**:31-37

[46] Ilizarov GA. The principles of the Ilizarov method. Bulletin of the Hospital for Joint Diseases Orthopaedic Institute. 1988;**48**:1-11

[47] Li G, Berven S, Simpson H, Triffitt JT. Expression of BMP-4 during distraction osteogenesis in rabbits. Acta Orthopaedica Scandinavica. 1998;**69**:420-425

[48] Sato M, Ochi T, Nakase T, Hirotam S, Kitamura Y, Nomura S, et al. Mechanical tension-stress induces expression of bone morphogenetic protein (BMP)-2 and BMP-4, but not BMP-6, BMP-7, and GDF-5 mRNA, during distraction osteogenesis. Journal of Bone and Mineral Research. 1999;**14**:1084-1095

[49] Lammens J, Liu Z, Aerssens J, Dequeker J, Fabry G. Distraction bone healing versus osteotomy healing: A comparative biochemical analysis. Journal of Bone and Mineral Research. 1988;**13**:279-286

[50] Farhadieh RD, Dickinson R, Yu Y, Gianoutsos MP, Walsh WR. The role of transforming growth factor-beta, insulin- like growth factor 1, and basic fibroblast growth factor in distraction osteogenesis of the mandible. The Journal of Craniofacial Surgery. 1999;**10**:80-86

[51] Raschke MJ, Bail H, Windhagen HJ, Kolbeck SF, Weiler A, Raun K, et al. Recombinant growth hormone accelerates bone regenerate consolidation in distraction osteogenesis. Bone. 1999;**24**:81-88

[52] Tee BC, Sun Z. Mandibular distraction osteogenesis assisted by cell-based tissue engineering: A systematic review. Orthodontics and Craniofacial Research. 2015;**18**(Suppl1):39-49

[53] Hu J, Qi MC, Zou SJ, Li JH, Luo E. Callus formation enhanced by BMP-7 ex vivo gene therapy during distraction osteogenesis in rats. Journal of Orthopaedic Research. 2007;**25**:241-251

[54] Zhang WB, Zheng LW, Chua DT, Cheung LK. Treatment of irradiated mandibles with mesenchymal stem cells transfected with bone morphogenetic protein 2/7. Journal of Oral and Maxillofacial Surgery. 2012;**70**:1711-1716

[55] Long J, Li P, Du HM, Liu L, Zheng XH, Lin YF, et al. Effects of bone morphogenetic protein 2 gene therapy on new bone formation during mandibular distraction osteogenesis at rapid rate in rabbits. Oral Surgery, Oral Medicine, Oral Pathology, Oral Radiology, and Endodontics. 2011;**112**:50-57

[56] Castro-Govea Y, Cervantes-Kardasch VH, Borrego-Soto G, Martinez-Rodriguez HG, Espinoza Juarez M, Romero-Diaz V, et al. Human bone morphogenetic protein 2-transduced mesenchymal stem cells improve bone regeneration in a model of mandible distraction surgery. The Journal of Craniofacial Surgery. 2012;**23**:392-396

[57] Jiang X, Zou S, Ye B, Zhu S, Liu Y, Hu J. bFGF-modified BMMSCs enhance bone regeneration following distraction osteogenesis in rabbits. Bone. 2010;**46**:1156-1161

[58] Kroczek A, Park J, Birkholz T, Neukam FW, Wiltfang J, Kessler P. Effects of osteoinduction on bone regeneration in distraction: Results of a pilot study. Journal of Cranio-Maxillo-Facial Surgery. 2010;**38**:334-344

[59] Lai QG, Yuan KF, Xu X, Li DR, Li GJ, Wei FL, et al. Transcription factor osterix modified bone marrow mesenchymal stem cells enhance callus formation during distraction osteogenesis. Oral Surgery, Oral Medicine, Oral Pathology, Oral Radiology, and Endodontics. 2011;**111**:412-419

[60] Lai QG, Sun SL, Zhou XH, Zhang CP, Yuan KF, Yang ZJ, et al. Adipose-derived stem cells transfected with pEGFP-OSX enhance bone formation during distraction osteogenesis. Journal of Zhejiang University. Science. B. 2014;**15**:482-490

[61] Sun JJ, Zheng XH, Wang LY, Liu L, Jing W, Lin YF, et al. New bone formation enhanced by ADSCs overexpressing hRunx2 during mandibular distraction osteogenesis in osteoporotic rabbits. Journal of Orthopaedic Research. 2014;**32**:709-720

[62] Djasim UM, Wolvius EB, van Neck JW, Weinans H, van der Wal KG. Recommendations for optimal

distraction protocols for various animal models on the basis of a systematic review of the literature. International Journal of Oral and Maxillofacial Surgery. 2007;**36**(10):877-883

[63] Ehrhart N. Longitudinal bone transport for treatment of primary bone tumors in dogs: Technique description and outcome in 9 dogs. Veterinary Surgery. 2005;**34**:24-34

[64] Bella B, Lara-Garcia A, Lafuente P. Canine appendicular osteosarcoma. Veterinary Ireland Journal. 2016;**6**(4):207-216

[65] Dernell WS. Treatment of severe orthopedic infections. The Veterinary Clinics of North America. Small Animal Practice. 1999;**29**:1261-1274

[66] Asada N, Tsuchiya H, Kitaoka K, et al. Massive autoclaved allografts and autografts for limb salvage surgery: A 1-8 year follow-up of 23 patients. Acta Orthopaedica Scandinavica. 1997;**68**:392-395

[67] Dernell WS, Withrow SJ, Straw RC. Clinical response to antibiotic impregnated methylmethacrylate bead implantation of dogs with severe infections after limb sparing surgery and allograft replacement: 18 cases (1994-1998). Veterinary and Comparative Orthopaedics and Traumatology. 1998;**11**:94-99

[68] Ortiz-Cruz E, Gebhardt MC, Jennings LC, et al. The results of transplantation of intercalary allografts after resection of tumors. A long-term follow-up study. The Journal of Bone and Joint Surgery. American Volume. 1997;**79**:97-106

[69] Cao J, Tan MH, Yang P, Li WL, Xia J, Du H, et al. Effects of adjuvant chemotherapy on bone marrow mesenchymal stem cells of colorectal cancer patients. Cancer Letters. 2008;**263**(2):197-203

[70] Fan C, Cool JC, Scherer MA, Foster BK, Shandala T, Tapp H, et al. Damaging effects of chronic low-dose methotrexate usage on primary bone formation in young rats and potential protective effects of folinic acid supplementary treatment. Bone. 2009;**44**(1):61-70

[71] Kemp K, Morse R, Wexler S, Cox C, Mallam E, Hows J, et al. Chemotherapy-induced mesenchymal stem cell damage in patients with hematological malignancy. Annals of Hematology. 2010;**89**(7):701-713

[72] Banfi A, Podesta M, Fazzuoli L, Sertoli MR, Venturini M, Santini G, et al. High-dose chemotherapy shows a dose-dependent toxicity to bone marrow osteoprogenitors: A mechanism for post-bone marrow transplantation osteopenia. Cancer. 2001;**92**(9):2419-2428

[73] Kapukaya A, Subasi M, Arslan H, Tuzuner T, Selek S. Technique and complications of callus distraction in the treatment of bone tumors. Archives of Orthopaedic and Trauma Surgery. 2006;**126**(3):157-163

[74] Watanabe K, Tsuchiya H, Sakurakichi K, Yamashiro T, Matsubara H, Tomita K. Treatment of lower limb deformities and limb-length discrepancies with the external fixator in Ollier's disease. Journal of Orthopaedic Science. 2007;**12**(5):471-475

[75] Lesensky J, Prince D. Distraction osteogenesis reconstruction of large segmental bone defects after primary tumor resection: Pitfalls and benefits. European Journal of Orthopaedic Surgery and Traumatology. 2017;**27**(6):715-727

[76] Rohde RS, Puhaindran ME, Morris CD, Alektiar KM, Schupak KD, Healey JH, et al. Complications of radiation therapy to the hand after soft

tissue sarcoma surgery. The Journal of Hand Surgery. 2010;**35**(11):1858-1863

[77] Sheplan LJ, Juliano JJ. Use of radiation therapy for patients with soft-tissue and bone sarcomas. Cleveland Clinic Journal of Medicine. 2010;**77**(Suppl 1):S27-S29

[78] Mahmoud O, Wolfson A. Perioperative irradiation in extremity soft tissue sarcoma. Expert Review of Anticancer Therapy. 2011;**11**(8):1233-1241

[79] Al-Absi E, Farrokhyar F, Sharma R, Whelan K, Corbett T, Patel M, et al. A systematic review and meta-analysis of oncologic outcomes of pre- versus postoperative radiation in localized resectable soft-tissue sarcoma. Annals of Surgical Oncology. 2010;**17**(5):1367-1374

[80] Tsuchiya H, Uehara K, Sakurakichi K, Watanabe K, Matsubara H, Tomita K. Distraction osteogenesis after irradiation in a rabbit model. Journal of Orthopaedic Science. 2005;**10**(6):627-633

[81] Ma Y, Shen G. Distraction osteogenesis after irradiation in rabbit mandibles. The British Journal of Oral and Maxillofacial Surgery. 2012;**50**:662-667

[82] Paley D. Problems, obstacles, and complications of limb lengthening by the Ilizarov technique. Clinical Orthopaedics and Related Research. 1990;**250**:81-104

[83] Makarov MR, Delgado MR, Samchukov ML, et al. SSEP evaluation of acute nerve injury associated with external fixation procedures. Clinical Orthopaedics. 1994;**306**:49-56

[84] Stogov MV, Emanov AA, Stepanov MA. Muscle metabolism during tibial lengthening with regular and high distraction rates. Journal of Orthopaedic Science. 2014;**19**(6):965-972

[85] Eldridge J, Bell D. Problems with substantial limb lengthening. The Orthopedic Clinics of North America. 1991;**22**:625-631

[86] Kwan TW, Marcellin-Little DJ, Harrysson OL. Correction of biapical radial deformities by use of bi-level hinged circular external fixation and distraction osteogenesis in 13 dogs. Veterinary Surgery. 2014;**43**(3):316-329

[87] Petazzoni M. Contralateral bone widening and transfer for limb sparing in a cat. Veterinary and Comparative Orthopaedics and Traumatology. 2016;**29**(2):174-180

[88] Gomi A, Sunaga A, Kamochi H, Oguma H, Sugawara Y. Distraction osteogenesis update: Introduction of multidirectional cranial distraction osteogenesis. Journal of Korean Neurosurgical Association. 2016;**59**(3):233-241

Section 3

Bone-Related Diseases

Chapter 7

Thyroid Disorders and Osteoporosis

Ayotunde Oladunni Ale

Abstract

Adequate amount of thyroid hormone is an essential requirement for normal development and maturity of bones in the early life as well as for the maintenance of the skeletal system (bone remodeling). Osteoporosis, one of the most common metabolic bone disorders, is strongly associated with hyperthyroidism (endogenous and exogenous), whereas association of the same disease with hypothyroidism is not quite established. Most of the data describing the association between osteoporosis and hyperthyroidism are collected among elderly population (especially postmenopausal women), and only a few studies in literature researched into osteoporosis and hyperthyroidism in <50 years of age; hence further studies are required in the younger population (including premenopausal women and younger males).

Keywords: bone remodeling, hyperthyroidism, hypothyroidism, postmenopausal women

1. Introduction

The skeletal system maintains a dynamic characteristic throughout its life by continuously undergoing bone modeling and bone remodeling processes [1–7]. Both bone modeling and remodeling processes include bone resorption mediated by osteoclasts and bone formation mediated by osteoblasts. Bone modeling is the predominant event during childhood, whereas in adults bone remodeling is the principal event [8]. In the case of bone modeling, both bone resorption and bone formation lead to major cur independently of one another at different sites of the skeletal system and lead to major change in the skeletal framework, whereas in the case of bone remodeling, both the processes of bone resorption and formation are closely related both in terms of time and site so that bone volume and density both remain more or less unchanged. The continuous process of bone remodeling repairs micro fractures, prevents formation of brittle bones, and balances calcium and phosphate homeostasis [6–8].

A number of systemic and local factors regulate the process of bone remodeling. Whenever the tightly coupled processes of bone resorption and bone formation in bone remodeling are disturbed, bone mineral diseases occur, excessive bone resorption leads to osteoporosis, and excessive bone formation leads to osteopetrosis [9].

Osteoblasts and osteoclasts are the two key players of bone remodeling; other cells involved in the process are osteocytes (derived from osteoblasts and acting as mechanosensor) and the bone lining cells [9]. The process of bone remodeling increases with aging; in both perimenopausal and menopausal women, the remodeling is faster than premenopausal women [9].

IntechOpen

There are a number of factors which are responsible for the development, maturation, and normal functioning of the skeletal system; these are genetic factors, maintenance of hormonal and metabolic harmony, adhering to balanced diet, exercise, etc. Any change in the abovementioned factors might lead to skeletal abnormality including restricted stature, deformity, osteoporosis, etc. [8, 10].

Osteoporosis leads to poor bone mass along with increased risk of fracture. Osteoporosis has emerged as a global healthcare problem with an estimated huge economic burden. Around 40% of women and 13–22% of men above 50 years will experience at least one episode of fracture (usually of spine, femur, or forearm) due to underlying osteoporosis in his or her lifetime [11]. Besides postmenopausal women and men above 50 years of age, the risk of secondary osteoporosis has increased in younger people as well [11].

Due to the increase in the number of patients with osteoporosis, all the secondary risk factors attributed to osteoporosis should be thoroughly investigated.

A number of factors are responsible for maintenance and development of the skeletal system; these are genetic factors, adequate hormonal and metabolic functions, intake of balanced diet, and exercise (mechanical load) [11]. Any type of imbalance among the abovementioned factors might lead to severe consequences like short stature, bony deformities, and fractures. The final outcome depends upon age, type, severity, and duration of the underlying imbalance. Although not all of the abovementioned factors can be modified (like genetic factors), some of them can be modified [11, 12].

A rising number of new osteoporosis cases both in elderly and in young patients warrant the need for thorough investigations to identify all other secondary conditions that might affect the disease negatively. Of all the secondary conditions, hormonal conditions are the most important ones that can lead to or aggravate osteoporosis [12]. Most commonly implicated endocrinological conditions are Cushing's syndrome, hyperthyroidism, hypogonadism, acromegaly, diabetes mellitus, etc. Fortunately, majority of the negative effects of these hormonal disorders on the skeletal system can be modified [10–12].

1.1 Osteoblasts

Osteoblasts, the bone-forming cells in bone remodeling process, are derived from the pluripotent mesenchymal stem cells. Osteoblasts are also responsible for the secretion of Type I collagen which in turn is the major bone matrix protein. Besides the abovementioned functions, osteoblasts are also responsible for adequate mineralization of the new bone (osteoid). Bone mineralization occurs due to the locally released phosphates from the osteoblast-derived vesicles located within the osteoid. Extracellular calcium also contributes to the process of bone formation by the production of hydroxyapatite crystals. Maintenance of correct balance between bone matrix and minerals is the key factor for ensuring the right amount of rigidity and flexibility of the skeletal structure. Adult human cortical bones consist of 60% mineral, 20% organic material, and 20% water [8, 9].

1.2 Osteoclasts

These are micronucleated cells that are derived from the mononuclear monocyte-macrophage cells. Osteoclasts, the only bone-resorbing cells, depend on two cytokines, colony-stimulating factor-1 or the macrophage colony-stimulating factor (CSF-1) and receptor activator of NF-kB ligand (RANKL), for production, expansion, and survival. Osteoprotegerin (OPG) acts as a decoy receptor for RANKL and inhibits the action of RANKL; hence the ration of RANKL to OPG determines the extent of osteoclast maturation and expansion [8, 9].

2. Physiology of thyroid hormones

The level of thyroid hormones in the circulation is controlled by the hypothalamic-pituitary-thyroid axis (HPT axis) [13]. Thyrotropin-releasing hormone (TRH) is produced and secreted from the medial neurons of the paraventricular nucleus (PVN) of the hypothalamus. TRH in turn regulates both production and secretion of thyroid-stimulating hormone (TSH) from the anterior pituitary cells. Next, TSH through action on its receptor (TSHR) located on the follicular cells of the thyroid gland stimulates synthesis and secretion of the thyroid hormones. There are two types of thyroid hormones, 3,5,30,50-L-tetraiodothyronine (T4), the pro-hormone, and 3,5,30-L-triiodothyronine (T3), the active hormone [14].

Thyroid hormones exert negative feedback effect on TRH and TSH and thus inhibit own synthesis and secretion.

Thus the HPT axis maintains a balanced relationship between the circulating thyroid hormones and their regulators like TSH and TRH. The set point for adequate functioning of the HPT axis is partly determined by genetic factors; there is an estimated genetic variation of 45–65% [13, 14].

2.1 Intracellular T3 supply

Circulating concentrations of both T4 and T3 along with target tissue uptake of the same and local activation or inactivation determine the intracellular supply of T3 (the active hormone). The thyroid gland secretes the pro-hormone T4 in larger proportions which is converted to the active form T3 in the liver and kidney through deiodination of T4 by type 1 iodothyronine deiodinase enzyme (DIO1). A major part (around 90%) of the circulating thyroid hormone remains bound to plasma proteins, and the concentration of free T3 (fT3) exceeds that of free T4 (fT4) by three to four times [13, 14].

There are specific membrane transporters associated with target tissue uptake of thyroid hormones; considered as monocarboxylate transporters (MCT8, MCT10), and organic acid transporter protein-1c1 (OATP1C1) [15]. Activity of T3 inside the cell is regulated by DIO2 and DIO3, as DIO2 converts T4 to T3 and DIO3 blocks the activation of T3 by producing reverse T3 [16].

Thyroid hormones mediate their actions through interaction with thyroid receptors (TRs). Unbound TRs bind with corepressor proteins and bind with thyroid response elements located at the promoter regions of the target genes and suppress transcription. Once thyroid hormone binds with its receptor, the receptor undergoes a conformational change with the unbinding of the corepressor proteins and facilitation of gene transcription following binding with the thyroid response elements at the target genes [14–16].

3. Thyroid hormone and the skeletal system

Action of T3 hormone on the skeletal system is rather complex and not completely understood. T3 mediates its action on the bones via direct and indirect pathways and affects the different phases of bone remodeling. T3 facilitates both osteoblastic (bone formation) and osteoclastic actions (bone resorption). T3 facilitates osteoblastic activity by promoting production and differentiation of osteoblasts and also increases the expression of osteocalcin, collagen (Type 1), metalloproteins, alkaline phosphatase, etc. Similarly, T3 also facilitates differentiation of osteoclasts through increased expression of interleukin-6 and prostaglandins. It also exhibits synergistic action with hormones facilitating osteoclastic activity (like parathyroid hormone and vitamin D). Moreover, T3 promotes the expression of mRNA of RANKL, stimulates RANK, and thus facilitates osteoclast production [14–16].

Majority of the TRs expressed in the skeletal system (bone marrow, chondrocytes, osteoblasts, and osteoclasts) are TRβ1 and TRα1. Molecular studies have shown that the expression of TRα1 is far greater than that of TRβ1 in the skeletal system, indicating that T3-mediated action on the skeleton system is mostly carried out through TRα1 receptor [17]. There were no changes in the bone mass following the treatment of adult female rats with TRβ-selective agonist 3,5-dimethyl-4-(4-hydroxy-3-isopropylbenzyl)phenoxy acetic acid (GC-1); however, the administration of supraphysiological dose of T3 led to significant loss of bone mass in the adult female rats [18]. These findings suggest that T3-mediated bone resorption occurs through TRα1 receptors [18]. Animal models with genetic modifications (for TRs) have led to better understanding of the actions of T3 on the skeletal systems. All these studies showed that mice with mutation of either both TRα1 and TRβ1 or only TRα1 had delayed bone growth due to delayed ossification and decreased bone mineralization in early life, whereas increased bone mineralization in later years of life is similar to the effects of hypothyroidism in humans. However, mice with mutation of only TRβ1 receptors had skeletal phenotype similar to thyrotoxic patients characterized by increased mineralization and faster ossification during early life and decreased bone mineralization and poor bone mass in adult life [18].

3.1 Hyperthyroidism and osteoporosis

Thyroid hormones are known to a play key role in the linear growth of the skeletal system, and these hormones are essential to achieve the expected bone mass [19]. However, hyperthyroidism or thyrotoxicosis, a rather rare occurrence in children, if present, leads to accelerated ossification (both intramembranous and endochondral) and rapid linear growth [17]. This accelerated increase in bone age often results in early epiphyseal closure and short stature. In younger children severe degree of thyrotoxicosis might lead to premature closure of cranial sutures and craniosynostosis (impaired growth of brain and skull) with neurological complications [17, 20]. Sometimes severe untreated thyrotoxicosis in mother might lead to craniosynostosis in the growing fetus [20].

In adults hyperthyroidism shorten the bone turnover and poor bone mineralization [11, 17]. Finally there is loss of bone mineral density by around 10–20% especially in the cortical bones [11]. The increased concentration of circulating thyroid hormones causes significant shortening of bone remodeling cycle by about 50%. Normally the average bone remodeling cycle lasts for 200 days; however, with hyperthyroidism it is shortened to an average of 113 days [11, 21, 22]. Hence the balance between bone resorption and bone formation is disturbed; the bone formation phase is severely compromised (the duration is decreased by 2/3) and is ultimately responsible for poor mineralization (loss of about 10% of mineralization of bone per cycle) [11]. All these effects lead to increased risk of osteoporosis and increased chance of fracture.

Another contributory factor for increased risk of osteoporosis in patients of hyperthyroidism is that there is increased circulatory concentration of IL-6 in these patients; IL-6 is known to be an activator for osteoclast production and facilitates action of parathyroid hormone in bones [11, 23]. Hyperparathyroidism is also known to cause negative calcium balance due to hypercalcemia and hypercalciuria. Negative calcium balance further increases the risk of osteoporosis in these already vulnerable patients.

Many researchers since Von Recklinghausen have been conducting researches on the effects of thyroid dysfunction on bones. Svare A and his colleagues conducted a cross-sectional study to assess the relationship between BMD of forearm and TSH level in Norwegian female population (HUNT2 Study) [24]. They found that women with lower TSH (<0.5 mU/L) had lower forearm BMD than the reference category. Similarly, the prevalence of osteoporosis was found to be higher in women with osteoporosis than those without any history of thyroid disorder.

Again, the occurrence of osteoporosis secondary to hyperthyroidism (thyrotoxicosis) is more common in postmenopausal women than premenopausal women. Ercolano MA and his colleagues conducted a non-interventional and cross-sectional study on euthyroid (who had euthyroid for the past 6 months) pre- and postmenopausal women with past history of hyperthyroidism due to Graves' disease [25]. It was found that BMD was significantly affected only in the postmenopausal group of women who remained euthyroid for the past 6 months and have a past history of Graves' disease. Again, Tuchendler and Bolanowski conducted a study on premenopausal women with hyper- and hypothyroidism to assess the effects of thyroid dysfunction on osteoporosis [26]. They found that only hyperthyroidism and not hypothyroidism can significantly affect BMD (measured at the femoral neck), and following the treatment for 12 months, a statistically significant increase in BMD in femoral neck was observed in premenopausal women with hyperthyroidism and not hypothyroidism.

Similar study was conducted in men by El Hadidy and his colleagues [27]. The study included males between 23 and 65 years with hyperthyroidism (Graves' disease or toxic nodular goiter). The researchers found that the men with hyperthyroidism had a significant fall in BMD compared to age-matched healthy men without any thyroid dysfunction. Besides this, the severity and the duration of hyperthyroidism were directly related to the increase in bone turnover markers and the degree of bone loss.

Similar study was conducted by Ale and her colleagues [28]. This cross-sectional study included females and males between 22 and 50 years. It was found that BMD measured in hyperthyroidism was significantly reduced compared to age- and sex-matched healthy controls. Osteoporosis was documented in hyperthyroidism but not in the controls.

Again a systematic review and meta-analysis of cohort studies by Yang and his fellow researchers documented that although both subclinical hypo- and hyperthyroidism are associated with increased risk of fracture, only subclinical hyperthyroidism and not subclinical hypothyroidism showed significant association with low BMD (osteoporosis) [29].

3.1.1 Subclinical hyperthyroidism and osteoporosis

Although medical data describing the relation between subclinical hyperthyroidism and osteoporosis is not much, still there are studies which have explored the relationship between the two. Segna and his colleagues published a study exploring the association between subclinical hyperthyroidism and osteoporosis [30]. They included all the prospective cohort studies (published between 1946 and 2016) in the electronic database (MEDLINE/EMBASE) which provided baseline thyroid hormone status and repeated measurements of BMD. The study found that in adult patients subclinical hyperthyroidism is significantly associated with bone loss in the femoral neck region leading to increased risk of osteoporosis and fracture.

However, some earlier studies as the one conducted by Földes and his colleagues have described that although in premenopausal women with subclinical hyperthyroidism BMD in femoral neck, lumbar spine, and in the midshaft of radius did not decrease significantly, the same condition might contribute to osteoporosis in postmenopausal women especially in the cortical bones [31]. Another study published by Lee and his fellow researchers revealed that both subclinical hypo- and hyperthyroidism are associated with increased risk of hip fracture in elderly men; however, no such association was found with women [32].

Vadiveloo and his colleagues published a retrospective study exploring the long-term consequences of subclinical hyperthyroidism (TEARS study) [33]. The researchers identified suitable patients using population record linkage technology retrospectively between January 1, 1993 and December 31, 2009. They found that patients with endogenous subclinical hyperthyroidism showed an increased risk of osteoporosis-related fracture (hazard ratio being 1.25) when compared with reference population; however, once these patients developed overt hyperthyroidism or euthyroidism and are excluded from the study, this association is lost.

Again, Saler and his colleagues described in their study that in contrast to exogenous subclinical hyperthyroidism, endogenous subclinical hyperthyroidism does not compromise BMD in premenopausal women and therefore do not pose a risk for either osteoporosis or osteopenia [34]. However, Tauchmanovà and her colleagues found that BMD of the femoral neck was significantly decreased in both pre- and postmenopausal women with endogenous subclinical hyperthyroidism (greater in in postmenopausal women). Study of lumbar spine BMD revealed bone loss only in postmenopausal women. Similar findings were documented by Rosario and his colleagues [35].

Thus it can be suggested that the threat of osteoporotic fracture is greater with exogenous subclinical hyperthyroidism especially in postmenopausal women.

3.2 Overt hypothyroidism and osteoporosis

Hypothyroidism is a rather common condition in children and is characterized by delay in the development of the skeletal system, poor growth, and impaired and early endochondral ossification leading to short stature and defective bone maturation. Patients often present with patent skull sutures (delay in closure of skull fontanelles) and typical facial characteristics like flattened nasal bridge and broad face due to defective ossification.

In severe cases postnatal growth can be completely arrested, impaired with skeletal growth characterized by epiphyseal dysgenesis, dislocation of hip joints, scoliosis, persistent patency of the fontanelles, and delay in eruption of tooth. Thyroid hormone replacement therapy in these children leads to "catch-up" growth with achievement of skeletal maturity and improved bone mineralization. Finally in most of the children, normal adult height and bone mineral density are achieved. However, in severely affected children and those with significant delay in receiving thyroid hormone replacement therapy, expected adult stature might not be achieved.

Several studies were conducted in adults to understand the effect of thyroid hormone disorder on adult skeletal system [11]. But several factors like heterogeneity of the study population, the presence of different confounding factors, and different end points for different studies have led to the uniform interpretation of the results obtained from these studies.

Earlier histomorphometric studies have shown that hypothyroidism in adults led to slow bone turnover with both poor bone formation by osteoblasts and decreased bone resorption by osteoclasts. Also increase in the bone remodeling time led to prolonged secondary mineralization of the bone without any change in the existing bone volume. However, all the abovementioned changes are very slow to occur, and there are hardly any clinical data to suggest these findings in adult patients [11].

Although the exact mechanism is not known, hypothyroidism is considered to increase the risk of fracture. Vestergaard and his fellow researchers documented in their study that following diagnosis of primary idiopathic hypothyroidism, the risk of fracture (in forearm) was significantly increased in patients above 50 years [36].

However, González-Rodríguez and his colleagues while assessing the prevalence of thyroid dysfunction in adult female population, from the data collected in the Latin American Vertebral Osteoporosis Study (LAVOS), documented that although there was a high prevalence of hypothyroidism in these females, no association between loss of bone mineral density and hypothyroidism was found [37]. They also found that there was no association between fractures (vertebral or nonvertebral) and hypothyroidism.

3.3 Prolonged treatment with TSH suppressive therapy with supraphysiological dose of levothyroxine (synthetic form of T4) and osteoporosis

Supraphysiological doses of levothyroxine are prescribed in patients of thyroid cancer following surgery and radioactive iodine therapy. Prolonged exposure to levothyroxine therapy might increase the risk of secondary osteoporosis [11].

Heemstra and his colleagues described that, although long-term thyroxine therapy increased the risk of poor BMD and thus osteoporosis, it was not seen in men and in premenopausal women [38].

In the year 2018, Mazziotti and his colleagues published a cross-sectional study conducted mainly on postmenopausal women (178 women were postmenopausal out of 179 of the study participants) [39]. These women underwent thyroidectomy for differentiated thyroid carcinoma and were receiving levothyroxine therapy. Radiological vertebral fractures (VF) are considered as an early indicator of bone fragility. The researchers found that the prevalence of VF was significantly greater in patients with TSH level <1.0 mU/L, duration of levothyroxine therapy, and densiometric diagnosis of osteoporosis.

Thus it can be suggested that the risk of osteoporosis increases with suppression of TSH therapy.

4. Conclusion

Osteoporosis is considered to be one of the most common skeletal disorders affecting both elderly and young patients. Besides the few primary causes (aging and menopause), in most of the cases, osteoporosis occurs due to underlying secondary causes. Common secondary risk factors for osteoporosis include hormonal disorders like Cushing's disease, hyperthyroidism, diabetes mellitus, hypogonadism, etc. Several studies have established that hyperthyroidism both endogenous (due to Graves' disease or toxic nodular goiter) and exogenous (due to prolonged levothyroxine therapy especially in patients with differentiated thyroid cancer) increases the risk of osteoporosis profoundly in postmenopausal women. Even subclinical hyperthyroidism especially the exogenous ones might lower BMD and increases the risk of osteoporosis, more commonly in postmenopausal women. Hypothyroidism, on the other hand, although responsible for an array of bone disorders, does not usually contribute to osteoporosis.

Most of the studies, exploring the association between hyperthyroidism (exogenous or endogenous) and osteoporosis, are usually conducted among elderly population (postmenopausal women and elderly men). Hence further studies are to be conducted to explore the association of hyperthyroidism and osteoporosis in younger population (premenopausal women and younger males).

Author details

Ayotunde Oladunni Ale
Department of Medicine, Obafemi Awolowo College of Health Sciences, Faculty of Clinical Sciences, Olabisi Onabanjo University, Sagamu campus, Ogun State, Nigeria

*Address all correspondence to: ayoale2004@yahoo.com

IntechOpen

© 2019 The Author(s). Licensee IntechOpen. This chapter is distributed under the terms of the Creative Commons Attribution License (http://creativecommons.org/licenses/by/3.0), which permits unrestricted use, distribution, and reproduction in any medium, provided the original work is properly cited.

References

[1] Clarke B. Normal bone anatomy and physiology. Clinical Journal of the American Society of Nephrology: CJASN. 2008;**3**(Suppl 3):S131-S139

[2] Oldknow KJ, MacRae VE, Farquharson C. Endocrine role of bone: Recent and emerging perspectives beyond osteocalcin. Journal of Endocrinology. 2015;**225**:R1-R19

[3] DiGirolamo DJ, Clemens TL, Kousteni S. The skeleton as an endocrine organ. Nature Reviews Rheumatology. 2012;**8**:674-683

[4] Mera P, Laue K, Ferron M, et al. Osteocalcin signaling in myofibers is necessary and sufficient for optimum adaptation to exercise. Cell Metabolism. 2017;**25**:218

[5] Mosialou I, Shikhel S, Liu JM, et al. MC4R-dependent suppression of appetite by bone-derived lipocalin 2. Nature. 2017;**543**:385-390

[6] Seeman E, Delmas PD. Bone quality: The material and structural basis of bone strength and fragility. New England Journal of Medicine. 2006;**354**:2250-2261

[7] Manolagas SC. Birth and death of bone cells: Basic regulatory mechanisms and implications for the pathogenesis and treatment of osteoporosis. Endocrine Reviews. 2000;**21**:115-137

[8] Kenkre JS, Bassett J. The bone remodelling cycle. Annals of Clinical Biochemistry. 2018;**55**:308-327. DOI: 10.1177/0004563218759371. Epub 2018 Mar 4

[9] Katsimbri P. The biology of normal bone remodelling. European Journal of Cancer Care. 2017;**26**:e12740. Available from: https://onlinelibrary.wiley.com/doi/10.1111/ecc.12740. DOI: 10.1111/ecc.12740. Epub 2017 Aug 8

[10] Nicholls JJ, Brassill MJ, Williams GR, Bassett JH. The skeletal consequences of thyrotoxicosis. The Journal of Endocrinology. 2012;**213**:209-221. DOI: 10.1530/JOE-12-0059. Epub 2012 Mar 27

[11] Tuchendler D, Bolanowski M. The influence of thyroid dysfunction on bone metabolism. Thyroid Research. 2014;7:12. DOI: 10.1186/s13044-014-0012-0. eCollection 2014

[12] Fitzpatrick LA. Secondary causes of osteoporosis. Mayo Clinic Proceedings. 2002;**77**:453-468

[13] Cardoso LF, Maciel LM, Paula FJ. The multiple effects of thyroid disorders on bone and mineral metabolism. Arquivos Brasileiros de Endocrinologia e Metabologia. 2014;**58**:452-463

[14] Biondi B, Wartofsky L. Treatment with thyroid hormone. Endocrine Reviews. 2014;**35**:433-512. DOI: 10.1210/er.2013-1083. Epub 2014 Jan 16

[15] Van der Deure WM, Peeters RP, Visser TJ. Molecular aspects of thyroid hormone transporters, including MCT8, MCT10, and OATPs, and the effects of genetic variation in these transporters. Journal of Molecular Endocrinology. 2010;**44**(1):1-11. DOI: 10.1677/JME-09-0042. Epub 2009 Jun 18

[16] Bianco AC, Kim BW. Deiodinases: Implications of the local control of thyroid hormone action. The Journal of Clinical Investigation. 2006;**116**:2571-2579

[17] Williams GR, Bassett JHD. Thyroid diseases and bone health. Journal of Endocrinological Investigation. 2018;**41**:99-109. DOI: 10.1007/s40618-017-0753-4. Epub 2017 Aug 29

[18] Freitas FR, Moriscot AS, Jorgetti V, Soares AG, Passarelli M, Scanlan TS, et al. Spared bone mass in rats treated

with thyroid hormone receptor TRβ-selective compound GC-1. American Journal of Physiology. Endocrinology and Metabolism. 2003;**285**:E1135-E1141

[19] Bassett JH, Williams GR. Role of thyroid hormones in skeletal development and bone maintenance. Endocrine Reviews. 2016;**37**:135-187. DOI: 10.1210/er.2015-1106. Epub 2016 Feb 10

[20] Hüffmeier U, Tietze HU, Rauch A. Severe skeletal dysplasia caused by undiagnosed hypothyroidism. European Journal of Medical Genetics. 2007;**50**:209-215. Epub 2007 Mar 12

[21] Harvey C, O'Shea P, Scott A, Robson H, Siebler T, Shalet S, et al. Molecular mechanisms of thyroid hormone effects on bone growth and function. Molecular Genetics and Metabolism. 2002;**75**:17-30

[22] Murphy E, Williams G. The thyroid and the skeleton. Clinical Endocrinology. 2004;**61**:285-298

[23] Reddy P, Harinarayan C, Sachan A, Suresh V, Rajagopal G. Bone disease in thyrotoxicosis. The Indian Journal of Medical Research. 2012;**135**:277-286

[24] Svare A, Nilsen T, Bjoro T, Forsmo S, Schei B, Bjoro T, et al. Hyperthyroid levels of TSH correlate with low bone mineral density: The HUNT 2 study. European Journal of Endocrinology. 2009;**161**:779-786

[25] Ercolano M, Drnovsek M, Croome M, Moos M, Fuentes AM, Viale F, et al. Negative correlation between bone mineral density and TSH receptor antibodies in long-term euthyroid postmenopausal women with treated graves' disease. Thyroid Research. 2013;**6**:11

[26] Tuchendler D, Bolanowski M. Assessment of bone metabolism in premenopausal females with hyperthyroidism and hypothyroidism. Endokrynologia Polska. 2013;**64**:40-44

[27] El Hadidy M, Ghonaim M, El Gawd S, El Atta M. Impact of severity, duration, and etiology of hyperthyroidism on bone turnover markers and bone mineral density in men. BMC Endocrine Disorders. 2011;**11**:15

[28] Ale AO, Ogbera AO, Ebili HO, Adeyemo OL, Afe TO. Prevalence, predictive factors, and characteristics of osteoporosis in hyperthyroid patients. International Journal of Endocrinology. 2018;**3**:1-7. DOI: 10.1155/2018/3540256

[29] Yang R, Yao L, Fang Y, Sun J, Guo T, Yang K, et al. The relationship between subclinical thyroid dysfunction and the risk of fracture or low bone mineral density: A systematic review and meta-analysis of cohort studies. Journal of Bone and Mineral Metabolism. 2018;**36**:209-220. DOI: 10.1007/s00774-017-0828-5. Epub 2017 Mar 29

[30] Segna D, Bauer DC, Feller M, Schneider C, Fink HA, Aubert CE, et al. Thyroid Studies Collaboration. Association between subclinical thyroid dysfunction and change in bone mineral density in prospective cohorts. Journal of Internal Medicine. 2018;**283**:56-72. DOI: 10.1111/joim.12688. Epub 2017 Oct 16

[31] Földes J, Tarján G, Szathmari M, Varga F, Krasznai I, Horvath C. Bone mineral density in patients with endogenous subclinical hyperthyroidism: Is this thyroid status a risk factor for osteoporosis? Clinical Endocrinology. 1993;**39**:521-527

[32] Lee J, Buzková P, Fink HA, Vu J, Carbone L, Chen Z, et al. Subclinical thyroid dysfunction and incident hip fracture in older adults. Archives of Internal Medicine. 2010;**170**:1876-1883

[33] Vadiveloo T, Donnan P, Cochrane L, Leese G. The thyroid epidemiology, audit, and research study (TEARS):

Morbidity in patients with endogenous subclinical hyperthyroidism. The Journal of Clinical Endocrinology and Metabolism. 2011;**96**:1344-1351

[34] Saler T, Ahbab S, Sağlam ZA, Keşkek ŞÖ, Kurnaz S. Endogenous subclinical hyperthyroidism may not lead to bone loss in premenopausal women. Hippokratia. 2014;**18**(3):240-244

[35] Tauchmanovà L, Nuzzo V, Del Puente A, Fonderico F, Esposito-Del Puente A, Padulla S, et al. Reduced bone mass detected by bone quantitative ultrasonometry and DEXA in pre- and postmenopausal women with endogenous subclinical hyperthyroidism. Maturitas. 2004;**48**:299-306

[36] Vestergaard P, Weeke J, Hoeck H, Nielsen H, Rungby J, Rejnmark L, et al. Fractures in patients with primary idiopathic hypothyroidism. Thyroid. 2000;**10**:335-340

[37] Gonzalez-Rodriguez L, Felici-Giovanini M, Haddock L. Thyroid dysfunction in an adult population: A population-based study of Latin American vertebral osteoporosis study (LAVOS): Puerto Rico site hypothyroidism in LAVOS-Puerto Rico site. Health Sciences. 2013;**32**:57-62

[38] Heemstra K, Hamdy N, Romijn J. The effects of thyrotropin-suppressive therapy on bone metabolism in patients with well-differentiated thyroid carcinoma. Thyroid. 2006;**16**:583-591

[39] Mazziotti G, Formenti AM, Frara S, Olivetti R, Banfi G, Memo M, et al. High prevalence of radiological vertebral fractures in women on thyroid-stimulating hormone-suppressive therapy for thyroid carcinoma. The Journal of Clinical Endocrinology and Metabolism. 2018;**103**:956-964. DOI: 10.1210/jc.2017-01986

Chapter 8

Relation between Vitamin K and Osteoporosis

Sawsan Jaghsi

Abstract

Vitamin K is an essential fat-soluble vitamin. The role of vitamin K as a cofactor involved in blood coagulation is well demonstrated. In the past two decades, vitamin K has been receiving more attention due to its role in bone health and metabolism. Vitamin K plays a role in activation of vitamin K-dependent proteins, which are involved not only in blood coagulation but in bone metabolism and the inhibition of arterial calcification. Numerous studies have exhibited the importance of vitamin K in bone health. The bone mineral density (BMD) does not remain steady with age, particularly declining after menopause. Osteoporosis is a metabolic bone disease of reduced bone density, fragile bone, and elevated susceptibility to fracture. A greater understanding of the biological linkages between vitamin K and bone may conduce to new treatment for osteoporosis that may improve bone density and prevent the adverse outcomes of osteoporosis.

Keywords: vitamin K, phylloquinone, menaquinone, bone mineral density, osteoporosis, Gla protein

1. Introduction

Vitamin K is an important fat-soluble vitamin. The discovery of vitamin K was in Germany in 1929 by Henrik Dam in his research on sterol metabolism, and he suggested the name vitamin K on the basis of its role in coagulation (koagulation in German spelling).

The exact function of vitamin K in the human body was discovered in the 1970s with the discovery of γ-carboxyglutamic acid (Gla), an amino acid found in all vitamin K proteins [1].

Gamma glutamyl carboxylase is an enzyme that located in the endoplasmic reticulum and mediates the posttranslational conversion of glutamyl to γ-carboxyglutamyl residues in vitamin K-dependent proteins; this enzyme needs vitamin K as a cofactor for this conversion; thus the important role of vitamin K appears in tissues that contain vitamin K-dependent protein to make them a functional protein [2].

During the last two decades, the researches have focused on the role of vitamin K in osteoporosis [3], cardiovascular disease [4], diabetes [5], and cancer [6] besides its role on coagulation [7].

In the liver there are several vitamin K-dependent proteins which all play a role in hemostasis. In addition to the hepatic tissue, bone tissue contains vitamin K-dependent proteins such as osteocalcin (bone Gla protein) and matrix Gla protein (MGP). Mineral binding capacity of osteocalcin needs vitamin K for adding mineral to the bone matrix in normal bone growth and development [8].

 IntechOpen

Studies have reported that vitamin K plays a role in bone metabolism in other mechanisms. There is an evidence that vitamin K positively affects calcium balance and increase of calcium retention [9]. Vitamins K and D work synergistically on bone metabolism, the form of osteocalcin that osteoblasts produce is undercarboxylated osteocalcin, and this process is upregulated by vitamin D, while carboxylation of osteocalcin is mediated by vitamin K [10].

Vitamin K is shown to decrease bone resorption by osteoclasts and inhibits production of bone-resorbing agents such as interleukin-6 [11] and prostaglandin E2 [12].

Osteoporosis is a metabolic bone disease of reduced bone density, fragile bone, and elevated susceptibility to fracture. Genetic factors, age, sex, race, general health, exercise, cigarette smoking, alcohol abuse, hormone replacement therapy, and nutrition are some of the factors that influence an individual's risk of osteoporosis [13].

The aim of the present paper is to summarize the present knowledge on vitamin K and bone metabolism, emphasize the role of vitamin K in bone health, and evaluate vitamin K as a diagnostic and therapeutic marker in osteoporosis.

2. Types of vitamin K

Vitamin K refers to a family of compounds with a common chemical structure of 2-methyl-1,4-naphthoquinone (**Figure 1**) [14].

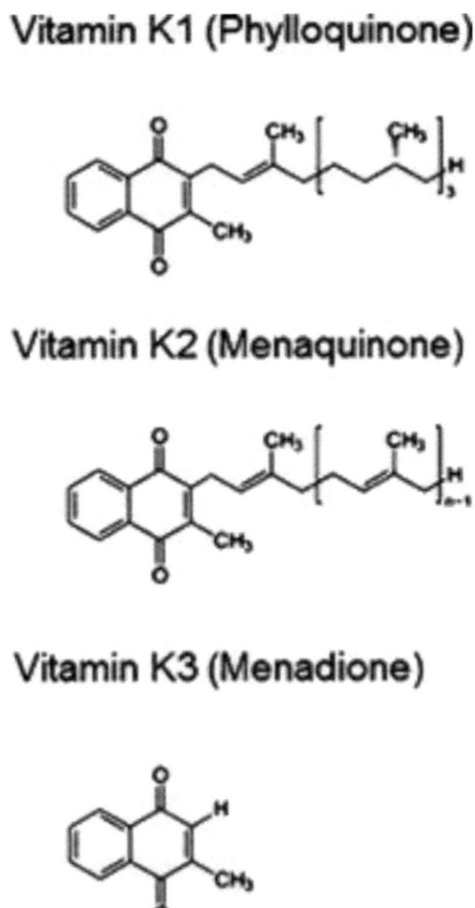

Figure 1.
Structure of the main forms of vitamin K.

These compounds include:

1. Vitamin K1 (phylloquinone)

2. Vitamin K2 (menaquinones)

3. Vitamin K3 (menadione) [7]

3. Sources of vitamin K

Vitamin K1 (phylloquinone) comes from vegetables, especially green leafy vegetables such as spinach, vegetable oils, broccoli, and some fruits [1].

Vitamin K2 (menaquinone) forms a subfamily in which it has an unsaturated isoprenyl side chain (may range from 1 to 13 isoprene residues). The various menaquinones are generally denoted as MK-n, where n symbolizes the number of isoprene residues in the side chain and is designated as MK-4 through MK-13, established upon the length of their side chain. The most well-studied menaquinones are MK-4, MK-7, MK-8, MK-9, and MK-10 that all occur in the human diet.

Menaquinones (except MK-4) are of microbial origin, and relatively high concentrations are only found in a few food items. Natto (a traditional Japanese food made from fermented soybeans) has high amounts of menaquinones (almost exclusively MK-7). Other fermented foods, such as cheese, also contain menaquinones. However, the forms and amounts of vitamin K in these foods likely vary relying on the strains of bacteria utilized to make the foods.

Bacteria in the human gut produce most of the menaquinones, especially the long-chain menaquinones; the amount of vitamin K that the body acquires in this manner is unclear.

Menadione is a synthetic form of vitamin K. It has increased toxic risk, so it is not a commonly supplemented form of vitamin K [1, 15].

4. Absorption and transport of vitamin K

In the intestine vitamin K is incorporated into mixed micelles, and it is absorbed by enterocytes. From there, vitamin K is combined into chylomicrons, released into the lymphatic capillaries, transported to the liver, and then packed again into very-low-density lipoproteins. In the circulation, vitamin K is carried mainly in lipoproteins [16].

5. Recommended intake

The AI for vitamin K1 is 120 mcg/day for men and 90 mcg/day for women as it was determined by the Institute of Medicine in the United States in 2001 [17].

These current AI values are established upon the hepatic vitamin K demanded for activation of coagulation factor and absence of abnormal bleeding. There was not any DRI for vitamin K2 or an upper limit intake level for vitamin K1 at that time. Clinical trials have used vitamin K supplements at doses much higher than the DRI levels (10 mg for vitamin K1 and 45 mg for vitamin K2) and found no evidence of toxic effects. However, trials which have used supplements of 45 mg/day of MK-4 demonstrate incidences of skin appendage lesions [18, 19].

6. Serum vitamin K concentration

Vitamin K is being absorbed via chylomicrons; in addition it is distributed via lipoproteins. The menaquinones with longer side chain are partitioned into LDL, whereas others including vitamin K1 are in the triglyceride rich fragment [20]. Vitamin K does appear to bioaccumulate in various tissues following oral ingestion, and it appears to have a relatively short time in the body prior to being excreted in comparison with the fat-soluble vitamins [16].

The major form of vitamin K in serum is vitamin K1, and it has a relative rapid half-life relative to MK-4, whereas MK-7 and other long-chain menaquinones have a very extended half-life and greater bioactivity [21].

The normal range of circulating concentrations of vitamin K1 is 05–2.5 nM/L (0.22–1.22 ng/ml) without taking any supplements [22]. However the range of vitamin K1 in patients and healthy adults was 0,22–8.88 nM/L (0.09–3.96 ng/ml) as reported in several clinical studies [23].

7. Bone uptake

Osteoblasts appear to take vitamin K which is transported via lipoproteins, and this uptake is facilitated by the LDL receptor which is expressed on these bone cells (LRP1 and, to a fewer degree, VLDLR) with the competence of the triglyceride fraction in giving its phylloquinone being greater than HDL but less than LDL, and the uptake is relying on ApoE. Hence it is thought that genetic variations in ApoE can affect vitamin K status. This region contains several Gla proteins such as matrix Gla protein and osteocalcin which need vitamin K to be effective [24].

Delivery of vitamin K to the bone tends to be less than in the liver, as in instances where vitamin K-dependent proteins (Gla) are totally γ-carboxylated in the liver, while they are not in the bone [20].

8. Vitamin K functions

Vitamin K plays a biological role as a cofactor of gamma glutamyl carboxylase, which mediates γ- carboxylation of glutamic acid residues (Glu) to γ-carboxyglutamic acid (Gla) on vitamin K-dependent protein. The Y-carboxylation of the vitamin K-dependent proteins Gla proteins is essential for their function.

Gla proteins or vitamin K-dependent proteins are a group of proteins that have calcium-binding characteristics and are existing in the extracellular matrix or in body fluids.

These proteins are included in blood clotting, bone mineralization, cartilage, and other soft tissues; and they have an important role in supporting the health of bones, joints, and blood vessels [3]. Some studies have suggested that vitamin K has anticancer [6], anti-inflammatory, and antioxidant characteristics [25].

There are seven different vitamin K-dependent proteins which all regulate coagulation; prothrombin (Factor II) is the most well-known target protein which was the first protein to be discovered to be γ-carboxylated by vitamin K. Afterwards factors VII, IX, and X as well as proteins C, S, and Z were discovered [8].

9. Vitamin K deficiency

There are not enough studies to determine a limit or threshold for concentration of vitamin K in serum that indicate deficiency or insufficiency [24].

Vitamin K deficiency is rare among adults, and it is determined clinically by bleeding because of low activation of coagulation proteins and is often estimated by measurement of undercarboxylated prothrombin concentration in serum released from the liver. Its concentration increases with the degree of severity of vitamin K deficiency [26].

Vitamin K deficiency is usually limited to people with liver and pancreas disease, cystic fibrosis, digestive disorders, disorders of fat malabsorption, chronic malnutrition, and alcohol dependency or those taking drugs that interfere with vitamin K metabolism such as vitamin K antagonist anticoagulants, bile acid sequestrants, certain types of antibiotics, and anticonvulsants [27].

The more common condition is subclinical vitamin K deficiency that results in increased levels of undercarboxylated or even uncarboxylated Gla proteins in serum. This occurs when serum vitamin K concentration is ≤0.5 nM/L [28] or serum undercarboxylated osteocalcin is ≥4.0 ng/mL [26].

Gla proteins that are not fully carboxylated are not activated and do not execute their role in the bone, cartilage, and soft tissue mineralization. Low vitamin K intake and low serum vitamin K concentrations are associated with increased risk of osteoporosis, cancer, and aortic calcification as observed by several studies [27–29].

10. The role of vitamin K in the bone

10.1 Mechanisms dependent on the ϒ-carboxylation via GGCX enzyme

Several vitamin K-dependent proteins have been verified. Some of them exist in the skeleton and cartilage such as osteocalcin, matrix Gla protein, Gla-rich protein, protein S, and gas 6 [30].

Osteocalcin is the first Gla protein discovered that originated from extrahepatic tissues. It is mainly produced by osteoblasts and has been suggested to affect bone metabolism by regulating osteoblast activity and bone mineralization [31].

Osteocalcin has three glutamic acid (Gla) residues which undergo gamma carboxylation by a process dependent on vitamin K; the ϒ-carboxylation of osteocalcin is necessary for its function. ϒ-carboxylated osteocalcin shows a high affinity to hydroxyapatite and bone matrix, contributing to bone formation. It has been shown that decarboxylated osteocalcin cannot bind calcium, thus emphasizing the importance role of vitamin K in the activation protein [32].

The percentage of overall osteocalcin that remained uncarboxylated (% ucOC) is a biomarker of vitamin K status (more carboxylation indicates a better status, less carboxylation indicates a worse status), and osteocalcin continually gets carboxylated up until a daily intake of around 1000mcg phylloquinone. Dietary recommendations (120 μg/day for men, 90 μg/day for women) are based on saturation of the coagulation system. Requirements to maintain bone Gla protein function and bone formation might be higher [33, 34].

Some studies have demonstrated that elevated concentration of undercarboxylated osteocalcin in serum is a predictor of fractures [35, 36].

MGP is included in the organic matrix and mobilization of calcium in the skeleton. It is mainly synthesized in the bone, cartilage, dentine, and soft tissues, including blood vessels, and is also found in the brain, heart, kidney, liver, lung, and spleen [37, 38].

10.2 Mechanisms independent of the ϒ-carboxylation via GGCX enzyme

Studies also reported that vitamin K prevents bone resorption through a mechanism totally different from that of ϒ-carboxylation. Vitamin K is shown to improve bone mineralization and decrease bone resorption by osteoclasts [39]. Other vitamin K roles have also been reported such as it can promote fracture reparation by stimulating bone formation and decrease calcium excretion by urine [3]. These results confirm the significant role of vitamin K in bone metabolism.

Vitamin K also functions as a ligand of steroid and xenobiotic receptor (SXR) and its murine homolog, pregnane X receptor (PXR), which after heterodimerization with the vitamin A receptor (RXR) induces the target genes including tsukushi (*Tsk*), matrilin-2 (*Matn2*), and *CD14*. *Tsk* encodes a protein that has a collagen-accumulating effect, and Matn2 is a protein comprising an extracellular matrix like collagen, whereas *CD14* regulates osteoblastogenesis and osteoclastogenesis.

Msx2 is another vitamin K-induced SXR-dependent gene identified, which induces osteoblast differentiation. Induction of these genes is not repressed by warfarin treatment, indicating a GGCX-dependent mechanism is not involved [30].

It has been reported that osteoporosis is linked with oxidative stress. Moreover, supplementation of vitamin K as an antioxidant vitamin could effectively reduce levels of oxidative stress, with possibly advantageous influence on bone, as displayed in several experimental models [27].

It is possible that higher levels of vitamin K suppress IL-6 secretion from inflammatory stressors, although the mechanisms underlying this are not currently known [11]. In addition, vitamin K also represses osteoclast activity, therefore averting the breakdown of bone [40].

11. Studies on vitamin K and the bone

Osteoporosis is a metabolic bone disease of reduced bone density, fragile bone, and elevated susceptibility to fracture [41]. Risk factors for osteoporosis contain genetic, nutrition, and hormone [3].

It is a common disease affecting 1 in 3 women and 1 in 12 men, resulting in substantial morbidity, excess mortality, and health and social services spending. It is therefore important to improve strategies for prevention and treatment osteoporosis in both men and women [42].

Some studies showed that the administration of vitamin K led to an increase of bone mineral density (BMD) in osteoporotic patients (Vermeer et al. [43]). In addition, administration of vitamin K was found to prevent bone loss and reduce the incidence of fractures (Shiraki et al. [44]).

A survey investigating vitamin K intake data from the fifth Korea National Health and Nutrition Examination Survey reported that low dietary vitamin K intake was related to low bone mineral density in subjects who were included (2785 men, 4307 women aged over 19 years). In addition, there was a reduction in risk for osteoporosis as vitamin K intake increased in women, but this effect was not continued after adjusting factors. This survey recommended increasing the dietary VK intakes for preserving BMD [45].

A study by Fujita et al. [46] observed that high intake of natto, fermented soybean high in phylloquinone, and MK-7 was associated with higher BMD, which was also demonstrated in a study by Ikeda et al. [47].

A cross-sectional study (3199 middle-aged Scottish females included) reported that females in the highest quartile of dietary intake of vitamin K1 (162 mcg/day) have a significantly higher lumbar spine (L2–L4) BMD and left femoral neck BMD against the lowest quartile (59 mcg/day) [48]. In vitro experiments by Hara et al. showed that vitamin K inhibits bone resorption induced by IL-la, PGE, PTH, and vitamin D3 in a dose-dependent manner [12].

Several studies have shown the relation between vitamin K and bone mineral density; a study by Kanai et al. reported that postmenopausal women with decreased bone mineral density (mean BMD, 0.73 g/cm2) had significantly lower levels of vitamin K1 and MK-7 than women with normal bone density (mean BMD, 0.99 g/cm^2) [49].

In our study we found that serum vitamin K1 level was significantly lower in the postmenopausal osteoporotic women group than in the normal control group, the mean serum vitamin k1 level was significantly lower in the postmenopausal osteoporotic women group than in the normal control group (mean = 0.794 vs. 3.61 ng/ml, $P < 0.0001$), and serum vitamin k1 concentration was positively correlated with lumbar spine BMD among postmenopausal osteoporotic women ($R = 0.533$, $p = 0.009$) and in postmenopausal healthy control ($R = 0.563$, $p = 0.02$). Diagnostic sensitivity and specificity of vitamin k1 for osteoporosis were 90 and 98%, respectively (cutoff value: 0.853 ng/ml). The area under the ROC curve (AUC) value for vitamin k1 was 0.984; the odd ratio result was 18.66 [50]. The same result was reported also by Heiss et al. [51].

These findings may suggest a role of vitamin K in bone metabolism. And therefore it has been thought that it might be effective for treating osteoporosis. Furthermore, Booth et al. [52] found that low plasma vitamin K1 concentrations were associated with low spine BMD among postmenopausal women not using estrogen replacement. These findings suggest a protective role of vitamin K in the skeleton in women. In addition, poor vitamin K nutritional status (low plasma phylloquinone concentrations and high serum %ucOC) was correlated with low BMD at the hip among men.

High incidence of vertebral fractures has reported to be contrarily correlated with BMD of lumbar spine and vitamin k1 concentration in the study on 379 Japanese women of 30–88 years to 4 years [53].

Vitamin K was found to increase bone mineral density in an in vivo osteoporosis model. A study by Hodges et al. deduced that osteoporotic patients had decreased levels of vitamin K and increased levels of non Υ-carboxylated osteocalcin [54].

The relations between vitamin K intake and bone mineral density are not coherent in observational studies [27].

Fang et al. showed that vitamin K supplements did not have influence on BMD at the femoral neck, but there was an increase in mean lumbar spine BMD by 1.3% (95% CI: 0.5–2.1) after supplementation for 6–36 months.

In this meta-analysis, seven studies utilized vitamin K1 with portions ranging from 0.2 to 10 mg/day. Ten studies utilized vitamin K2 (eight used MK-4 with portions of 15–45 mg/day, and two studies utilized MK-7 with portions of 0.2–3.6 mg/day), and after studies with high risk of bias have been excluded, the writer deduced that supplementation with vitamin K did not have significant effect on lumbar spine BMD in their subgroup analysis; they found that supplementation with vitamin K2 increased mean lumber spine BMD by 1.8% (95% CI, 0.9–2.8). No such influence was realized for studies with vitamin K1 supplementation [19].

It has been reported that osteoporosis is related to oxidative stress. Moreover, supplementation of vitamin K, as an antioxidant vitamin, could effectively decrease levels of oxidative stress, with possibly beneficial effect on the bone, as displayed in several experimental models [55].

Vitamin K is necessary for bone health. In fact, low vitamin K intake, low vitamin K circulating levels, and high undercarboxylated osteocalcin levels are all related with excessive hip fractures risk in observational studies [15].

More studies are required regarding the influences of vitamin K on diagnosis and management of osteoporosis and similarly on BMD.

12. Conclusion

Studies suggest that vitamin K has a role in bone metabolism and it may contribute in maintaining BMD and diagnosing osteoporosis. Studies have demonstrated that in the healthy population, all clotting factors are synthesized in their active form, whereas the synthesis of other Gla proteins is sub-optimal in non-supplemented subjects. Prolonged subclinical vitamin K deficiency is a risk factor for osteoporosis. Present recommendations for dietary intake are based on the daily dose required to prevent bleeding. Scientific data suggests that new, higher recommendations for vitamin K intake should be formulated.

Author details

Sawsan Jaghsi
Department of Biochemistry and Microbiology, Faculty of Pharmacy, Damascus University, Damascus, Syria

*Address all correspondence to: jaghsisph@gmail.com

IntechOpen

© 2019 The Author(s). Licensee IntechOpen. This chapter is distributed under the terms of the Creative Commons Attribution License (http://creativecommons.org/licenses/by/3.0), which permits unrestricted use, distribution, and reproduction in any medium, provided the original work is properly cited.

References

[1] Ferland G. The discovery of vitamin K and its clinical applications. Annals of Nutrition & Metabolism. 2012;**61**(3):213-218

[2] Booth SL. Roles for vitamin K beyond coagulation. Annual Review of Nutrition. 2009;**29**:89-110

[3] Heiss C, Hoesel LM, Wehr U, Wenisch S, Drosse I, Alt V, et al. Diagnosis of osteoporosis with vitamin k as a new biochemical marker. Vitamins and Hormones. 2008;**78**:417-434

[4] Geleijnse JM, Vermeer C, Grobbee DE, Schurgers LJ, Knapen MH, van der Meer IM, et al. Dietary intake of menaquinone is associated with a reduced risk of coronary heart disease: The Rotterdam study. The Journal of Nutrition. 2004;**134**:3100-3105

[5] Manna P, Kalita J. Beneficial role of vitamin K supplementation on insulin sensitivity, glucose metabolism, and the reduced risk of type 2 diabetes: A review. Nutrition. 2016;**32**(7-8):732-739

[6] Fan XV, Chen J, Duan L, Li S. Research progress on the anticancer effects of vitamin K2. Oncology Letters. 2018;**15**(6):8926-8934

[7] Stafford DW. The vitamin K cycle. Journal of Thrombosis and Haemostasis. 2005;**3**(8):1873-1878

[8] Price PA, Otsuka AA, Poser JW, Kristaponis J, Raman N. Characterization of a gamma-carboxyglutamic acid-containing protein from bone. Proceedings of the National Academy of Sciences of the United States of America. 1976;**73**(5):1447-1451

[9] Sakamoto N, Nishiike T, Iguchi H, Sakamoto K. The effect of diet on blood vitamin K status and urinary mineral excretion assessed by a food questionnaire. Nutrition and Health. 1999;**13**(1):1-10

[10] Masterjohn C. Vitamin D toxicity redefined: Vitamin K and the molecular mechanism. Medical Hypotheses. 2007;**68**(5):1026-1034

[11] Novotny JA, Kurilich AC, Britz SJ, Baer DJ, Clevidence BA. Vitamin K absorption and kinetics in human subjects after consumption of 13C-labelled phylloquinone from kale. The British Journal of Nutrition. 2010;**104**(6):858-862

[12] Hara K, Akiyama Y, Tajima T, Shiraki M. Menatetrenone inhibits bone resorption partly through inhibition of PGE2 synthesis in vitro. Journal of Bone and Mineral Research. 1993;**8**(5):535-542

[13] Czeczuk A, Huk-Wieliczuk E, Michalska A, Bylina D, Sołtan J, Zofia D. The effect of menopause on bone tissue in former swimmers and innon-athletes. Advances in Clinical and Experimental Medicine. 2012;**21**(5):645-652

[14] Azuma K, Inoue S. Multiple Modes of Vitamin K Actions in Aging-Related Musculoskeletal Disorders. International Journal of Molecular Sciences. 11 Jun 2019;**20**(11)

[15] Vermeer C. Vitamin K: The effect on health beyond coagulation–an overview. Food & Nutrition Research. 2012;**56**:1-9

[16] Shearer MJ, McBurney A, Barkhan P. Studies on the absorption and metabolism of phylloquinone (vitamin K1) in man. Vitamins and Hormones. 1974;**32**:513-542

[17] Food and Nutrition Board, Institute of Medicine. Dietary Reference Intakes for Vitamin a, Vitamin K, Arsenic, Boron, Chromium, Copper, Iodine, Iron, Molybdenum, Nickel, Silicon, Vanadium and Zinc. Chapter 5.

Washington, DC: National Academy Press; 2001. pp. 162-196

[18] Braam LA, Knapen MH, Geusens P, Brouns F, Vermeer C. Factors affecting bone loss in female endurance athletes: A two-year follow-up study. The American Journal of Sports Medicine. 2003;**31**(6):889-895

[19] Fang Y, Hu C, Tao X, Wan Y, Tao F. Effect of vitamin K on bone mineral density: A meta-analysis of randomized controlled trials. Journal of Bone and Mineral Metabolism. 2012;**30**(1):60-68

[20] Kohlmeier M, Salomon A, Saupe J, Shearer MJ. Transport of vitamin K to bone in humans. The Journal of Nutrition. 1996;**126**(4 Suppl):1192S-1196S

[21] Erkkila AT, Lichtenstein AH, Dolnikowski GG, Grusak MA, Jalbert SM, Aquino KA, et al. Plasma transport of vitamin K in men using deuterium-labeled collard greens. Metabolism. 2004;**53**(2):215-221

[22] Sadowski JA, Hood SJ, Dallal GE, Garry PJ. Phylloquinone in plasma from elderly and young adults: Factors influencing its concentration. The American Journal of Clinical Nutrition. 1989;**50**(1):100-108

[23] Shea MK, Booth SL. Concepts and controversies in evaluating vitamin K status in population-based studies. Nutrients. 2016;**8**(1):2-4

[24] Shearer MJ, Fu X, Booth SL. Vitamin K nutrition, metabolism, and requirements: Current concepts and future research. Advances in Nutrition. 2012;**3**(2):182-195

[25] Kidd PM, Vitamins D. K as pleiotropic nutrients: Clinical importance to the skeletal and cardiovascular systems and preliminary evidence for synergy. Alternative Medicine Review. 2010;**15**:199-222

[26] Kaneki M, Hosoi T, Ouchi Y, Orimo H. Pleiotropic actions of vitamin K: Protector of bone health and beyond? Nutrition. 2006;**22**(7-8):845-852

[27] Hamidi MS, Cheung AM. Vitamin K and musculoskeletal health in postmenopausal women. Molecular Nutrition & Food Research. 2014;**58**(8):1647-1657

[28] Misra D, Booth SL, Tolstykh I, Felson DT, Nevitt MC, Lewis CE, et al. Vitamin K deficiency is associated with incident knee osteoarthritis. The American Journal of Medicine. 2013;**126**(3):243-248

[29] Ducy P, Desbois C, Boyce B, Pinero G, Story B, Dunstan ESC, et al. Increased bone formation in osteocalcin-deficient mice. Nature. 1996;**382**(6590):448-452

[30] Azuma K, Ouchi Y, Inoue S. Vitamin K: Novel molecular mechanisms of action and its roles in osteoporosis. Geriatrics & Gerontology International. 2014;**14**(1):1-7

[31] Kidd PM. Vitamins D and K as pleiotropic nutrients: Clinical importance to the skeletal and cardiovascular systems and preliminary evidence for synergy. Alternative Medicine Review. 2010;**15**(3):199-222

[32] Szulc P, Chapuy MC, Meunier PJ, Delmas PD. Serum undercarboxylated osteocalcin is a marker of the risk of hip fracture: A three year follow-up study. Bone. 1996;**18**(5):487-488

[33] Gundberg CM, Nieman SD, Abrams S, Rosen H. Vitamin K status and bone health: An analysis of methods for determination of undercarboxylated osteocalcin. The Journal of Clinical Endocrinology and Metabolism. 1998;**83**(9):3258-3266

[34] Binkley NC, Krueger DC, Kawahara TN, Engelke JA, Chappell RJ, Suttie JW. A high phylloquinone intake is required to achieve maximal osteocalcin gamma-carboxylation. The American Journal of Clinical Nutrition. 2002;**76**(5):1055-1060

[35] Bügel S. Vitamin K and bone health in adult humans. Vitamins and Hormones. 2008;**78**:393-416

[36] Vergnaud P, Garnero P. Meunier P J, Breart G, Kamihagi K, and Delmas P D, Undercarboxylated osteocalcin measured with a specific immunoassay predicts hip fracture in elderly women: The EPIDOS study. The Journal of Clinical Endocrinology and Metabolism. 1997;**82**(3):719-724

[37] Price PA. Gla-containing proteins of bone. Connective Tissue Research. 1989;**21**(1-4):51-57; discussion 57-60

[38] Shea MK, Holden RM. Vitamin K status and vascular calcification: Evidence from observational and clinical studies. Advances in Nutrition. 2012;**3**(2):158-165

[39] Price PA. Vitamin K-dependent formation of bone Gla protein (osteocalcin) and its function. Vitamins and Hormones. 1985;**42**:65-108

[40] Falcone TD, Kim SS, Cortazzo MH. Vitamin K: Fracture prevention and beyond. PM&R. 2011;**3**(6 Suppl 1):S82-S87

[41] Lorentzon M, Cummings SR. Osteoporosis: The evolution of a diagnosis. Journal of Internal Medicine. 2015;**277**(6):650-661

[42] Tuck SP, Francis RM. Osteoporosis. Postgraduate Medical Journal. 2002 Sep;**78**(923):526-532

[43] Vermeer C, Jie KS, Knapen MH. Role of vitamin K in bone metabolism. Annual Review of Nutrition. 1995;**15**:1-22

[44] Shiraki M, Shiraki Y, Aoki C, Miura M. Vitamin K2 (menatetrenone) effectively prevents fractures and sustains lumbar bone mineral density in osteoporosis. Journal of Bone and Mineral Research. 2000;**15**(3):515-521

[45] Kim MS, Kim ES, Sohn CM. Dietary intake of vitamin K in relation to bone mineral density in Korea adults: The Korea National Health and nutrition examination survey (2010-2011). Journal of Clinical Biochemistry and Nutrition. 2015;**57**(3):223-227

[46] Fujita Y, Iki M, Tamaki J, et al. Association between vitamin K intake from fermented soybeans, natto, and bone mineral density in elderly Japanese men: The Fujiwara-kyo osteoporosis risk in men (FORMEN) study. Osteoporosis International. 2012;**23**(2):705-714

[47] Ikeda Y, Iki M, Morita A, et al. Intake of fermented soybeans, natto, is associated with reduced bone loss in postmenopausal women: Japanese population-based osteoporosis (JPOS) study. The Journal of Nutrition. 2006;**136**(5):1323-1328

[48] Macdonald HM, McGuigan FE, Lanham-New SA, Fraser WD, Ralston SH, Reid DM. Vitamin K1 intake is associated with higher bone mineral density and reduced bone resorption in early postmenopausal Scottish women: No evidence of gene-nutrient interaction with apolipoprotein E polymorphisms. The American Journal of Clinical Nutrition. 2008;**87**(5):1513-1520

[49] Kanai T, Takagi T, Masuhiro K, Nakamura M, Iwata M, Saji F. Serum vitamin K level and bone mineral density in post-menopausal women. International Journal of Gynaecology and Obstetrics. 1997;**56**(1):25-30

[50] Jaghsi S, Hammoud T, Haddad S. Relation between circulating vitamin K1 and osteoporosis in the lumbar spine in Syrian post-menopausal

women. Open Rheumatology Journal. 2018;**12**:1-9

[51] Heiss C, Hoesel LM, Wehr U, et al. Vitamin K in combination with other biochemical markers to diagnose osteoporosis. Biomarkers. 2004;**9**(6):479-488

[52] Booth SL, Broe KE, Peterson JW, et al. Associations between vitamin K biochemical measures and bone mineral density in men and women. The Journal of Clinical Endocrinology and Metabolism. 2004;**89**(10):4904-4909

[53] Tsugawa N, Shiraki M, Suhara Y, et al. Low plasma phylloquinone concentration is associated with high incidence of vertebral fracture in Japanese women. Journal of Bone and Mineral Metabolism. 2008;**26**(1):79-85

[54] Hodges SJ, Akesson K, Vergnaud P, Obrant K, Delmas PD. Circulating levels of vitamins K1 and K2 decreased in elderly women with hip fracture. Journal of Bone and Mineral Research. 1993;**8**(10):1241-1245

[55] Palermo A, Tuccinardi D, D'Onofrio L, et al. Vitamin K and osteoporosis: Myth or reality? Metabolism. 2017;**70**:57-71

Chapter 9

Metabolic Disorders in Patients with Chronic Osteomyelitis: Etiology and Pathogenesis

Archil Tsiskarashvili, Nikolay Zagorodny, Svetlana Rodionova and Dmitry Gorbatyuk

Abstract

In this study, we discuss the peculiarities of metabolic disorders that follow the development of chronic osteomyelitis. For the purposes of this study, we analyzed the available data as well as results of our own clinical and scientific research. Chronic osteomyelitis leads not only to the destruction of bone tissue by pathogen but also to the shift of equilibrium between osteogenesis and bone resorption in the locus of bone infections. Such shift leads to additional damage not only to the bone cells (primarily osteoblasts) but also to the bone matrix. The final complications include difficulties with bone consolidation and prolongation of therapy, even when the patient is treated using an external fixation method like Ilizarov or similar techniques. Etiopathogenetic therapy, aimed at correction of metabolic disorders, allows to shorten the bone consolidation time (and respectively, the treatment time), preventing different pathogenetic processes that exacerbate and enhance each other's effects. This study emphasizes the importance of etiopathogenetic therapy of metabolic disorders in patients with chronic osteomyelitis. Etiopathogenetic therapy should be combined with other necessary methods of the patient's treatment, such as surgical debridement of the infection locus and antibiotic therapy.

Keywords: chronic osteomyelitis, metabolic disorders, bone tissue

1. Introduction

The empirical experience of surgeons operating patients with orthopedic infection shows that the mechanical properties of the bone (including strength) differ from physiological ones. The bone in or near the infected area tends to be more fragile and soft. Proper mechanical strength of the bone tissue is one of the key factors for completing successful osteosynthesis as the mechanical strength of the bone directly influences the stability of fixators, treatment of bone tissues in the surgery process, and other technical but pivotal aspects of the treatment.

Despite some empirical data, the change of mechanical properties of the bone in orthopedic infection remained practically unresearched for a long time. The change of the mechanical properties of the bone in inflamed areas had been connected to tissue destruction or lysis caused by bacterial pathogen. In other words, this change of the mechanical properties of the bone happening in the inflamed area was viewed similarly as the complications in soft tissues in the purulent surgery, widely known for a long period of time.

Consequently, this falsely simplified view of the problem has led to a shortage of publications. For example, the search query in the PubMed database based on Mesh terms “Osteomyelitis” and “Bone mineral density” (latest access time: December 08, 2019, 0:01 UTC +3) has provided only 30 search results, the earliest of them is signed as published in February 1991. Most publications refer to dentistry and maxillofacial surgery but not to traumatology and/or orthopedics. Another search based on Mesh terms “Osteomyelitis” and “Metabolic disorders” (latest access time: December 08, 2019, 0:03 UTC +3) has provided 596 results, but most papers refer to other topics and problems: “combinations” of chronic osteomyelitis and diabetes mellitus [1, 2], chronic osteomyelitis and bisphosphonate-induced necrosis of the jaw [3, 4]; less papers refer to the problem of treating chronic osteomyelitis in patients with genetic, systemic, neuropathic, and oncological diseases [5–8]. In several papers, the accent is put on the clinical aspects of bone infection with particular pathogens only [9–11]. Some papers can be considered of a relatively good quality but the accent is put on clinical results themselves and not on the pathogenesis of metabolic bone tissue disorders in the presence of bone infection [12, 13].

Numerous clinical guidelines and publications on osteoporosis and related disorders have much to offer about the pathophysiology of these diseases, but have a rather serious common disadvantage: they do not describe or poorly describe the interaction of pathogen and bone tissue, although the infectious and purely osteoporotic metabolic processes have similar mechanisms.

Lack of understanding of the metabolic bone tissue disorders as a result of its interaction with bacterial pathogen during orthopedic infection practically eliminated the possibility of providing adequate etiological treatment; in most cases, the treatment methods were limited to surgical treatment (necrectomy, debridement, external fixation, and related methods) and antibiotic therapy. Despite being approved and reliable, these methods themselves are not enough to treat chronic osteomyelitis. The correction of the impaired bone tissue metabolism is also needed. For this purpose, a clinician should be familiar with the aspects of biochemistry, physiology, and pathophysiology of the bone affected by orthopedic infections.

At this moment, several fundamental papers in the domain of bone tissue and pathogen interaction are available [14, 15], which can be evaluated as a positive trend. These works can be useful to systematize the knowledge cumulated by the scientific community.

Within this chapter, we made an attempt to synergize the knowledge in pathophysiology of the disorders described, as well as illustrate the importance of correction of impaired bone tissue metabolism using the results of our own work published in 2019 [16].

2. Pathogenesis of metabolic bone tissue disorders at the site of orthopedic infection

Current views on chronic osteomyelitis allow its understanding not simply as a “bone-lytic” or “infectious” process, but also as a condition associated with bone metabolism alteration. Understanding the nature of these alterations is one of the key points in treating chronic osteomyelitis. Without this understanding, the process of treatment may not succeed or may be less successful even if supported by superb surgery and antibiotic therapy (**Figure 1**).

As an attempt to describe the links between changes in bone tissue metabolism during orthopedic infection, we created a scheme displayed above. From our point of view, deep understanding of the pathogenesis is of paramount importance for a clinician.

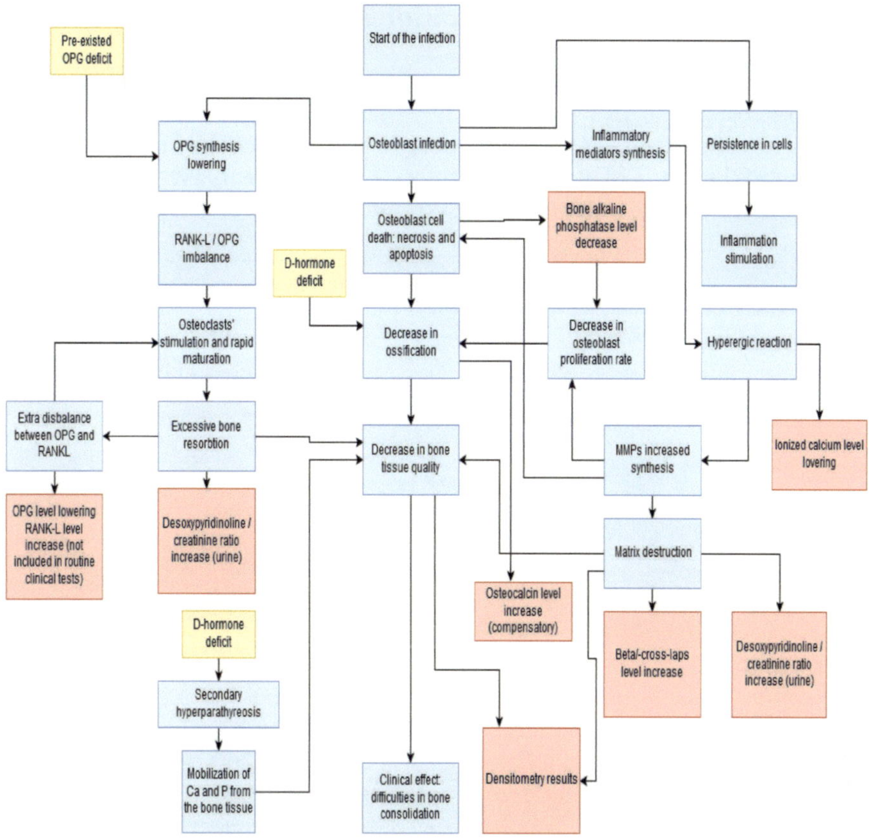

Figure 1.
Pathogenesis of metabolic disorders of the bone tissue, influence of the background factors and laboratory diagnostic markers (figure credits: Gorbatyuk D.S., Tsiskarashvili A.V., Rodionova S.S.).

The overall scheme can be divided into three major parts, which represent main pathogenetic pathways enforcing and exacerbating each other while developing at the same time:

1. Osteoblast cell death and proliferation lowering.

2. Bone remodeling shift to the resorption prevalence.

3. Matrix destruction.

These parts will be discussed separately to make them easier for understanding, even though the pathogenic processes described would influence each other in a "crossing-over" manner. De facto, it is hardly possible to separate them because all of the components take part in general bone metabolism and remodeling process.

The color of the blocks is associated with their aim:

- Blue blocks represent the stages of pathophysiological processes.

- Red blocks represent the "final" changes in the levels of the markers (e.g., beta-cross-laps (C-terminal telopeptide) increase). These changes can be detected using laboratory methods and are used by a clinician during the diagnostics.

- Yellow blocks represent the background factors (markers and their levels) that also can be measured with methods of laboratory diagnostics.

3. Osteoblast cell death and proliferation lowering

One of the most obvious effects of bacterial pathogen on a bone tissue is the destruction of osteoblasts.

Destruction of osteoblasts includes necrotic and apoptotic pathways. Papers contributing to the study of *S. aureus'* influence on the osteoblast culture show that these two pathways work independently. Apoptosis is triggered by ligand TRAIL

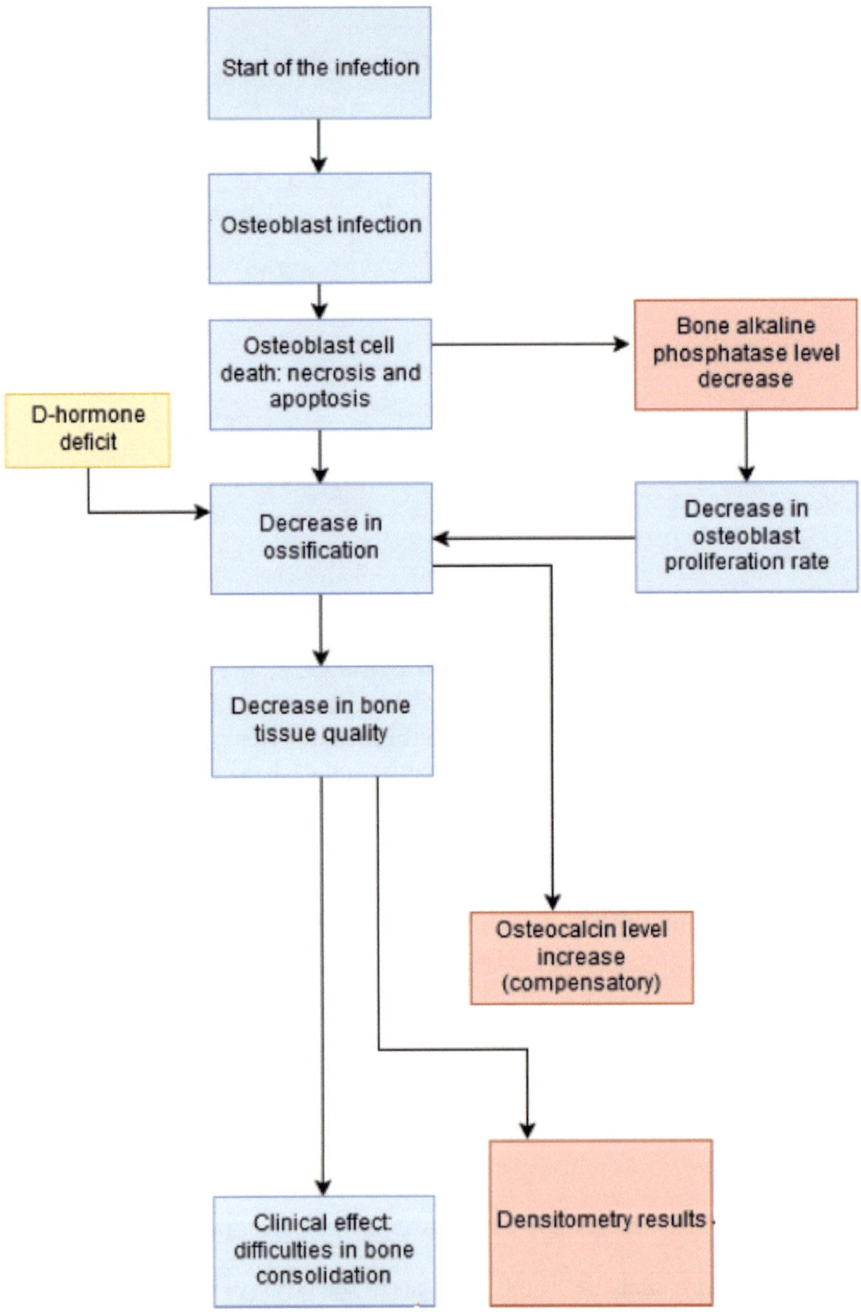

Figure 2.
Pathogenetic stages and processes associated particularly with osteoblast cell death and proliferation lowering. The link between bone matrix destruction processes and associated decrease in osteoblast proliferation rate (will be shown and illustrated in the corresponding part of the chapter).

linking with "death receptors" DR4 and DR5, and necrosis is triggered by *S. aureus* toxins PSMα и PSMβ that destroy the osteoblast cell membrane [15, 17, 18].

Lowering of the osteoblast number leads to slowing of ossification and mineralization of the bone. The level of bone resorption can remain stable or be increased at the same time (see "Bone remodeling shift").

As a result, the production of bone alkaline phosphatase lowers [15]. We must say that alkaline phosphatase itself is not very convenient as a marker: it is produced by different cell types in four different forms. In this case, we have an interest in bone alkaline phosphatase that is coded with ALPL gene [19]. For precise diagnostics, a laboratory should have a specially trained personnel and corresponding equipment. A clinician should note that children and adolescents have normally elevated levels of bone alkaline phosphatase in comparison to adults, and the association between age and serum level of BAP is inverse [20] (**Figure 2**).

Deficit of D hormone is a background factor that lowers ossification and is therefore marked as yellow block [21–23]. It is well known that low level of hormone D leads to increase in PTH level and lowering of bone mineral density [24]. Presence of generalized osteoporosis can additionally intensify this negative trend [25].

4. Bone remodeling (bone turnover) shift

Orthopedic infection and excessive production of pro-inflammatory cytokines [15] influence the bone remodeling balance. Such hyperproduction can be triggered by infection itself and can increase when the pathogen persists inside the osteoblasts. Furthermore, some pathogens can additionally increase the inflammatory response because of paracrine action of their factors, interfering with the cytokine balance [26]. As it will be shown later, the inflammatory response tends to turn into a hyperergic response because of excessive activation of the cell immunity, which is an important factor for chronization of the process.

One of the most well-studied bacterial pathogens that is convenient for illustration is *S. aureus*. Many authors [14, 15, 27] show that *S. aureus* influences both parts of the bone turnover-bone resorption and ossification. During infection, *S. aureus* not only destroys (damages) osteoblasts through necrosis and apoptosis, but also lowers their proliferation rate. Influence on bone resorption is based on rapid maturation and additional activation of the osteoclasts by this pathogen. This mechanism is based on excessive synthesis of prostaglandin E2 (PGE2) by osteoblasts and persisting of *S. aureus* inside the osteoblasts, as well as auto and paracrine regulatory mechanisms in which PGE2 plays its biochemical role. The synthesis of osteoprotegerin (OPG) is also impaired because of lowering of the level of corresponding mRNA; [28] as a result, more RANK-ligand (RANKL) molecules remain unbound and act as osteoclast activators. Excessive activation of the osteoclasts and lowering of the number and proliferation rate of the osteoblasts lead to obvious shift of the bone turnover to bone resorption. As a result, the loss of bone tissue and impairment of its mineralization at the site of orthopedic infection (bone infection) can lead to difficulties in bone consolidation in patients with bone defects and/or fractures (**Figure 3**).

"Red blocks" of this part include the OPG and RANK-ligand (RANKL) level changes.

"Yellow blocks" include the pre-existing low level of the osteoprotegerin. An example is a case of chronic osteomyelitis development in a patient with pre-existing low-speed bone turnover and associated osteoporosis with OPG synthesis impairment.

These markers are rarely used in routine clinical practice but can be of a certain value when an appropriate laboratory is available.

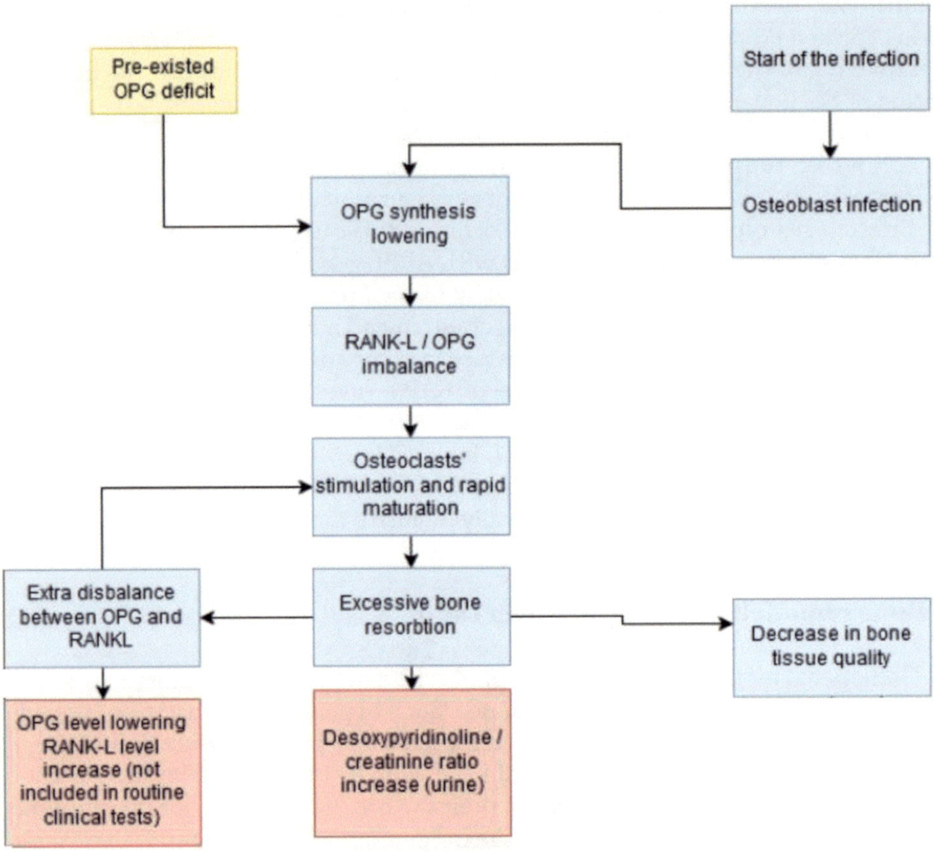

Figure 3.
Pathogenetic stages and processes associated particularly with bone turnover shift.

OPG is a soluble glycoprotein synthesized by different cell types, including osteoblasts [29]. This compound can be found in monomeric (50 kDa) or dimeric (120 kDa) form (the dimeric form contains disulfide bonds between monomers). Dimeric form has a higher affinity to RANKL than a monomeric one, and the chemical analogues of OPG should have the features of dimeric form.

RANKL (RANK-ligand) is a compound synthesized by several cell types. It can be expressed in three different molecular forms: transmembrane trimer, primary (secreted) form, and cell ectodomain [30]. RANKL serves as a ligand for RANK receptor that activates osteoclasts. RANKL is a target for osteoprotegerin; if OPG is secreted in low amounts, more RANKL remains unbound and the intensity of resorption increases.

Therefore, a "pathogenetic chain" is as follows: infection-osteoblast cell death and proliferation rate decrease-OPG synthesis decrease-RANKL inhibition decrease-osteoclastogenesis activation-bone resorption increase-shift of bone remodeling toward a resorption prevalence-decrease in bone tissue quality and quantity in the infection site. The resulting clinical effect is slowing of the consolidation of the bone tissue defects, pseudarthroses, and related conditions.

5. Matrix destruction

The matrix destruction in infection can be explained by several factors. The "starting point" in pathogenesis is the infection itself. *S. aureus* is, as shown by several authors [14, 31, 32], capable of persisting in osteoblasts and that leads to additional stimulation of inflammatory process that stepwise turns into local hyperergic reaction. It is important to take into account that pathogens also play a role in matrix destruction—particularly *S. aureus* can adhere to matrix elements and destroy them [33].

The hyperergic reaction leads to excessive synthesis of matrix metalloproteases (MMPs). Among them, MMP-2 (gelatinase A) and MMP-9 (gelatinase B) [34] play the main role. Excessive synthesis of MMP is a key point in the process because it has two major effects:

- Osteoblast cell death and lowering of the proliferation rate; this effect weakens the regenerative potential of bone tissue.

- MMPs damage the matrix by themselves, being synthesized in excessive amounts [34, 35].

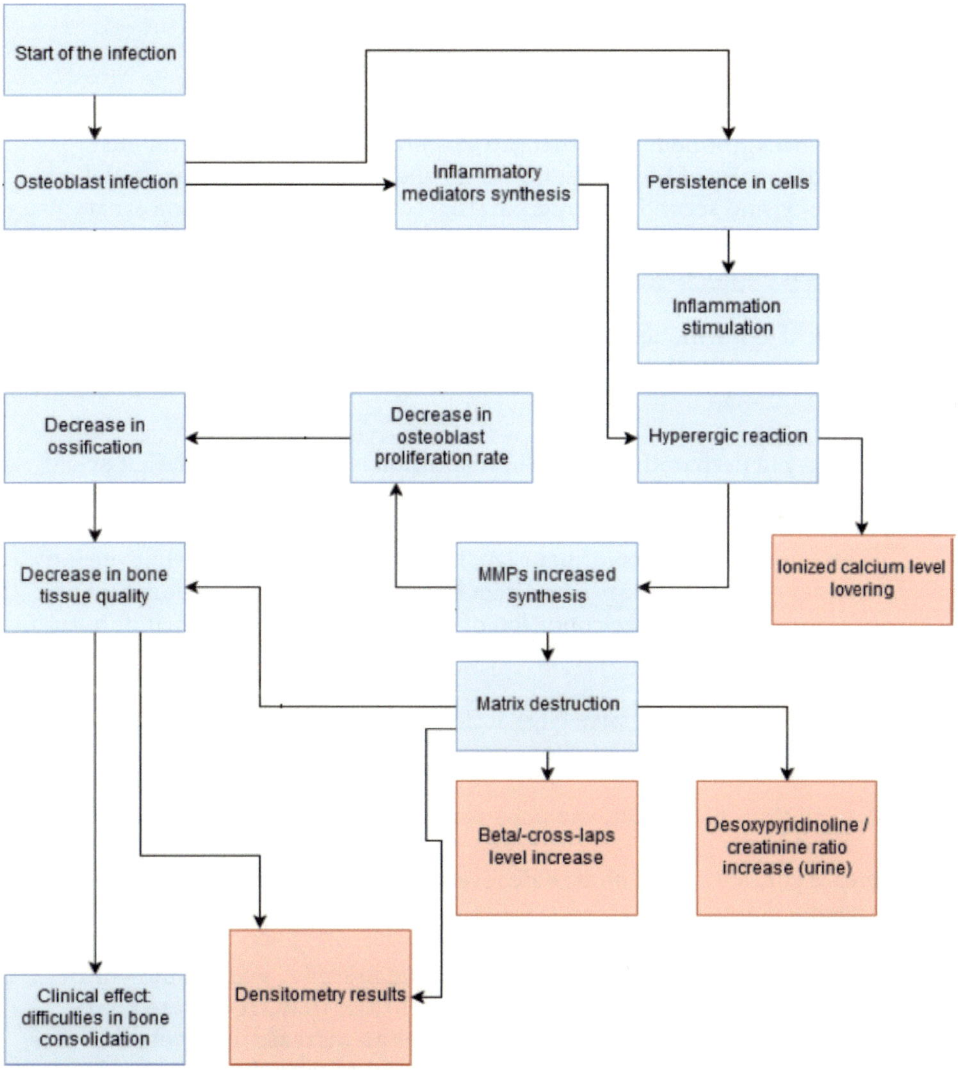

Figure 4.
Pathogenetic stages and processes associated particularly with bone matrix destruction.

The matrix destruction leads to increase in following resorption markers: B-cross-laps (C-terminal telopeptide) and desoxypyridinoline/creatinine ratio.

- B-cross-laps: This marker is a product of collagen destruction that is a basis of bone tissue matrix. B-cross-laps have two octapeptide fragments in structure, which are linked with a transverse molecular bond. Its level can be evaluated using the immunoassay method [36].

- Increase in the desoxypyridinoline/creatinine ratio: Desoxypyridinoline is a molecular basis for transverse bonds between collagen I type molecules in bone tissue matrix. Its level increases while the matrix is destroyed. It is important to note that this factor can be increased as a result of not only osteoclast activation, but also of a MMP action.

A clinician should note that the destruction of the matrix is combined with lowering of its synthesis by osteoblasts. Therefore, both processes act in a synergic way and occur at the same time, which negatively influences the treatment (**Figure 4**).

6. Background factors

The main background factors that can exacerbate bone tissue metabolism impairment at the site of bone infection are: generalized osteoporosis, D-deficit, D-insufficiency, and secondary hyperparathyreosis. These factors exacerbate also the condition of patients with bone infection, lowering the regenerative potential of bone tissue. On the scheme, these factors are marked as yellow blocks.

- The lack of D hormone leads to lowered absorption of calcium in the intestine, lowered mineralization of the bone, and consequent decrease of the osteoblast function [21–23].

- Secondary hyperparathyreosis: This condition is a result of D-deficit or D-insufficiency and is actually a compensative reaction. It has rather complex pathogenetic action mechanism [37]. It is shown that during short-term increase in PTH level, its influence on bone tissue is anabolic, while during a long-term constant increase, its effect becomes catabolic with bone loss as a result, for example, at the condition of chronic hormone D-deficit or hormone D-insufficiency [37].

Thus, because of the excessive PTH action on bone tissue, two major effects, that can be "found out" using markers, occur [38–40]:

- "Mobilization" of calcium and phosphates from the bones.

- Increase in calcium and phosphate levels in the urine because of relatively high secreted amounts.

As a result, calcium and phosphates are being literally "washed out" of the bone in amounts more than physiological. After that, they are secreted out of the organism through urine. A bright example is an increase in vertebral bodies fractures risk in patients with primary hyperparathyreosis. Even simple densitometry can help to diagnose the lowered bone density and trabecular thinning.

Removal of calcium and phosphates exceeds not only the physiological values or amounts, but also the compensative intake with the food leading to progressive lowering of bone tissue quality in general and its mineralization in particular. To cope successfully with these changes, the secondary parathyreosis should be treated and compensative therapy, including calcium, phosphates, and hormone D medication, introduced.

7. Summary of scheme review

In this part of the chapter, the etiopathogenetic mechanisms of bone tissue metabolism impairment are discussed, as well as reasons for change of laboratory-measured bone metabolism markers and their levels.

The mentioned markers have a direct link with metabolic impairments of a certain type. Such impairments can be found in different diseases, especially in patients with chronic osteomyelitis and other forms of bone infection.

The therapy of metabolic bone tissue impairments due to bone (orthopedic) infection should combine etiopathogenetic and compensating approaches. For example, bisphosphonates can be recommended for use in addition to antibiotic therapy and surgery, as well as calcium, D hormone, and other drugs because of the bisphosphonates' ability to decrease the osteoclasts' activity.

8. Our experience

Nowadays, the published data on epidemiology of metabolic diseases in healthy volunteers and orthopedic patients without bone infection (except patients with osteoporosis and related diseases) are scarce. Therefore, these data cannot serve as statistical material for comparison with data in patients with bone infection.

Accordingly, our work is limited to patients with bone infection (chronic osteomyelitis and related diseases) already diagnosed. The dynamics of the parameters was studied with addition of metabolic disorders therapy and without it.

In 2019, we published a retrospective study; the aim was to evaluate dynamics and values of markers and parameters of bone metabolism [16], which included 112 patients with infected pseudarthroses of long bones (humerus, femur, tibia) developing as an exacerbation of chronic osteomyelitis. The study had three main purposes:

- Gaining the whole "picture" of metabolic bone tissue disorders in these patients.
- Studying the dynamics of corresponding marker level and parameters.
- Comparing the duration of consolidation of pseudarthroses after surgical treatment, antibiotic treatment, and using external fixation apparatus (with and without bone metabolism correction therapy).

We formed two groups of 56 patients each using anatomical segment-stratified randomization. The main group received not only surgery and antibiotic therapy but also medication for correction of impaired bone metabolism. The control group received the same therapy except correction of bone metabolism.

The dynamics of parameters was evaluated only in the main study group. Data from the control group patients were used to evaluate the duration of bone consolidation and comparing them between groups.

To form a "picture" of a bone tissue metabolism, we evaluated the following parameters:

- Homeostasis of Ca and P-values: blood Ca, ionized Ca, blood P, PTH, transportation form of D hormone (25(OH)D3).

- Ossification markers: bone alkaline phosphatase, osteocalcin.

- Resorption markers: beta-cross-laps (C-terminal telopeptide).

- Ca and P (daily amount secreted with urine); deoxypyridinoline/creatinine ratio.

For therapy, we used calcium medicaments (Ca carbonate, ossein-hydroxyapatite complex) and active metabolite of D hormone (alfacalcidol). Dosage was set individually for each patient according to a patented way [41] on the basis of the following key parameters:

- Sex and age.

- Densitometry results.

- Values of the parameters listed above.

As an anti-resorptive drug, the ibandronate acid was administered (with the dosage of 3 mg (3 ml) one time in 3 months).

The described therapy was empirically proved to be effective not only against osteoporosis in patients that underwent arthroplasty but also in cases of osteoporosis connected with low intensity of ossification; that was the key reason why it was selected for treatment.

The numerical data of patients are described using descriptive statistics. To compare the changes in metabolic values after 3 months and before treatment, we used the Wilcoxon test. To compare the consolidation duration in main and control groups, we used Mann-Whitney U-test. The threshold p-value in all cases was set as $p < 0.05$. The software used was IBM SPSS Statistics 22. All values, including theoretically possible outliers, were considered in the statistics (**Table 1** and **Figure 5**).

Routine screening of the whole population described above exceeds the ranks of this study.

We found statistically significant changes after 3 months in osteocalcin level (decrease), PTH (decrease), and desoxypyridinoline/creatinine ratio (decrease) (respectively: $p = 0.043$, $p = 0.043$, $p = 0.041$). Changes in daily amounts of calcium and phosphate secreted with urine, as well as beta-cross-laps were not statistically significant but, in our opinion, the follow-up tie of 3 months can be insufficient. We suppose that the following mechanisms can take part in forming this "picture":

- Lowering of the resorption because of ibandronic acid use leads to decrease in desoxypyridinoline/crcatinine ratio.

Metabolic marker	Value[1], median ± SD	Range[1]	Units	Test p-value[2]	Threshold p-value	Plot[3]
Ca—0 months[4]	2.4 ± 0.1	2.1–2.71	mmol/l	0.172	0.05	A
Ca—3 months[5]	2.5 ± 0.6	2.38–2.63				
P—0 months	1.2 ± 0.2	0.7–1.6	mmol/l	0.180		B
P—3 months	1.2 ± 0.147	1.0–1.39				
Ca^{2+}—0 months	1.2 ± 0.2	0.96–2.2	mmol/l	0.807		C
Ca^{2+}—3 months	1.2 ± 0.1	1.11–1.33				
Bone alkaline phosphatase—0 months	123.5 ± 65.7	60.3–373.0	U/l	0.893		D
Bone alkaline phosphatase—3 months	113.7 ± 24.3	90.0–148.0				
B-cross-laps—0 months	0.7 ± 0.3	0.1–1.1	ng/ml	0.18		E
B-cross-laps—3 months	0.7 ± 0.3	0.2–1.0				
Osteocalcin—0 months	22.6 ± 11.1	2.0–46.0	ng/ml	**0.043**		F
Osteocalcin—3 months	24.9 ± 11.5	11.5–39.0				
PTH—0 months	12.5 ± 15.5	1.8–60.0	mol/l	**0.043**		G
PTH—3 months	2.6 ± 1.0	1.0–4.2				
P (urine, day amount)—0 months	24.0 ± 9.6	10.50–42.5	mmol/day	0.180		H
P (urine, day amount)—3 months	9.9 ± 5.3	3.5–17.1				
25-OH-D3—0 months	17.8 ± 10.2	6.6–40.0	ng/ml	0.715		I
25-OH-D3—3 months	19.0 ± 10.8	5.0–33.0				
Deoxypyridinoline/creatinine—0 months	11.6 ± 6.4	5.0–38.4	nmol/mmol Cre	**0.041**		J
Deoxypyridinoline/creatinine—3 months	8.6 ± 3.3	3.5–17.5				
Ca (urine, day amount)—0 months	3.7 ± 1.5	1.00–6.34	mmol/day	0.180		K
Ca (urine, day amount)—3 months	2.5 ± 0.8	1.4–3.6				

Data represent the study group (56 patients). Control group is quantitatively equal (56 patients).
[1]Rounded to first decimal place.
[2]Wilcoxon signed-rank test. Values are rounded to the third decimal place.
*[3]Letters represent the particular plots at **Figure 5A-K** for the information to be easily to followed.*
[4]0 months—value before operative treatment.
[5]3 months—value at 3 months after the operative treatment.
Statistically significant values ($p < 0.05$) are labeled as bold.

Table 1.
Comparative data of patients before and after 3-month therapy of metabolic bone disorders.

- Decrease in osteocalcin level can be explained by lowering of the earlier increased (in a compensative way) osteoblast activity that at least partially normalized.
- Decrease of PTH level can be explained by administration of D hormone and elimination of D deficit, which also led to decrease in blood calcium. In other words, the immediate mechanism of secondary hyperparathyreosis was eliminated.

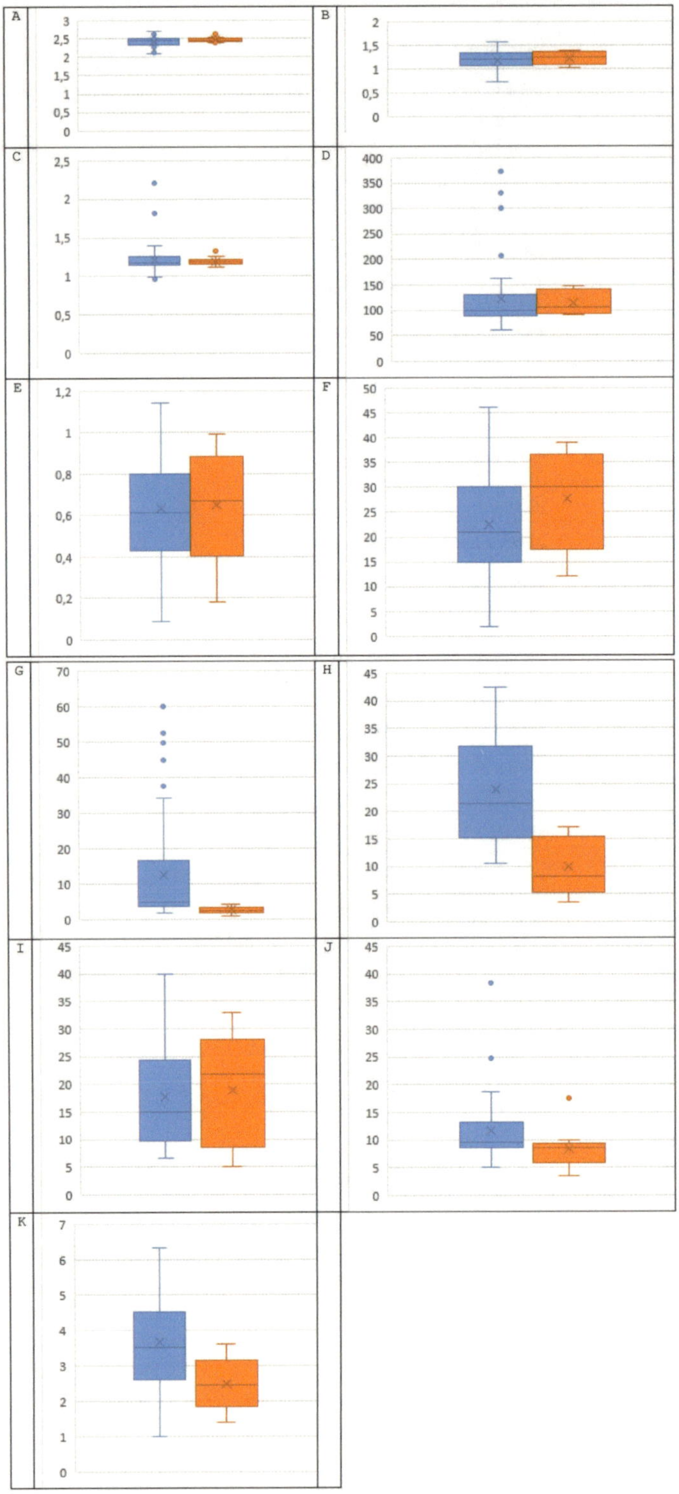

Figure 5.
(A-K) "Box and whiskers" plots illustrating the data provided in ***Table 1****. Blue box and whiskers (left at all figures) represent data of patients before therapy. Orange boxes and whiskers represent data of the same patients after 3 months of therapy. A: blood calcium. B: phosphate of the blood. C: ionized calcium, D: bone alkaline phosphatase levels, E: beta-cross-laps (C-terminal telopeptide), F: osteocalcin, G: PTH. H: phosphate (urine, day amount), I: 25 (OH) D3, J: deoxypyridinoline/creatinine, K: calcium (urine, daily amount). Units: see* ***Table 1****.*

- Decrease of Ca and phosphates in blood and their daily amounts secreted with urine is not statistically significant at 3-month follow-up (p = 0.172 for Ca, p = 0.18 for phosphates, p = 0.18 for both daily secreted amounts of Ca and phosphates in urine), but we can potentially explain these changes as an effect—even statistically insignificant—of PTH level decrease (partial normalization).

The rationale of metabolic bone tissue impairment correction is proved by clinical results (decrease of fracture consolidation type in the main group that received corresponding therapy). In each group (56 patients), the "anatomical distribution" of patients according to a treated segment was as follows:

- Humerus—6 patients
- Femur—25 patients
- Tibia—25 patients

The software used was SPSS Statistics 22. All values, including theoretically possible outliers, were considered in the statistics. Statistically significant changes between groups were found in all studied segments (**Table 2** and **Figure 6**).

As shown, the additional therapy of metabolic disorders of bone tissue has a statistically significant effect on shortening the duration of bone consolidation in patients treated by external fixation apparatus.

In our opinion, the next step should be a comparative analysis of bone metabolism aspects in orthopedic patients with and without bone infection and a study of the dynamics of mentioned parameters during a long follow-up period (more than 3 months).

Anatomical segment/study group	No. of patients	Consolidation duration[1], days, mean ± SD	Range	Test p-value[2]	Threshold p-value	Plot[3]
Humerus, main group	6	199.9 ± 31.6	147–243	0.041	0.05	A
Humerus, control group	6	254.2 ± 45.1	196–321			
Femur, main group	25	266.9 ± 52.7	190–399	0.009		B
Femur, control group	25	338.0 ± 107.1	197–559			
Tibia, main group	25	235.0 ± 49.3	154–351	0.041		C
Tibia, control group	25	270.0 ± 61.1	189–427			

Both groups received "standard" surgery and antibiotic therapy.
[1]Rounded to first decimal place.
[2]Mann-Whitney U-test. Values are rounded to the third decimal place.
*[3]Letters represent particular plots in **Figure 6A–C**.*

Table 2.
Comparison of consolidation time in patients with (main group) or without (control group) bone tissue metabolism correction therapy.

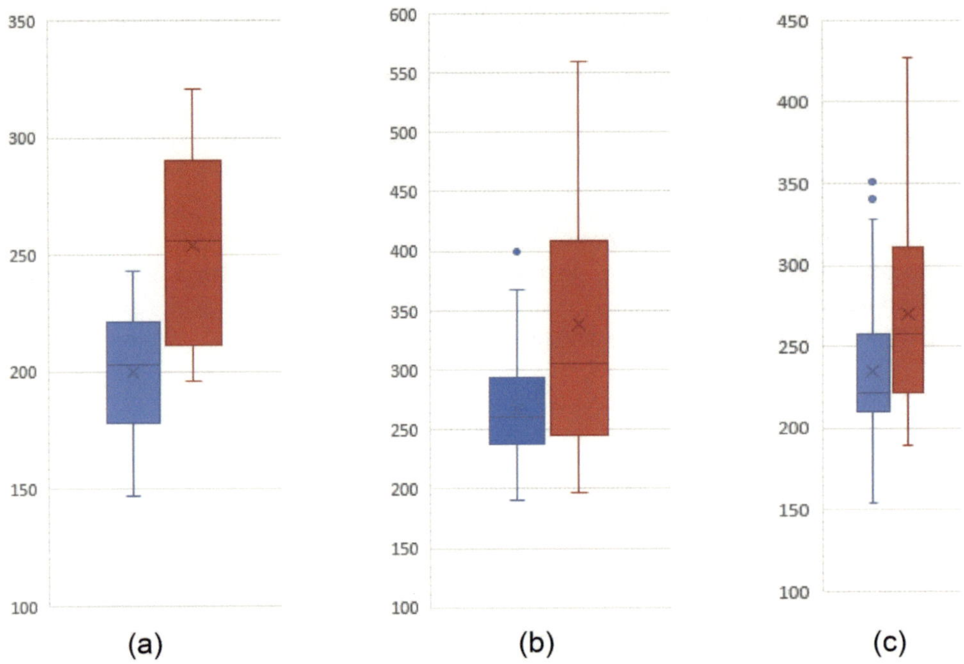

Figure 6.
(a-c) "Box-and-whiskers" plots illustrating the duration (in days) of bone consolidation in patients that underwent treatment of the fractures of different segments exacerbated by orthopedic infection using the external fixation apparatus. Left (a): humerus; in the middle (b): femur; right (c): tibia. Blue box and whiskers (at the left at all figures) represent data for the main study group that received surgery, antibiotic and etiologic metabolism impairment therapy; red box and whiskers (at the right at all figures) represent the control group that received surgery and antibiotic therapy, but no treatment of bone metabolism impairment.

9. Conclusion

In this chapter, we attempted to describe the basic pathophysiology of metabolic processes at the site of orthopedic infection. Knowledge of peculiarities of such processes is important for an orthopedic surgeon because the general success of treatment relies not only on surgery and antibiotic therapy but also etiologic therapy of bone metabolism impairment. This thesis is supported not only by pathophysiological rationale but also by the results of our study.

Metabolic disorders of bone tissue associated with orthopedic infection are complex and yet poorly understood. Research of this topic will improve not only the existing treatment strategy but also the philosophy of it and will greatly contribute to development of traumatology and orthopedics.

Author details

Archil Tsiskarashvili*, Nikolay Zagorodny, Svetlana Rodionova
and Dmitry Gorbatyuk
National Medical Research Center of Traumatology and Orthopedics, Moscow,
Russia

*Address all correspondence to: archil.tsiskarashvili@gmail.com

IntechOpen

© 2020 The Author(s). Licensee IntechOpen. This chapter is distributed under the terms of the Creative Commons Attribution License (http://creativecommons.org/licenses/by/3.0), which permits unrestricted use, distribution, and reproduction in any medium, provided the original work is properly cited.

References

[1] Garg S, Gupta M, Choundry P. A rare case of emphysematous osteomyelitis of spine in uncontrolled diabetes mellitus. Medicina Intensiva. 2019;**43**(2):127-128

[2] Liao D, Xie L, Han Y, Du S, Wang H, Zeng C, et al. Dynamic contrast-enhanced magnetic resonance imaging for differentiating osteomyelitis from acute neuropathic arthropathy in the complicated diabetic foot. Skeletal Radiology. 2018;**47**(10):1337-1347

[3] Yamazaki T, Yamori M, Tanaka S, Yamamoto K, Sumi E, Nishimoto-Sano M, et al. Risk factors and indices of osteomyelitis of the jaw in osteoporosis patients: Results from a hospital-based cohort study in Japan. PLoS One. 2013;**8**(11):e79376

[4] Doll C, Hartwig S, Nack C, Nahles S, Nelson K, Raguse J. Dramatic course of osteomyelitis in a patient treated with immediately placed dental implants suffering from uncontrolled diabetes: A case report. European Journal of Oral Implantology. 2015;**8**(4):405-410

[5] Mikosch P, Hughes D. An overview on bone manifestations in Gaucher disease. Wiener Medizinische Wochenschrift (1946). 2010;**160**(23-24):609-624

[6] Ndip A, Jude E, Whitehouse R, Prescott M, Boulton A. Charcot neuroarthropathy triggered by osteomyelitis and/or surgery. Diabetic Medicine. 2008;**25**(12):1469-1472

[7] de Oliviera E, de Arruda J, Nascimento P, Neiva I, Mesquita R, Souza L. An update on osteomyelitis treatment in a pycnodysostosis patient. Journal of Oral and Maxillofacial Surgery. 2018;**76**(10):2136.e1-2136.e10

[8] Morbach H, Hedrich C, Beer M, Girschick H. Autoinflammatory bone disorders. Clinical Immunology. 2013;**147**(3):185-196

[9] Verma R, Morrad S, Wirtz JJ. *Peptoniphilus asaccharolyticus*-associated septic arthritis and osteomyelitis in a woman with osteoarthritis and diabetes mellitus. BMJ Case Reports [Internet]. BMJ; 2 June 2017:bcr–2017-219969. Available from: http://dx.doi.org/10.1136/bcr-2017-219969

[10] Herman T, Siegel M. Osteopenia of prematurity, staphylococcal rib osteomyelitis. Journal of Perinatology. 2009;**29**(3):254-255

[11] Khan I, Murfi A, Khan M, Khan A, Afridi H, Jan H. Salmonella osteomyelitis of ribs. Journal of Ayub Medical College, Abbottabad. 2018;**30**(4):605-607

[12] Jiang N, Liu G, Yang J, Lin Q, Hu Y, Yu B. Is hypercalcemia a frequent complication following local use of calcium sulfate with antibiotics for the treatment of extremity posttraumatic osteomyelitis? A preliminary study. BioMed Research International [Internet]. Hindawi Limited; 31 March; **2019**:1-7. Available from: http://dx.doi.org/10.1155/2019/7315486

[13] Kim J, Kim S, Lee S, Kim T, Jung J. Bone mineral density in osteoporotic patients with pyogenic vertebral osteomyelitis: Effect of early versus late treatment for osteoporosis. Osteoporosis International. 2018;**29**(12):2761-2770

[14] Thwaites G, Gant V. Are bloodstream leukocytes Trojan horses for the metastasis of *Staphylococcus aureus*? Nature Reviews. Microbiology. 2011;**9**(3):215-222

[15] Josse J, Velard F, Gangloff SC. *Staphylococcus aureus* vs osteoblast: Relationship and consequences in

osteomyelitis. Frontiers in Cellular and Infection Microbiology. 2015;**5**:1-17

[16] Tsiskarashvili A, Rodionova S, Mironov S, Bukhtin K, Gorbatiuk D, Taraskin A. Metabolic bone tissue disorders in patients with long bone fractures complicated by chronic osteomyelitis. Genij Ortopedii. 2019;**25**(2):149-155

[17] Tucker KKA, Reilly SSS, Leslie CCS, Hudson MCM. Intracellular *Staphylococcus aureus* induces apoptosis in mouse osteoblasts. FEMS Mictrobiological Letters. 2000;**186**:151-156

[18] Valour F, Rasigade JP, Trouillet-Assant S, Gagnaire J, Bouaziz A, Karsenty J. Delta-toxin production deficiency in *Staphylococcus aureus*: A diagnostic marker of bone and joint infection chronicity linked with osteoblast invasion and biofilm formation. Clinical Microbiology and Infection. 2015;**21**:568.e1-568.e11

[19] Millan J. Alkaline phosphatases: Structure, substrate specificity and functional relatedness to other members of a large superfamily of enzymes. Purinergic Signal. 2006;**2**(2):335-341

[20] Reiss I, Inderrieden D, Kruse K. Bestimmung der knochenspezifischen alkalischen Phosphatase bei Störungen des Kalziumstoffwechsels im Kindesalter. Monatschrift Kinderheilkd. 1996;**144**(9):885-890

[21] Elmaataoui A, Elmachtani Idrissi S, Dami A, Bouhsain S, Chabraoui L, Ouzzif Z. Association entre les marqueurs du remodelage osseux, la densité minérale osseuse et le statut vitaminique D chez des femmes ménopausées d'origine marocaine. Pathologie et Biologie. 2014;**62**(1):49-54

[22] Nakamura K, Saito T, Oyama M, Oshiki R, Kobayashi R, Nishiwaki T. Vitamin D sufficiency is associated with low incidence of limb and vertebral fractures in community-dwelling elderly Japanese women: The Muramatsu study. Osteoporosis International. 2011;**22**(1):97-103

[23] Ardawi M, Qari M, Rouzi A, Maimani A, Raddadi R. Vitamin D status in relation to obesity, bone mineral density, bone turnover markers and vitamin D receptor genotypes in healthy Saudi pre- und postmenopausal women. Osteoporosis International. 2011;**22**:463-475

[24] Cosman F, de Beur SJ, LeBoff MS, Lewiecki EM, Tanner B, Randall S, et al. Clinician's Guide to Prevention and Treatment of Osteoporosis. Osteoporosis International [Internet]. Berline, Germany: Springer Science and Business Media LLC. 15 August 2014;**25**(10):2359-2381. Available from: http://dx.doi.org/10.1007/s00198-014-2794-2

[25] Kuchuk N, van Schoor N, Pluijm S. Vitamin D status, parathyroid function, bone turnover, and BMD in postmenopausal women with osteoporosis: Global perspective. Journal of Bone and Mineral Research. 2009;**24**:693-701

[26] Lukens JR, Gross JM, Calabrese C, Iwakura Y, Lamkanfi M, Vogel P, et al. Critical role for inflammasome-independent IL-1b production in osteomyelitis. PNAS. 2013:1-6

[27] Claro T, Widaa A, O'Seaghda M. *Staphylococcus aureus* protein A binds to osteoblasts and triggers signals that weaken bone in osteomyelitis. PLoS One. 2011;**6**(4):e18748

[28] Johansen LK, Iburg TM, Nielsen OL, Leifssin PS, Dahl-Petersen K, Koch J. Local osteogenic expression of cyclooxygenase-2 and systemic response in porcine models ofosteomyelitis.

Prostaglandins & Other Lipid Mediators. 2012;**97**:103-108

[29] Schneeweis L, Willard D, Milla M. Functional dissection of protegerin and its interaction with receptor activator of NF-kappaB ligand. The Journal of Biological Chemistry. 2005;**280**(50):41155-41164

[30] Findlay D, Atkins G. Relationship between serum RANKL and RANKL in bone. Osteoporosis International. 2011;**22**(10):2597-2602

[31] Alexander E, Hudson M. Factors influencing the internalization of *Staphylococcus aureus* and impacts on the course of infections in humans. Applied Microbiology and Biotechnology. 2001;**56**:361-366

[32] Garzoni C, Kelley W. *Staphylococcus aureus*: New evidence for intracellular persistence. Trends in Microbiology. 2009;**17**(2):59-65

[33] Flock J. Extracellular-matrix-binding proteins as targets for the prevention of *Staphylococcus aureus* infections. Molecular Medicine Today. 1999;**5**(12):532-537

[34] Rogova LN, Shesternina NV, Zamechnik TV, Fastova IA. Matrix metalloproteinases, their role in physiological and pathological processes (review). Bulletin of New Medical Technologies. 2011;**18**(2):86-89

[35] Protasov MV, Smagina LV, Galibin OV, Pinaev GP, Voronkina IV. The dependence of Mmp-2 and Mmp-9 activity in wound fluid on the wound tissue state at initial stages of wound healing process. Cytology. 2008;**50**(10):882-886

[36] Hanson D, Weis M, Bollen A-M, Masian S, Singer F, Eyre D. A specific immunoassay for monitoring human bone resorption: Quantitation of type I collagen cross-linked N-telopeptides in urine. Journal of Bone and Mineral Research. 1992;**7**:1251-1258

[37] Bellido T, Saini V, Paola DP. Effects of PTH on osteocyte function. Bone. 2013;**54**(2):250-257

[38] Hansen S, Beck Jensen J, Rasmussen L, Hauge E, Brixen K. Effects on bone geometry, density, and microarchitecture in the distal radius but not the tibia in women with primary hyperparathyroidism: A case-control study using HR-pQCT. Journal of Bone and Mineral Research. 2010;**25**(9):1941-1947

[39] Stein E, Silva B, Boutroy S, Zhou B, Wang J, Udesky J. Primary hyperparathyroidism is associated with abnormal cortical and trabecular microstructure and reduced bone stiffness in postmenopausal women. Journal of Bone and Mineral Research. 2013;**28**(5):1029-1040

[40] Liu M, Williams J, Kuo J, Lee JA, Silverberg SH, Walker MD. Risk fractures for vertebral frature in primary hyperparathyroidism. Endocrine. 2019. Available from: https://link.springer.com/article/10.1007%2Fs12020-019-02099-1

[41] Rodionova S, Popova T, Balberkin A, Kolondaev A, Kliushnichenko I. Sposob profilaktiki poteri kostnoi tkani vokrug implantatov pri endoprotezirovanii [The way to prevent bone tissue loss around implants in arthroplasty]. Patent RF, no. 2176519. Russian Federation. 2001

Chapter 10

Immunological Monitoring of Osteogenesis Disorder

Olga Viktorovna Berdyugina and
Kirill Alexandrovich Berdyugin

Abstract

The study of immune responses of peripheral blood in bone regeneration for bone formation predicting complications is relevant. Studies were carried out on patients with the facial skeleton injury before and after stable osteosynthesis of the mandible in a fixing device for external fixation. Of the 136 patients, 17 people's bone tissue regeneration has been slow. Laboratory tests were carried out before and after the operation. The studies included the study of cellular immunity, humoral immunity, phagocytosis, acute phase proteins and cytokine status. The obtained data were processed using variation statistics methods and the modified theorem of T. Bayes. The study revealed that alternating stages of regeneration of bone tissue (inflammation, proliferation of osteoblasts, collagenogenesis and ossification) are accompanied by changes in the immunological status. A comparative study of the dynamics of immunological parameters at normal and slow osteogenesis had made it possible to establish criteria for delayed consolidation of bone tissue. Prognostic criteria before the operations include increasing the concentration of IgM and decreasing the concentration of C-reactive protein, in the early postoperative period-increasing the number of leukocytes, the concentration of tumor necrosis factor, IgM, as well as reducing the number of $CD45^{+}CD3^{+}$-cells, the complement activity and the amount of lactoferrin.

Keywords: monitoring of osteogenesis, prognostic criteria, nitro blue tetrazolium test, tumor necrosis factor, IgM, C-reactive protein

1. Introduction

Regulation of bone formation when damaged is regulated by a complex set of factors, including mechanical conditions for the formation of high-grade regeneration, vascular reactions, the influence of the neuroendocrine system, effects of metabolites and growth factors [1]. A reflection of the processes becomes dynamic of blood parameters, among which the most important are the changes in the immune status.

It is known that the immune system and bone tissue have broad functional and structural connections. The heterogeneity of cell population included in the immune system and the variety of regulators produced determine its ambiguous participation in the regulation of bone tissue regeneration.

Both macrophages and osteoclasts develop from the same progenitor cell of the monocytic line [2]. Both of these cells have the ability to destroy tissues, which leads to the activation of repair processes carried out by cells of mesenchymal origin, fibroblasts or osteoblasts. From stromal cells expressing the most important regulators of osteoclastogenesis and being a natural microenvironment for normal hematopoiesis, osteoblasts develop [3].

Quantitative and qualitative changes in immunocompetent cells are due to lymphocyte-macrophage regulation of osteogenesis and are reflected regeneration of the bone-favorable or delayed.

An important role in the regulation of bone tissue regeneration belongs to immune cells-lymphocytes. In an animal experiment, it was shown that thymectomy leads to a significant delay in osteogenesis after a bone fracture [4]. Different lymphocyte populations influence the regulation of bone tissue regeneration ambiguously: when analyzing the cellular composition of the regeneration zone in difficultly fused fractures, a significant decrease in the number of T cells, the absence of mast cells and the predominance of fibroblasts and mononuclear cells was revealed [5]. There are reports that with severe mechanical polytrauma, deep disturbances of the cellular immunity are observed in the form of inhibition of the expression of $CD2^{-}DR^{+}$ receptors and a decrease in the absolute number of cells with $CD4^{+}$ and $CD8^{+}$ phenotypes [6]. It was also shown that the activity of NK cells is significantly reduced among the patients in the fracture zone, as well as in peripheral blood [7]. A number of authors have found that in animals with a deficiency of mature T lymphocytes, physiological metabolism in bone tissue is not disturbed [8]. However, under conditions when there was a need to increase bone metabolism (in trauma and after surgery), deficiency of T-lymphocyte function led to the formation of demineralized bone matrix and loss of density of existing bone tissue [9]. Clinical studies had also confirmed the role of T lymphocytes in the regulation of bone density. It was revealed that both $CD4^{+}$ and $CD8^{+}$ cells can produce factors that affect osteoclastogenesis [10]. There are a number of studies that show the inhibitory role of T lymphocytes in relation to the formation of osteoclasts and resorptive changes in the bone [11]. It is indicated that activated T lymphocytes can reduce osteoclastogenesis by producing INF-γ. In vitro, the removal of $CD8^{+}$ T lymphocytes from a cell culture containing both osteoclast precursors and bone marrow cells significantly increases the formation of mature osteoclasts [12]. Some in vivo data indicate the involvement of the prostaglandin mechanism in this process [13]. In various pathological conditions, the nature of the influence of T lymphocytes on osteoclastogenesis is determined by both a set of locally secreted cytokines and the degree of differentiation of T lymphocytes [14]. Bone resorption caused by some cytokines secreted by T lymphocytes is often accompanied by further increased bone tissue formation, which leads to an increase in bone metabolism [15]. The direct molecular mechanisms of influence, as well as the conditions that determine the stimulating or inhibitory role of T lymphocytes in the regulation of bone tissue regeneration, are under study.

B lymphocytes are also involved in the regulation of bone tissue regeneration. In the bone marrow, the earliest precursors of B lymphocytes are in close contact with the endosteal surface of the bone, and the most mature cells of this series are located in the center of the bone marrow. Such a spatial organization of B lymphopoiesis in the bone marrow suggests that the cells of the osteoblastic germ located in the endosteum, as well as stromal cells located in the connective tissue stroma of the bone marrow, produce factors that influence the early precursors of B lymphocytes. It has been suggested that molecules like vascular cell adhesion molecules (VCAMs), expressed on the surface of stromal cells, mediate the binding of lymphocyte precursors, predominantly B lymphocytes, since the latter form an essential part of the entire lymphoid component of the bone marrow. It was also revealed that this molecule plays an important role in the phenomenon of homing of lymphocytes into the bone marrow [16]. These cells and bone tissue molecules, as it turned out, ultimately realize their effect on B lymphocytes through the transcription factor Pax5 (B-cell specific activator). In the absence of this factor, maturation of B lymphocytes does not occur. In this case, immature pre-B cells can differentiate into other cells of bone marrow origin, for example, into macrophages, osteoclasts and other cells [17]. The lack of mature lymphocytes in bone tissue is reliably associated with an increased volume of trabecular bone tissue [18]. It is interesting to note that under physiological conditions [19], as well as under the conditions of ontogenesis [20], the lack of mature B lymphocytes practically does not affect the cellular balance and metabolism in bone tissue. However, under pathological conditions or external stimuli, the absence of mature B lymphocytes does not allow bone tissue to adequately respond to changing conditions [21].

An important role in the regulation of bone tissue regeneration belongs to neutrophils. The impact of a damaging factor on the tissues leads to the development of acute inflammation, the main effectors of which are these cells. The outcome of the process largely depends on the reactivity of neutrophils [22]. Neutrophils, while not playing a key role in the repair phase, at the same time have an effect on collagenosis and remodeling of the extracellular matrix of bone tissue. They produce factors that activate fibroblasts and metalloproteinases (collagenases, gelatinases and stromalysin), which can catabolize all the main products of extracellular matrix and play an important role in remodeling of bone matrix [23]. When studying the state of non-specific protection among the victims of severe mechanical polytrauma, it was found that regardless of the nature of the traumatic agent, the degree and severity of the damage, in almost all cases, certain changes in the immune system were observed. For example, in the first week after an injury, the polymorphonuclear neutrophil system was functionally inferior [6]. Currently, researchers are inclined to believe that the complex interactions between individual cells of the immune system during the entire post-traumatic period have not been sufficiently studied. However, it is widely known that bone damage, like any other traumatic effect, leads to an increase in the migratory ability of polymorphonuclear neutrophils [24]. At the same time, the mechanism, according to which a sharp decrease in this migratory ability is noted several times throughout the post-traumatic period, remains unclear [25]. A study of the role of polymorphonuclear leukocytes by other scientists showed that a decrease in the number of cells led to a significant decrease in the mechanical strength of the regeneration. This, according to the authors, was associated with the outflow of neutrophils into the focus of inflammation (hematoma revascularization), which was accompanied by the release of a large number of inflammatory mediators (serotonin, bradykinins and histamine). This process violated the revascularization of the forming bone callus and led to a decrease in its mechanical strength [26].

When bone tissue is damaged, reactive changes are noted not only in the cellular but also in the humoral component of the immune system. It was found that activated lymphocytes responded with a significant reduction in proliferation when interacting with the main component of the extracellular matrix-collagen both in vitro and in vivo [27]. It is also interesting to note that bone tissue injury leads to the production of autoantibodies to oxidized low-density lipoproteins, and the concentration of these autoantibodies is quite strongly related to the intensity of post-traumatic osteogenesis [28]. In the framework of the study of immunoregulation of osteogenesis, a violation of the synthesis of immunoglobulins by lymphocytes with damage to bone tissue was established [29]. Some authors also obtained data on a decrease in the synthesis of immunoglobulins class G in severe mechanical polytrauma [6].

Lactoferrin is an important regulator of osteocyte activity that increases bone formation in vivo [30]. Usually, lactoferrin is secreted under the influence of stimuli caused by inflammation, as it is contained in neutrophil secretory granules [31]. Lactoferrin affects the synthesis of chemokines, plays an important immunomodulatory function to reduce the high concentration of osteolytic cytokines such as TNF-α and IL-1α [32] and stabilizes binding complexes [33]; therefore, its direct effects on the activity and development of osteocytes are apparently supplemented by these intermediary effects [30]. Reliable data have now been obtained, and it shows that lactoferrin stimulates osteoblastic growth and acts as a powerful factor in the survival of osteoblasts, preventing cell apoptosis. In addition, lactoferrin enhances the function of differentiated osteoblasts [34]. The effect of lactoferrin on the development of osteoclasts was evaluated in mouse's bone marrow cultures; as a result, it was found to exceed the response to such strong growth factors as insulin, amylin, IL-18, adrenomedullin, C-terminal telopeptides and calcitonin [35]. After local injection of lactoferrin, active bone growth was established, as well as the fact that it is a powerful factor in osteoblast growth, which can reduce bone resorption [30]. Lactoferrin acts on preosteoclasts and a large number of mature cells of this origin; however, it has no effect on bone resorption by isolated mature osteoclasts [30]. There is also a report on the effects of lactoferrin leading to bone resorption, which demonstrates that lactoferrin reduces bone function: a mixed rabbit bone cell culture is resorbed in a manner independent of RANK (receptor activator of NF-kB)/RANKL (receptor activator of NF-kB ligand)/OPG (osteoprotegerin) system [36]. Obviously, the identification of the mechanisms by which lactoferrin acts on bone cells is important due to the revealed possibilities of the demonstrated effects, and therefore this direction is being actively studied. The putative lactoferrin receptor is known to have been identified [37]. There is evidence that lactoferrin acts through a receptor-bound protein related to the low-density lipoprotein family (LRP) [38]. Identification of the LRP1 receptor as a functional lactoferrin receptor in osteoblasts explains the interaction mechanism and makes it possible to regulate the physiological or pharmacological effects on the bone, as well as the introduction of vitamins and other necessary substances into the bone tissue [39]. The same applies to the revealed LRP5 and LRP6 receptors, structurally associated with LRP1, which are necessary regulators of osteoblast functions [40]. Thus, lactoferrin, on the one hand, provides bone growth and, on the other hand, can perform the therapeutic function of a local agent to restore bone integrity after damage.

Integrins for extracellular matrix proteins also take part in the regulation of bone tissue regeneration. These receptors are a substrate for adhesion, migration and differentiation of fibroblasts and osteogenic cells [41]. Receptors provide a link between the cytoskeleton and the extracellular matrix, transmitting information about stretching and compression of bone tissue through, the cell membrane [42] and activate certain signaling pathways, affecting gene expression [43]. It was found that during the recirculation process, when the cells of the immune system migrate through tissues and interact with one of the main components of the extracellular matrix (collagen), and integrins act as receptors, the activation signal is combined with an antigen-recognizing receptor and is able to change the direction of action of immunocompetent cells [44]. It is known that the metabolism of bone tissue during damage is provided by numerous cytokines-IL-1 (interleukin), IL-3, IL-4, IL-6, IL-11, TNF-α (tumor necrosis factor), TNF-β, colony stimulating factors, leukemia inhibitory factor, INF-γ (interferon), TGF-β (transforming growth factor) [45, 46]. There is no doubt that the study of blood immune responses in patients with damage to the bone will assess their relationship with the passage of bone formation and find the results obtained practical application. Thus, current is the study of blood immunological reactions during the regeneration of bone tissue to predict complications osteogenesis.

2. Material and methods

The study included 136 patients with lesions of the facial skeleton before and after stable osteosynthesis of the mandible in a fixing device for external fixation. Limitation of the injury was on average 12.0 ± 3.0 days. Indications for the use of external fixation devices in damaged bone were complicated by primary and secondary shifts: mandibular fractures, in 92 persons (67.6%); disjoint fractures, in 20 persons (14.7%); fused fractures, in 21 persons (15.4%); and gunshot defects, in 3 people (2.2%). A study was authorized by the Ethics Committee, guided by the order of operation, standard operating procedures and international instruments, which are based on "Declaration of Helsinki of the World Medical Association" and its subsequent editions, UN documents and of the Council of Europe documents relating to the rights of the patient, Consolidated Guideline for Good Clinical Practice and the National Russian Federation Standard "Good Clinical Practice" GOST R 52379-2005 from 01.04.2006. Informed consent to participate in a research project in accordance with the "Statement of Ethical Control" had been obtained from all surveyed participants in this test.

The diagnosis is based on clinical and instrumental learning techniques using X-ray data, orthopantomography and CT. The volume of surgical intervention determines the nature and localization of lesions. External or intraoral access was used. The second type of access was a priority, since its implementation in the postoperative period was excluded orostoma development. The inner edge of the subsystems was fixed at 1 cm from the skin surface to avoid damaging the soft tissue. An important moment during the use of external fixation device was to restore a fractured bone axis creating contact bone fragments across the fracture surface and compression at the junction of the bone fragments. Some patients have been diagnosed with osteomyelitis. When the osteomyelitis was detected, osteosynthesis was done by opening and draining the purulent chamber. Surgical treatment of purulent focus was conducted by conventional rules.

Permanent rigid fixation of bone fragments and permanent functional damage to the load of the lower jaw were created to organize the normal course of the recovery process and a successful fight against purulent infection. These conditions of bone tissue restoration were achieved by the periodic-every 5–7 days-tension of weakened rods and displacement of rings of external retainer relative to each other. When dressing wounds and fistulas, great importance had been attached to providing constant drainage of purulent separable. Medical dressings are replaced in a timely and high-quality manner, taking into account the nature and stage of wound healing, microbial composition of purulent discharge.

An apparatus for external fixation after treatment was taken off when the following clinical signs of coalescence bone appeared: disappearance of soft tissue swelling, lack of mobility at the junction of the bone fragments during the clinical trial on the motility and on the basis of radiographic criteria: identifying fuzziness of contour ends of the fragments and improving optical densities in the gap region of bone damage. Terms of use of metal structures averaged 15.0 ± 3.0 days. Long-term results of treatment patients were followed up to 4 years.

Of the total patients (136 people) based on retrospective analysis of data, a group with slow regeneration of bone tissue was isolated, because of osteomyelitis presence. It amounted to 17 people or 12.5% of all patients. Consolidation of bone tissue in this group was observed after an average 43.0 ± 1.0 postoperative day. The control group consisted of patients whose postoperative period was uneventful. Their consolidation of bone tissue occurs on average through 29.0 ± 2.0 days after the imposition of an external fixation device. It occurred somewhat earlier than in the treatment with the other ways. Usually, the terms of consolidation of mandibular fractures make 34.5–39.7 days.

The main clinical indicators are as follows: the ratio in the group of patients by gender and by age, the amount of intraoperative blood loss, presence of concomitant pathology of the cardiovascular, respiratory, urinary systems and the gastrointestinal tract, and the presence of allergies and operations, which were previously carried out using steel structures in both groups significantly did not differ. Laboratory studies were performed preoperatively and after 3 and 10 days and 1 and 3 months after its execution. Blood was obtained in the morning fasting from subclavian vein using the phlebotomy method and from the cubital vein or veins on the back of the hand, to receive physiotherapy.

To assess the lymphocyte population composition, whole blood with K_3EDTA anticoagulant (ethylenediaminetetraacetic acid) was used at a concentration of 1.6 mg/ml (tube S-Monovette® 2.7 ml, Sarstedt, Germany), for determining the phagocytic activity of the cells-the blood with the anticoagulant heparin Li (lithium heparin) at a concentration of 16 IU/ml (tube S-Monovette® 7.5 ml, Sarstedt, Germany). Serum was used for obtaining tubes S-Monovette® 7.5 ml (Sarstedt, Germany) with polystyrene beads as activators of coagulation.

To evaluate the immune status, a standard set of laboratory tests has been used complete with modern diagnostic methods [47]. The number of leukocytes was determined using hematology analyzer Cell-Dyn 1700 (Abbot, USA), reagents and equipment from the firm Abbott. Differentiation of population composition of leukocytes was carried out in the Romanovsky-Giemsa stained smears. Stab neutrophil and segmented neutrophil cell ratio was calculated [48]. Lymphocyte subpopulations were determined by flow cytometry on the device Coulter®Epics®XL (Beckman Coulter, USA), using a monoclonal antibody produced by Beckman Coulter. Lysis of erythrocytes was performed by using the sample preparation station Coulter®Q-Prep (Beckman Coulter, USA) and reagents Immunoprep, manufactured by Beckman Coulter. Quality control was performed using gauge particles Flow Check. In vitro activation of T lymphocytes with phytohemagglutinin was performed and evaluated in the reaction of inhibition of leukocyte migration [49]. The metabolic activity of neutrophils was evaluated in the reduction reaction of nitro blue tetrazolium peroxide radicals under the action of cells and evaluated by light microscopy [50]. Spontaneous and latex-stimulated activity was determined, their ratio was calculated (stimulation index). The ability of the neutrophils to kill was determined using cytochemical cell study data. Myeloperoxidase activity was determined by Grantham-Knoll [51], and the result was expressed by the average cytochemical coefficient of Kaplow [52]. The level of the lysosomal cationic cytoplasmic proteins was determined by reaction with bromophenol blue, and the results are also expressed as the average cytochemical factor [53]. The content of serum immunoglobulin classes A, M and G was determined by enzyme immunoassay. Lysozyme activity was evaluated by gel-diffusion test for the ability to lyse culture *M. lysodeikticus* [54], and the functional state of the complement system was adjusted to 50% by assessment of hemolysis of sheep erythrocytes [49]. Contents lactoferrin and cytokines (IL-1α, IL-8, TNF-α, IL-10 and IL-1ra) were determined using the method of two-site "sandwich" ELISA-variant using test systems from firms "Protein contour" (St. Petersburg, Russia), "Cytokine" (St. Petersburg, Russia), "Vector-Best" (Novosibirsk, Russia) and BioSourse International (USA) on immunoassay equipment Stat Fax (Awareness Technology Inc., USA). The concentration of C-reactive protein was determined by turbidimetric and ceruloplasmin - at Ravin [55].

The selection of antibiotic therapy in osteomyelitis was performed based on bacteriological examination of wound and aspirate purulent contents of the cavity. The evaluation included a microscopic examination of a Gram stain, inoculation of culture media production by bioMérieux (France). Identification of microorganisms and determination of their sensitivity to antibiotics were carried out by the analyzers Vitek 2-compact and ATB-Expression (bioMérieux, France). Bacteriological examination most frequently detected *Staphylococcus aureus* (92–95% of cases), among others were *Pseudomonas aeruginosa*, *Burkholderia cepacia*, *Acinetobacter baumannii*, *Enterococcus faecalis* and *Proteus vulgaris* (the proportion of each of them in the total number of cases was not more than 1%).

Statistical data processing was carried out using the "Microsoft Office Excel 2007" program and "Statistica for Windows v.6.1". It included an assessment of the data on the normality of the distribution in the test groups and was based on data on the mathematical expectation of 0 and the corresponding standard deviation equal to 1. Kolmogorov–Smirnov test, Lilliefors, Shapiro–Wilk and χ^2 were used to test the hypothesis that the sample has a Gaussian (normal) distribution. To compare the variance of the studied samples, F-Fisher criterion was used. Statistical hypothesis is considered confirmed with a significance level of $p < 0.05$. Modified theory of T. Bayes was used to identify the prediction criteria [56]. Calculation of diagnostic sensitivity, diagnostic specificity and diagnostic information content of immunological tests was performed using the following Eqs. (1)–(3) [57].

$$\text{Diagnostic sensitivity} = \left(\frac{TP}{TP + FN}\right) \times 100 \tag{1}$$

$$\text{Diagnostic specificity} = \left(\frac{TN}{TN + FP}\right) \times 100 \tag{2}$$

$$\text{Diagnostic informative laboratory test} = \left(\frac{TP}{TP + FP}\right) \times 100 \tag{3}$$

where TP is the true-positive results: the number of patients with complications who were correctly classified using this criterion; FP is the false-positive results: the number of patients without complications, which have been erroneously attributed to the number of patients with complications as a result of this test; TN is the true-negative results: the number of patients without the complications that were correctly classified with the help of this test; and FN is the false-negative results: the number of patients with complications who were misclassified using this test.

3. Results and discussion

As a model for studying the dynamics of immunological parameters in normal and complicated osteogenesis, the study used laboratory parameters in patients with lesions of the facial skeleton. Injury of facial skeleton, especially with slow consolidation of bone tissue, leads to disturbances of body functions and generating esthetic defects. Therefore, the creation of forecasting system complications of osteogenesis in the recovery of fractures of the lower jaw becomes important. To address the issue of participation of immunological reactions in the restoration of bone tissue, first consider the dynamics of the main laboratory parameters during normal consolidation lesions of the mandible. Before operation values, immunological parameters were compared to known literature data [58, 59].

3.1 Features of immune responses of peripheral blood in normal bone consolidation

Before surgery, along with a slight increase in the relative number of $CD45^{+}CD3^{+}$-, $CD45^{+}CD19^{+}$-cells revealed increased production of IgA and IgM (**Table 1**). There was also a decrease in the activity of oxygen-dependent (nitro blue

Laboratory parameters	Normal values	Before surgery	3 days	10 days	1 month	3 months
Total number of white blood cells, 10^9/l	4.0–9.0	6.85±0.33	6.68±0.45	7.30±0.51	7.35±0.55	7.30±0.48
Total number of neutrophils, 10^9/l	2.00–5.80	4.34±0.26	4.40±0.27	4.62±0.43	4.70±0.30	4.88±0.35
Ratio stab neutrophil/segmented neutrophils	0.02–0.06	0.03±0.01	0.02±0.01	0.02±0.01	0.03±0.01	0.03±0.01
Total number of monocytes, 10^9/l	0.09–0.60	0.54±0.05	0.45±0.05	0.69±0.05*	0.50±0.05	0.52±0.05
Total number of lymphocytes, 10^9/l	1.2–3.0	1.89±0.09	1.56±0.27	2.08±0.22	2.15±0.09*	2.10±0.09
$CD45^+CD3^+$-cells, %	46.0–56.0	60.00±2.00	63.33±1.67	51.29±6.36	62.40±7.17	62.33±0.88
$CD45^+CD19^+$-cells, %	4.0–8.0	9.50±1.50	9.67±1.17	9.71±0.64	9.20±1.98	7.33±0.33
Leukocyte migration inhibition test with phytohemagglutinin, %	0–30	8.03±0.24	23.02±1.25*	13.50±1.08*	5.06±1.03	22.09±1.11*
Nitro blue tetrazolium test spontaneous, %	10–20	34.05±9.10	23.67±4.77	31.50±6.36	32.40±9.05	24.00±9.64
Nitro blue tetrazolium test stimulated, %	50–100	31.00±4.00	35.56±5.59	37.13±5.94	52.20±4.46*	49.67±4.17*
Nitro blue tetrazolium test, stimulation index	>1.3	1.00±0.20	1.83±0.27*	1.52±0.26	1.73±0.14*	2.81±0.56*
Myeloperoxidase activity of neutrophils, average coefficient cytochemical	1.9–2.8	1.91±0.25	0.70±0.12*	2.28±0.33	2.10±0.08	0.69±0.09*
Activity cationic proteins neutrophilic granulocytes, average coefficient cytochemical	1.6–1.9	1.35±0.12	1.22±0.11	1.27±0.02	1.36±0.12	1.22±0.05
Lactoferrin, ng/ml	700–1500	825.10±12.60	501.09±12.65*	1250.90±18.34*	836.21±25.16	500.03±12.89*
IgA, g/l	1.38–2.50	2.89±0.23	2.69±0.31	2.89±0.45	3.18±0.18	2.03±0.29
IgM, g/l	0.92–2.10	2.27±0.03	1.41±0.23*	1.62±0.24*	1.60±0.22*	2.10±0.63
IgG, g/l	8.5–15.8	12.35±2.05	11.73±0.58	12.56±0.77	12.30±0.57	11.97±2.56
Lysozyme, mkg/ml	28.6–31.0	16.23±1.17	20.80±1.56*	12.25±2.37	8.02±1.88*	14.90±2.04
Total hemolytic complement activity, arbitrary units/ml	40.0–42.0	50.28±2.06	36.35±5.00*	45.30±2.28	48.06±2.26	36.71±13.38
IL-1α, pg/ml	0–50	22.06±2.04	21.03±1.54	625.18±12.36*	20.14±1.98	19.25±1.15
IL-1ra, pg/ml	0–500	35.24±0.22	40.08±1.45*	609.65±12.54*	81.07±2.59*	39.66±3.08
TNF-α, pg/ml	0–50	11.17±6.23	25.03±6.17	141.25±33.75*	39.50±2.98*	24.37±7.02

DOI: http://dx.doi.org/10.5772/intechopen.92099

Laboratory parameters	Normal values	Before surgery	3 days	10 days	1 month	3 months
IL-8, pg/ml	0–50	42.88±3.64	76.03±3.60*	415.12±11.98*	70.47±2.65*	39.74±2.99
IL-10, pg/ml	<1.0	2.31±0.08	0.07±0.02*	0.02±0.01*	0.09±0.03*	0.92±0.04*
Ceruloplasmin, g/l	0.24–0.42	0.53±0.02	0.40±0.05*	0.55±0.10	0.29±0.04*	0.33±0.07*
C-reactive protein, mg/l	0–8	11.50±5.50	7.50±2.95	30.84±13.40	1.40±0.25*	0.61±0.02*

*$p < 0.05$ compared with preoperative levels.

Table 1.
Immunological parameters of peripheral blood in the regeneration of bone tissue.

tetrazolium test) and oxygen-independent (neutrophil activity cationic proteins) killing mechanisms, lowering the concentration of serum lysozyme.

Major changes were detected due to the inflammatory reaction induced by damage to the bone tissue in the mandible fracture, which was evaluated on the basis of a complex of acute-phase proteins. Prior to surgery, in particular, it was revealed that there was an increase in the most sensitive C-reactive protein with increasing concentration of ceruloplasmin and complement activity, indicating the presence of acute inflammation (**Table 1**).

On day 10 after surgery, the number of monocytes increased by 27.8% ($p < 0.05$) compared to preoperative level, and at 1 month after surgery, the number of lymphocytes increased by 13.8% ($p < 0.05$); the composition of population lymphocytes did not change (**Table 1**). It is known that a recognized mitogen for assessing the activity of T cells is phytohemagglutinin. According to the stress tests with phytohemagglutinin, a gain in the functional activity of the cells during the early postoperative period was identified, that is, for 3–10 days after surgery (**Table 1**). In the same period, there was a decrease in the concentration of IgM by 37.9% ($p < 0.05$) with the subsequent restoration of its level in the peripheral blood (**Table 1**). Postoperatively, increased activity of "early" killing mechanisms was also observed: an increase in lactoferrin levels by 51.6% ($p < 0.05$) and the rise of total production of reactive oxygen species (nitro blue tetrazolium test) on 83.0% ($p < 0.05$). From the humoral immunity, a significant decrease in complement activity was revealed to be 27.7% ($p < 0.05$), followed by rapid recovery at 10 days. These changes appear to have been associated with the participation of complement in the elimination of foreign substance in the development of inflammatory response.

Due to the fact that not only cellular and humoral reactions played an important role in the regulation of immunological reactions, but also the effect of a number of low molecular weight peptides (cytokines) was noted, the dynamics of some of them was studied. In particular, it was found that in the postoperative period there was an increase in the concentration of IL-1α ($p < 0.05$), an activator of the initial stages of the immune response (**Table 1**). This is likely to determine the development and course of a large number of immunological reactions in the reduction of bone tissue. Simultaneously, the increasing concentrations of receptor antagonist IL-1–IL-1ra were revealed, which limited the development of systemic inflammatory response (**Table 1**).

Concentrations of IL-1α and IL-1ra were increased to respectively 28.4 times and 17.3 times to the 10th day of observation compared to preoperative values. A similar trend was also characteristic of TNF-α ($p < 0.05$), similar to having IL-1 phlogogenic properties. On day 10, there was a significant increase in the level of another factor inflammation-IL-8-whose concentration in the blood was increased 9.7 times as compared to preoperative values (**Table 1**). However, during the activation process, the decreased concentrations of IL-10 were revealed, which is a factor that inhibits the synthesis of most of the cytokines. Its concentration in the serum was reduced more than 100 times ($p < 0.05$). The inflammatory response in normal bone regeneration had little activity and duration.

It is known that the regeneration of bone tissue composed of several sequentially successive stages: inflammation, proliferation of osteoblasts, collagenogenesis and ossification. In this case, additional studies were conducted 3 months after the operation, at the last stage when the external fixing device was dismantled, reparative regeneration is completed, the bone tissue has formed and the mandible functioned normally. By the time of full functional bone formation, immunological parameters were within normal limits.

In a number of patients with osteomyelitis (17 people) based on clinical and radiographic data, delayed regeneration of bone tissue of the lower jaw was revealed. It occurs 1.5 times later than normal consolidation ($p < 0.05$).

3.2 Features of peripheral blood response in slow consolidation of the mandible

In this group of patients, before surgery, differences in immunological parameters from data obtained on the bone consolidation without complicating osteomyelitis were revealed. The number of monocytes (**Table 2**) was lower, than in the group with the slow regeneration of bone tissue by 59.3% ($p < 0.05$). There was a significant attenuation of the bactericidal activity of mechanisms: the level of lactoferrin was reduced 3.5 times ($p < 0.05$) was only 33.6% compared with the normal values. The same can be mentioned for complement activity-30.2% of the lower limit of normal and below 4.2 times ($p < 0.05$) than in the group with normal bone regeneration. Increased concentration of 37.4% IgM ($p < 0.05$) in peripheral blood also exceeded 49.0% and the normal values (**Table 2**). There was increased functional activity of $CD45^{+}CD3^{+}$-cells and it was more than 3.5 times ($p < 0.05$)-differences in the recorded response of leukocyte migration inhibition (**Table 2**). Serum lysozyme was reduced by 5.8 times. Interestingly, the concentration of the receptor antagonist of IL-1ra concentration was lower for IL-1α (**Table 2**) that was not observed in patients with normal bone consolidation. IL-8 levels were reduced by 1.8-fold ($p < 0.05$) (**Table 2**) in comparison with patients with the other group.

The postoperative period was characterized by leukocytogenesis activation: leukocytosis was marked with the change in the ratio of group cells to the segmented cells. On day 3, a reduction in the number of T cells was shown (according to the dynamics of $CD45^{+}CD3^{+}$-cells) 40.8% ($p < 0.05$), confirming previously published data [60]. Recovery of these cell populations occurred in 10 days (**Table 2**). Perhaps this change in the amount of T cells in the early postoperative period resulting, ultimately, in disruption of bone regeneration, because it is known that both by generating INF-γ, and through prostaglandin mechanism of these cells involved in suppressing bone destruction and the formation of osteoclasts. Decrease in the relative number of B cells (based on dynamics of $CD45^{+}CD19^{+}$-cells) by 55.6% ($p < 0.05$) was observed later, on day 10 (**Table 2**).

Important changes were noted by the indicators characterizing the phagocytic activity of neutrophils. Amplification reactions were detected at 3 days after surgery when the spontaneous and stimulated superoxide radical production by neutrophils' superior control values was in the subgroup of 1.6- to 1.7-fold ($p < 0.05$). It can be assumed that the changes in neutrophil phagocyte system in the blood reflect the processes occurring in bone tissue. Of interest for the study was the dynamics of the content of lactoferrin at the stages of bone tissue consolidation (**Table 2**). As noted earlier, prior to the operation, its level was significantly reduced. Due to the fact that lactoferrin causes proliferation of osteoblasts and bone growth, it is not excluded that lowering the level of lactoferrin in the blood is also one of the reasons for slow regeneration of bone tissue. Later, after the operation, the lactoferrin content was always significantly lower in patients with delayed bone formation compared with patients who have bone fusion that took place at the usual time.

Slow bone formation was accompanied by significant increase (72.0%) in IgM levels (**Table 2**). The revealed changes were statistically significant differences between these patients with normal bone tissue regeneration. Inflammatory response was characterized by pronounced dynamics of slow-reacting acute-phase proteins. Specifically, on day 3, after surgery, ceruloplasmin concentration was higher by 1.9-fold ($p < 0.05$) than in patients with normal bone regeneration. The functional activity of T cells throughout the observation period was 2.0- to 3.3-fold higher ($p < 0.05$) than in patients with normal consolidation, while it exceeds the normal value of 1.5 times (**Table 1**). Active cationic proteins and myeloperoxidase neutrophilic granulocytes were higher than in patients with complication of osteogenesis, respectively, by 33.6% ($p < 0.05$) and 3.1-fold ($p < 0.05$).

Laboratory parameters	Normal values	Before surgery	3 days	10 days	1 month	3 months
Total number of white blood cells, 10^9/l	4.0–9.0	7.08±0.50	9.08±0.66$^{*,\#}$	8.43±0.47*	6.13±0.38	7.50±0.51
Total number of neutrophils, 10^9/l	2.00–5.80	4.37±0.38	6.95±0.48$^{*,\#}$	5.17±1.01	3.63±0.39$^{\#}$	4.76±0.69
Ratio stab neutrophil/segmented neutrophils	0.02–0.06	0.04±0.01	0.08±0.01$^{*,\#}$	0.06±0.01$^{\#}$	0.04±0.01	0.02±0.01
Total number of monocytes, 10^9/l	0.09–0.60	0.32±0.07$^{\#}$	0.52±0.15	0.30±0.11	0.59±0.10*	0.58±0.18
Total number of lymphocytes, 10^9/l	1.2–3.0	2.09±0.20	1.40±0.22*	2.63±0.55	1.70±0.10$^{\#}$	1.94±0.22
$CD45^+CD3^+$-cells, %	46.0–56.0	63.77±3.24	38.50±3.51$^{*,\#}$	46.47±3.54*	63.61±2.98	47.74±3.64$^{*,\#}$
$CD45^+CD19^+$-cells, %	4.0–8.0	7.03±0.89	9.06±2.01	4.31±0.59$^{*,\#}$	5.88±0.47$^{\#}$	12.71±0.36$^{*,\#}$
Leukocyte migration inhibition test with phytohemagglutinin, %	0–30	28.45±5.46$^{\#}$	45.45±5.07$^{*,\#}$	44.73±6.98$^{\#}$	42.07±5.32$^{\#}$	91.09±12.34$^{*,\#}$
Nitro blue tetrazolium test spontaneous, %	10–20	41.12±5.96	37.02±3.99$^{\#}$	23.07±6.34*	45.23±5.87	25.31±5.34*
Nitro blue tetrazolium test stimulated, %	50–100	31.09±3.88	60.50±1.54$^{*,\#}$	38.18±4.67	68.34±5.46$^{*,\#}$	39.96±6.13
Nitro blue tetrazolium test, stimulation index	>1.3	0.75±0.21	1.64±0.24*	1.65±0.13*	1.51±0.22*	1.50±0.14$^{*,\#}$
Myeloperoxidase activity of neutrophils, average coefficient cytochemical	1.9–2.8	1.88±0.14	2.19±0.18$^{\#}$	2.12±0.15	1.37±0.19$^{\#}$	0.77±0.12*
Activity cationic proteins neutrophilic granulocytes, average coefficient cytochemical	1.6–1.9	1.42±0.07	1.63±0.08$^{*,\#}$	1.36±0.12	1.55±0.11	1.26±0.07
Lactoferrin, ng/ml	700–1500	235.14±22.63$^{\#}$	451.09±17.35$^{*,\#}$	956.88±16.44$^{*,\#}$	566.22±23.26$^{*,\#}$	355.84±14.87$^{*,\#}$
IgA, g/l	1.38–2.50	2.48±0.41	2.59±0.19	2.46±0.15	2.06±0.21$^{\#}$	2.68±0.31
IgM, g/l	0.92–2.10	3.12±0.38$^{\#}$	1.05±0.19*	2.80±0.25$^{\#}$	0.78±0.13$^{*,\#}$	2.86±0.34
IgG, g/l	8.5–15.8	15.30±2.36	11.26±2.20*	14.13±1.87	6.31±0.69$^{*,\#}$	14.51±1.45
Lysozyme, mkg/ml	28.6–31.0	2.78±0.49$^{\#}$	3.87±0.56$^{\#}$	14.21±2.33*	3.87±0.49$^{\#}$	13.41±2.17*
Total hemolytic complement activity, arbitrary units/ml	40.0–42.0	12.07±1.18$^{\#}$	44.93±2.51*	13.46±1.49$^{\#}$	44.03±2.66*	44.07±2.37*
IL-1α, pg/ml	0–50	30.24±3.08$^{\#}$	234.07±21.46$^{*,\#}$	604.26±18.29*	36.41±2.65$^{\#}$	18.33±2.14*
IL-1ra, pg/ml	0–500	18.36±1.17$^{\#}$	100.51±13.96$^{*,\#}$	321.61±15.96$^{*,\#}$	24.74±2.96$^{*,\#}$	13.22±1.74$^{*,\#}$

DOI: http://dx.doi.org/10.5772/intechopen.92099

Laboratory parameters	Normal values	Before surgery	3 days	10 days	1 month	3 months
TNF-α, pg/ml	0–50	22.65 ± 6.58	$62.50 \pm 11.54^{*,\#}$	$75.12 \pm 9.67^{*,\#}$	$100.33 \pm 9.89^{*,\#}$	$102.61 \pm 10.24^{*,\#}$
IL-8, pg/ml	0–50	$24.15 \pm 4.78^{\#}$	$90.32 \pm 3.66^{*,\#}$	$180.74 \pm 14.85^{*,\#}$	$55.41 \pm 6.74^{*,\#}$	$41.65 \pm 8.97^{*}$
IL-10, pg/ml	<1.0	2.19 ± 0.07	$0.08 \pm 0.02^{*}$	$0.04 \pm 0.01^{*}$	$0.04 \pm 0.01^{*}$	$0.85 \pm 0.06^{*}$
Ceruloplasmin, g/l	0.24–0.42	0.50 ± 0.02	$0.75 \pm 0.16^{\#}$	0.66 ± 0.08	0.51 ± 0.12	$0.99 \pm 0.09^{*,\#}$
C-reactive protein, mg/l	0–8	9.09 ± 0.22	$6.01 \pm 1.12^{*}$	$0.14 \pm 0.03^{*,\#}$	$0.12 \pm 0.03^{*,\#}$	$0.14 \pm 0.04^{*,\#}$

$^{*}p < 0.05$ compared with preoperative levels.
$^{\#}p < 0.05$ compared with uncomplicated osteogenesis.

Table 2.
Immunological parameters of peripheral blood at slowing bone formation.

The concentration of lysozyme in the same period was significantly reduced by 5.4 times (**Table 2**). The dynamics of cytokine concentrations also had differences: on day 3 after surgery significantly, namely more than 11-fold ($p < 0.05$), increased concentration of IL-1α, one of the stimulants of osteoclasts (**Table 2**). However similar changes were observed in patients with normal bone tissue regeneration. Most likely, the ratio between the level of IL-1α and IL-1ra after surgery (on day 10) played an important role in the violation of regeneration, when in patients with normal bone consolidation it was equal (**Table 1**), and at late bone consolidation, the level of IL -1ra was almost two times lower than the concentration of IL-1α (**Table 2** and **Figure 1**).

After one month, when the regeneration of bone tissue in the other group was completed, in patients with delayed consolidation, it was in the stage collagenogenesis. Features of the dynamics of immunological parameters are as follows: the number of neutrophils and lymphocytes in peripheral blood was reduced by 23.0% ($p < 0.05$) and 21.0% ($p < 0.05$) compared to those of patients with normal bone regeneration. Inhibition signs of humoral immunity were shown: IgA level was lower by 35.3% ($p < 0.05$), the concentration of IgM (**Table 2**), and IgG – 2.0 times ($p < 0.05$) was compared with the results in patients with the normal regeneration of the bone tissue. There was also a decrease in myeloperoxidase activity by 34.8% ($p < 0.05$) and lysozyme concentration by 2 times ($p < 0.05$) reduced (**Table 2**). One month after surgery, the receptor level antagonist of IL-1 was higher concentration of IL-1α (**Table 2**) and TNF-α content was increased by 2.5-fold ($p < 0.05$), while the functional activity of the $CD45^{+}CD3^{+}$-cells (**Table 2**), as already mentioned, was increased by 8.3-fold ($p < 0.05$).

It is interesting that in circumstances where bone regeneration has been completed, 3 months after the operation, the factors of immune responses, causing the growth of bone, are reduced. Thus, the concentration of lactoferrin was reduced by 40.5% ($p < 0.05$) and the number of T cells by 23.4% ($p < 0.05$). During this same period, the factors of immune reactions associated with the destruction of the bone tissue continue to maintain high concentrations. In particular, TNF-α level was increased by 4.2-fold ($p < 0.05$) (**Table 2**). The functional state of T cells in the neutrophil migration inhibition of the reaction was increased by 4.1 times (**Table 2**) metabolic functional activity of neutrophils to normal.

Based on the study, criteria were developed by predicting delayed bone consolidation in the treatment of injuries of the lower jaw (**Table 3**).

These criteria allow for different stages of treatment (before surgery, for 3 or 10 hours after surgery) to predict the development of delayed consolidation of bone

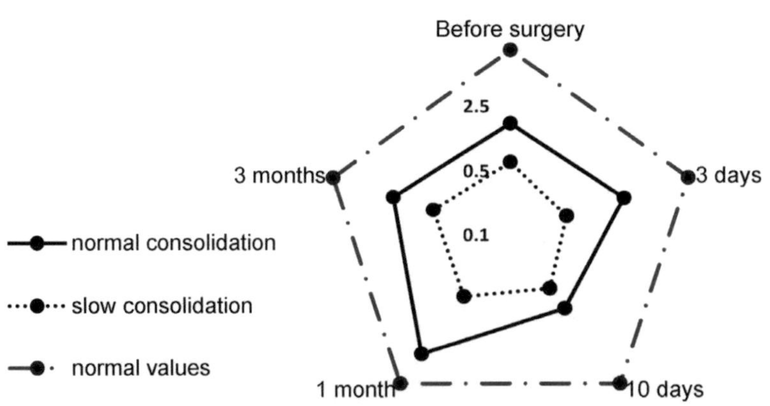

Figure 1.
The ratio of the concentration of IL-1α to IL-1ra, a logarithmic scale was used to represent the data.

DOI: http://dx.doi.org/10.5772/intechopen.92099

Prognostic criteria	Morbidity osteogenesis	Average for osteogenesis	The diagnostic sensitivity of the test laboratory	The diagnostic specificity of the test laboratory	Diagnostic informative laboratory test
		Before surgery			
IgM, g/l	↑ 2.4	0.9–2.3	85.4%	94.6%	87.3%
C-reactive protein, mg/l	↓ 9.3	9.4–17.0	79.2%	81.2%	83.2%
		3 days			
Total number of white blood cells, 10^9/l	↑ 6.9	4.0–6.8	92.3%	80.1%	93.1%
$CD45^+CD3^+$ -cells, %	↓ 45.0	46.0–70.0	90.4%	92.3%	91.7%
Nitro blue tetrazolium test spontaneous, %	↑ 33.0	10.0–32.0	91.4%	77.8%	96.3%
Lactoferrin, ng/ml	↓ 499.0	500.0–1500.0	81.3%	88.4%	86.2%
TNF-α, pg./ml	↑ 51.0	0–50.0	92.0%	90.9%	94.1%
		10 days			
Total hemolytic complement activity, arbitrary units/ml	↓ 36.0	37.0–54.0	91.5%	93.0%	92.6%
IgM, g/l	↑ 2.7	0.9–2.6	87.7%	88.3%	89.5%

Table 3.
The criteria for predicting delayed consolidation of bone tissue in the treatment of lesions of the mandible.

tissue. For each of the criteria, diagnostic sensitivity, diagnostic specificity and informative test are calculated, that is the ability to predict the possible development of delayed consolidation of bone tissue.

To test the statistical hypotheses were recruited separate independent test samples of 49 people. It included patients with the same embodiments of bone damage and with the same kind of surgical treatment as the two major groups of the study. The criteria developed in this study showed that the coefficient of determination in this independent test sample was in the range of 84.2–97.5%. The joint use of two or more prognostic indicators allowed to increase the value of a diagnostic test for 3–4%. This fact gives more opportunities to clinicians in predicting delayed bone formation.

4. Conclusion

The study revealed that the stages of regeneration of bone tissue (inflammation, proliferation of osteoblasts, collagenogenesis and ossification) are accompanied by changes in the immunological status. When delayed consolidation of bone tissue revealed differences of response of individual parts of the immune system, a comparative study of the immunological parameter dynamics at normal and slow osteogenesis is possible to establish criteria for delayed consolidation of bone tissue. Prognostic criteria to the operations include increasing the concentration of IgM and decreasing in concentration of C-reactive protein in the early postoperative period-increasing the number of leukocytes, the concentration of tumor necrosis factor, IgM, the production of superoxide anion in nitro blue tetrazolium test, as well as reducing the number of $CD45^{+}CD3^{+}$-cells, complement activity and the content of lactoferrin.

Acknowledgements

This work was carried out in the framework of the state task Institute of Immunology and Physiology, Ural Branch of Russian Academy of Sciences (topic number AAAA A18-118020590108-7).

Conflict of interest

The authors declare no conflict of interest.

Author details

Olga Viktorovna Berdyugina and Kirill Alexandrovich Berdyugin*
Institute of Immunology and Physiology, Ural Branch of Russian Academy of Sciences, Ekaterinburg, Russia

*Address all correspondence to: berolga73@rambler.ru

IntechOpen

© 2020 The Author(s). Licensee IntechOpen. This chapter is distributed under the terms of the Creative Commons Attribution License (http://creativecommons.org/licenses/by/3.0), which permits unrestricted use, distribution, and reproduction in any medium, provided the original work is properly cited.

References

[1] Partanen J, Heikkinen J, Jämsä T, Jalovaara P. Characteristics of lifetime factors, bone metabolism, and bone mineral density in patients with hip fracture. Journal of Bone and Mineral Metabolism. 2002;**20**(6):367-375. DOI: 10.1007/s007740200053

[2] Miyamoto T, Arai F, Ohneda O, Takagi K, Anderson DM, Suda T. An adherent condition is required for formation of multinuclear osteoclasts in the presence of macrophage colony-stimulating factor and receptor activator of nuclear factor kappa B ligand. Blood. 2000;**96**:4335-4343. DOI: 10.1182/blood.V96.13.4335.h8004335_4335_4343

[3] Ducy P, Schinke T, Karsenty G. The osteoblasts: A sophisticated fibroblast under central surveillance. Science. 2000;**289**:1501-1504. DOI: 10.1126/science.289.5484.1501

[4] Askalonov AA, Gordienko SM, Avdyunicheva OE, Bondarenko AV, Voronkov SF. The role of T-system immunity in reparatory regeneration of the bone tissue in animals. Journal of Hygiene, Epidemiology, Microbiology, and Immunology. 1987;**31**(2):219-224. PMID: 3497192

[5] Santavirta S, Konttinen YT, Nordstrom D, Mäkelä A, Sorsa T, Hukkanen M, et al. Immunologic studies of nonunited fractures. Acta Orthopaedica Scandinavica. 1992;**63**(6): 579-586. DOI: 10.1080/17453679209169713

[6] Zheklov AN, Petlenko SV, Bogdanov EG, Parfilova TV. Immunity changes and nonspecific factors of patient protection who have suffered from severe mechanical polytrauma [Izmeneniya immuniteta i faktorov nespecificheskoj zashchity u postradavshih ot tyazheloj mekhanicheskoj politravmy (in Russian)]. Journal of Medical Immunology [Medicinskaya Immunologiya]. 2002;**4**(2):327-328

[7] Hauser CJ, Joshi P, Jones Q, Zhou X, Livingston DH, Lavery RF. Suppression of natural killer cell activity in patients with fracture/soft tissue injury. The Archives of Surgery. 1997;**132**(12): 1326-1330. DOI: 10.1001/archsurg.1997.01430360072013

[8] Buchinsky FJ, Ma YF, Mann GN, Rucinski B, Bryer HP, Paynton BV, et al. Bone mineral metabolism in T lymphocyte-deficient and -replete strains of rat. Journal of Bone and Mineral Research. 1995;**10**:1556-1565

[9] Buchinsky FJ, Ma Y, Mann GN, Rucinski B, Bryer HP, Romero DF, et al. T-lymphocytes play a critical role in the development of cyclosporin A-induced osteopenia. The Journal of Endocrinology. 1996;**137**:2278-2285. DOI: 10.1210/en.137.6.2278

[10] Shevach EM, McHugh RS, Piccirillo CA, Thornton AM. Control of T-cell activation by $CD4^{+}CD25^{+}$ suppressor T-cells. Immunological Reviews. 2001;**182**:58-67. DOI: 10.1034/j.1600-065x.2001.1820104.x

[11] Takayanagi H, Ogasawara K, Hida S, Chiba T, Murata S, Sato K, et al. T-cell-mediated regulation of osteoclastogenesis by signaling cross-talk between RANKL and IFN. Nature. 2000;**408**:600-605. DOI: 10.1038/35046102

[12] John V, Hock JM, Short LL, Glasebrook AL, Galvin RJ. A role for CD8+ T-lymphocytes in osteoclast differentiation in vitro. The Journal of Endocrinology. 1996;**137**:2457-2463. DOI: 10.1210/endo.137.6.8641199

[13] Grèeviæ D, Lee SK, Marušiæ A, Lorenzo JA. Depletion of CD4 and CD8 T-lymphocytes in mice in vivo enhances

1,25-dihydroxyvitamin D3-stimulated osteoclast-like cell formation in vitro by a mechanism that is dependent on prostaglandin synthesis. Journal of Immunology. 2000;**165**:4231-4238. DOI: 10.4049/jimmunol.165.8.4231

[14] Sallusto F, Lanzavecchia A, Mackay CR. Chemokines and chemokine receptors in T-cell priming and Th1/Th2-mediated responses. The Journal of Immunology. 1998;**19**: 568-574. DOI: 10.1016/s0167-5699(98) 01346-2

[15] Marušiæ A, Raisz LG. Cortison modulates the actions of interleukin-1 on bone formation, resorption, and prostaglandin production in cultured mouse parietal bones. The Journal of Endocrinology. 1991;**129**:2699-2706. DOI: 10.1210/endo-129-5-2699

[16] Koni PA, Joshi SK, Temann UA, Olson D, Burkly L, Flavell RA. Conditional vascular cell adhesion molecule 1 deletion in mice: Impaired lymphocyte migration to bone marrow. The Journal of Experimental Medicine. 2001;**193**:741-753. DOI: 10.1084/ jem.193.6.741

[17] Smithson G, Couse JF, Lubahn DB, Korach KS, Kincade PW. The role of estrogen receptors and androgen receptors in sex steroid regulation of B-lymphopoiesis. Journal of Immunology. 1998;**161**:27-34. PMID: 9647203

[18] Miyaura C, Onoe Y, Inada M, Maki K, Ikuta K, Ito M, et al. Increased B-lymphopoiesis by interleukin 7 induces bone loss in mice with intact ovarian function: Similarity to estrogen deficiency. Proceedings of the National Academy of Sciences of the United States of America. 1997;**94**:9360-9365. DOI: 10.1073/PNAS.94.17.9360

[19] Onoe Y, Miyaura C, Ito M, Ohta H, Nozawa S, Suda T. Comparative effects of estrogen and raloxifene on B-lymphopoiesis and bone loss induced by sex steroid deficiency in mice. Journal of Bone and Mineral Research. 2000;**15**: 541-549. DOI: 10.1359/jbmr.2000.15.3.541

[20] Lorenzo JA, Grèeviæ D, Lee S, Kalinowski J, Jastrzebski S, Dougall W, et al. Murine osteoclasts and B-lymphocytes share a common progenitor cell whose abundance in bone marrow is regulated by estrogen. Journal of Bone and Mineral Research. 2000;**15**:1176. Researchgate.Net/Publica tion/296232519

[21] Marušiæ A, Grèeviæ D, Kataviæ V, Kovacic N, Lukic IK, Kalajzic I, et al. Role of B-lymphocytes in new bone formation. Laboratory Investigation. 2000;**80**:1761-1774. DOI: 10.1038/ LABINVEST.3780186

[22] Dolgushin II, Bukharin OV. Neutrophils and Homeostasis [Nejtrofily i Gomeostaz (in Russian)]. Ekaterinburg: Publishing House of the Ural Branch of the Russian Academy of Sciences; 2001. 277 p. ISBN: 5-7691-1096-1

[23] Fedorova MZ, Levin VN. Spontaneous migration of blood neutrophils in a mixed population of leukocytes and its changes under the influence of autoplasma substances for different functional conditions of the body [Spontannaya migpaciya nejtpofilov kpovi v smeshannoj populyacii lejkocitov i ee izmeneniya pod vliyaniem veshchestv autoplazmy ppi pazlichnyh funkcionalnyh sostoyaniyah opganizma (in Russian)]. Clinical Laboratory Diagnostics [Klinicheskaya Laboratornaya Diagnostika]. 2001;**5**:16-20

[24] Dolgushin II. The role of neutrophils in the regulation of antimicrobial resistance [pol nejtpofilov v pegulyacii antimikpobnoj pezistentnosti (in Russian)]. Bulletin of RAMS [Vestnik RAMN]. 2002;**3**:16-21

[25] Hofer HP, Egger G, Kukovetz EM, Bratschitsch G, Steindorfer P, Schaur RJ.

The influence of trauma on changes in neutrophil granulocyte function assessed by an analysis of granulocyte migration. Langenbeck's Archives of Surgery. 1996;**381**(3):148-154. DOI: 10.1007/bf00187619

[26] Grogaard B, Gerdin B, Reikeras O. The polymorphonclear leukocyte: Has it a role in fracture healing? Archives of Orthopaedic and Trauma Surgery. 1990; **109**(5):261-271. DOI: 10.1007/bf00419942

[27] Davydova HV, Kozlov IG, Sergei IG. Inhibition of proliferation of in vivo activated lymphocytes in interaction with fibrillar collagen [Ingibirovanie proliferacii aktivirovannyh in vivo limfocitov pri vzaimodejstvii s fibrillyarnym kollagenom (in Russian)]. Journal of Medical Immunology [Medicinskaya Immunologiya]. 2002; **4**(2):121

[28] Wildburger R, Borovic S, Zarkovic N, Tatzber F. Post-traumatic dynamic changes in the antibody titer against oxidized low density lipoproteins. Wiener Klinische Wochenschrift. 2000;**112**(18):798-803 c

[29] Richter M, Jodouin CA, Moher D, Barron P. Immunologic defects following trauma: A delay in immunoglobulin synthesis by cultured B-cells following traumatic accidents but not elective surgery. The Journal of Trauma. 1990; **30**(5):590-596. PMID: 2342144

[30] Naot D, Grey A, Reid IR, Cornish J. Lactoferrin—A novel bone growth factor. Journal of Clinical Medical Research. 2005;**2**(3):93-101. DOI: 10.3121/cmr.3.2.93

[31] Baveye S, Elass E, Mazurier J, Spik G, Legrand D. Lactoferrin: A multifunctional glycoprotein involved in the modulation of the inflammatory process. Clinical Chemistry and Laboratory Medicine. 1999;**37**:281-286. DOI: 10.1515/CCLM.1999.049

[32] Kimber I, Cumberbatch M, Dearman RJ, Headon DR, Bhushan M, Griffiths CE. Lactoferrin: Influences on Langerhans cells, epidermal cytokines, and cutaneous inflammation. The International Journal of Biochemistry & Cell Biology. 2002;**80**:103-107. DOI: 10.1139/o01-227

[33] He S, McEuen AR, Blewett SA, Li P, Buckley MG, Leufkens P, et al. The inhibition of mast cell activation by neutrophil lactoferrin: Uptake by mast cells and interaction with tryptase, chymase and cathepsin G. Biochemical Pharmacology. 2003;**65**:1007-1015. DOI: 10.1016/s0006-2952(02)01651-9

[34] Cornish J. Lactoferrin promotes bone growth. BioMetals. 2004;**17**: 331-335. DOI: 10.1023/B: BIOM.0000027713.18694.91

[35] Naot D, Callon KE, Grey AA, Cooper GJS, Reid IR, Cornish J. A potential role for adrenomedullin as a local regulator of bone growth. The Journal of Endocrinology. 2001;**142**:1849-1857. DOI: 10.1210/ENDO.142.5.8152

[36] Lorget F, Clough J, Oliveira M, Daury MC, Sabokbar A, Offord E. Lactoferrin reduces in vitro osteoclast differentiation and resorbing activity. Biochemical and Biophysical Research Communications. 2002;**296**:261-266. DOI: 10.1016/s0006-291x(02)00849-5

[37] Suzuki YA, Shin K, Lonnerdal B. Molecular cloning and functional expression of a human intestinal lactoferrin receptor. Journal of Biochemistry. 2001;**40**:15771-15779. DOI: 10.1021/bi0155899

[38] Grey A, Banovic T, Zhu Q, Watson M, Callon K, Palmano K, et al. The low-density lipoprotein receptor-related protein I is a mitogenic receptor for lactoferrin in osteoblastic cells. Journal of Molecular Endocrinology. 2004;**18**(9):2268-2278. DOI: 10.1210/me.2003-0456

[39] Niemeier A, Kassem M, Toedter K, Wendt D, Ruether W, Beisiegel U, et al. Expression of LRP1 by human osteoblasts: A mechanism for the delivery of lipoproteins and vitamin K1 to bone. Journal of Bone and Mineral Research. 2005;**20**:283-293. DOI: 10.1359/JBMR.041102

[40] Kato M, Patel MS, Levasseur R, Lobov I, Chang BH, Glass DA 2nd, et al. Cbfa1-independent decrease in osteoblast proliferation, osteopenia, and persistent embryonic eye vascularization in mice deficient in Lrp5, a Wnt coreceptor. The Journal of Cell Biology. 2002;**157**:303-314. DOI: 10.1083/jcb.200201089

[41] Nasr HF, Aichelmann-Reidy ME, Yukna RA. Bone and bone substitutes. Journal of Periodontology. 1999;**19**: 74-86. DOI: 10.1111/j.1600-0757.1999. tb00148.x

[42] Schoenwaelder SM, Burridge K. Bidirectional signaling between the cytoskeleton and integrins. Current Opinion in Cell Biology. 1999;**11**:274-286. DOI: 10.1016/S0955-0674(99)80037-4

[43] Giancotti FG, Ruoslahti E. Integrin signaling. Science. 1999;**285**:1028-1032. DOI: 10.1126/science.285.5430.1028

[44] Bolcato-Bellemin AL, Elkaim R, Abehsera A, Fausser JL, Haikel Y, Tenenbaum H. Expression of mRNAs encoding for α and β integrin subunits, MMPs, TIMPs in stretched human periodontal ligament and gingival fibroblasts. Journal of Dental Research. 2000;**79**:1712-1716. DOI: 10.1177/00220345000790091201

[45] Kobayashi Y, Hashimoto F, Miyamoto H. Force-induced osteoclast apoptosis in vivo is accompanied by elevation in transforming growth factor beta and osteoprotegerin expression. Journal of Bone and Mineral Research. 2000;**15**:1924-1934. DOI: 10.1359/jbmr.2000.15.10.1924

[46] Lorenzo JA. Interactions between immune and bone cells: New insights with many remaining questions. The Journal of Clinical Investigation. 2000; **106**:749-752. DOI: 10.1172/JCI11089

[47] Petrov RV, Khaitov RM, Pinegin BV. Evaluation of the immune status of the individual in mass surveys [Ocenka immunnogo statusa cheloveka pri massovyh obsledovaniyah (in Russian)]. Immunology [Immunologiya]. 1992;**6**:51-62

[48] Menshikov VV, editor. Clinical Laboratory Analytics [Klinicheskaya Laboratornaya Analitika (in Russian)]. Moscow: Agat-Med; 2003. p. 816. ISBN: 5-94419-008-6

[49] Fedoseyeva VN, Poryadin GV, Kovalchuk LV. Guide to Immunological and Allergological Methods in Hygienic Studies [Rukovodstvo po Immunologicheskim i Allergologicheskim Metodam v Gigienicheskih Issledovaniyah (in Russian)]. Moscow: Promedek; 1993. p. 320

[50] Shatrov VA, Kuznetsova LV, Belyanovskaya TI. Study of the ability of monocytes of patients with pulmonary tuberculosis restore NBT during phagocytosis of latex particles [Izuchenie sposobnosti monocitov bolnyh tuberkulezom legkih vosstanavlivat nitrosinij tetrazolij pri fagocitoze chastic lateksa (in Russian)]. Laboratory Science [Laboratornoe Delo]. 1985;**7**:408-410

[51] Menshikov VV, editor. Laboratory Methods in the Clinic [Laboratornye Metody Issledovaniya v Klinike (in Russian)]. Moscow: Medicine; 1987. p. 368

[52] Kaplow LS. A histochemical procedure for localizing and evaluating leukocyte alkaline phosphatase activity in smears of blood and marrow. Blood. 1955;**10**:1023-1029. PMID: 13260361

[53] Pigarevsky VE. Granular Leukocytes and Their Properties [Zernistye Lejkocity i ih Svojstva (in Russian)]. Moscow: Medicine; 1978. p. 128

[54] Fedortsov KK, Kuzmin CN, Kozlova NN, Pershyn BB. Standardization lysozyme activity determination by the method of diffusion in agar gel [Standartizaciya opredeleniya aktivnosti lizocima metodom diffuzii v agarovom gele (in Russian)]. Laboratory Science [Laboratornoe Delo]. 1981;**12**:735-736

[55] Kolb VG, Kamyshnikov VC. Handbook of Clinical Biochemistry [Spravochnik po Klinicheskoj Biohimii (in Russian)]. Belarus: Minsk; 1982. p. 290

[56] Medic VA, Tokmachev MS, Fishman BB, Komarov UM, editors. Statistics in Medicine and Biology [Statistika v Medicine i Biologii (in Russian)]. Moscow: Medicine; 2000. p. 412

[57] Tietz NU, Menshikov VV, editors. Encyclopedia Clinical and Laboratory Tests [Enciklopediya Klinicheskih i Laboratornyh Testov (in Russian)]. Moscow: Labinform; 1997. p. 942. ISBN: 5-89429-004-X

[58] Ketlinsky SA, Kalinina NM. Immunology for the Doctor [Immunologiya Dlya Vracha (in Russian)]. St. Petersburg: Hippocrates; 1998. p. 156. ISBN: 5-200929-18-3: 50.00

[59] Livshits VM, Sidelnikova VI. Laboratory Tests in Healthy Individuals (Reference Limits): A Handbook [Laboratornye Testy u Zdorovyh Lyudej (Referentnye Predely): Spravochnik (in Russian)]. Moscow: Triada-X; 2004. p. 128. ISBN: 5-8249-0087-6

[60] Melenberg TV, Zhestkov AB. Immunological aspects of non-united fractures of the lower jaw [Immunologicheskie aspekty nesrosshihsya perelomov nizhnej chelyusti (in Russian)]. Journal of Medical Immunology [Medicinskaya Immunologiya]. 2002;**2**(4):156

Section 4

Biologicals for Bone Tissue Regeneration

Chapter 11

Application of Adipose-Derived Stem Cells in Treatment of Bone Tissue Defects

Stevo Najman, Jelena Najdanović and Vladimir Cvetković

Abstract

Despite excellent self-regeneration capacity of bone tissue, there are some large bone defects that cannot be healed spontaneously. Numerous literature data in the field of cell-based bone tissue engineering showed that adipose-derived stem cells (ADSCs) after isolation could be subsequently applied in a one-step approach for treatment of bone defect, without previous in vitro expansion and osteoinduction. However, standard approaches usually involve in vitro expansion and osteoinduction of ADSCs as an additional preparation step before its final application. Bioreactors are also used for the preparation of ADSC-based graft prior application. The commonly used approaches are reviewed, and their outcomes, advantages, disadvantages, as well as their potential for successful application in the treatment of bone defects are discussed. Difficulty in spontaneous healing of bone defects is very often due to poor vascularization. To overcome this problem, numerous methods in bone tissue engineering (BTE) were developed. We focused on freshly isolated stromal vascular fraction (SVF) cells and ADSCs in vitro induced into endothelial cells (ECs) as cells with vasculogenic capacity for the further application in bone defect treatment. We have reviewed orthotopic and ectopic models in BTE that include the application of SVFs or ADSCs in vitro induced into ECs, with special reference to co-cultivation.

Keywords: stromal vascular fraction, adipose-derived stem cells, endothelial cells, in vitro-induced differentiation, bone tissue engineering, vascularization, osteogenic process stromal vascular fraction, adipose-derived stem cells, endothelial cells, in vitro-induced differentiation, bone tissue engineering, vascularization, osteogenic process

1. Introduction

Structure of the bone tissue is very dynamic due to environmental influence but also because of many factors that act inside the body [1]. The bone can regenerate and repair itself, but large fractures and bone defects fail to heal and repair successfully. In addition to other adverse factors, this results in delayed unions, malunions, or nonunions. To aid bone healing and repair in such situations, build bone-deficient areas, or replace missing bone as well as in purposes of joint reconstruction, bone grafting is used [2–5].

Bone grafting is one of the most common options for the treatment of major bone defects, and the use of bone grafts is among the most common procedures in orthopedic surgery and the second most frequent transplantation of tissue after blood. Over 2 million bone grafting procedures are performed annually in surgery [5, 6]. Bone graft material, alone or in combination with other materials, can perform bone healing function by having at least one of the features among osteogenicity, osteoinduction, and osteoconduction and therefore usually have one or more components—scaffold, as an osteoconductive matrix that supports bone growth, osteoinductive proteins and factors, and osteogenic cells [5, 7]. The main types of bone grafting materials are autografts, allografts, xenografts, synthetic and biological tissue engineering biomaterials, and combinations of these materials [2–6]. Bone grafts and graft substitutes may differ by material type, source, and origin and may also be categorized as osteogenic, osteoinductive, and osteoconductive agents [7]. The choice of bone graft depends on the condition of the bone tissue, defect size, surgical feasibility of the procedure, possible health complications, graft structure, its biological and mechanical characteristics, size and shape, cost, and ethical issues [5].

Each of the bone graft material and its substituents has its advantages and disadvantages, of which there is considerable agreement in surgical practice. Autografts are the best clinical solution among grafts because they have all the necessary properties to stimulate bone repair and regeneration—osteogenicity, osteoinductivity, and osteoconductivity—as they provide osteogenic cells, osteoinductive factors, and osteoconductive scaffold for bone growth. So far, autografts have proven superior in quality and time to bone healing. That is why in orthopedic practice, for the purpose of reconstruction of small defects and replacement of lost bone, autografts are the "gold standard" [3, 5–7]. Autografts can be of different types such as vascularized grafts, bone tissue, or bone marrow. They are usually obtained from the iliac crest, as well as from mandibular bone in dentistry, and by osteectomy and osteoplasty in various procedures. The vascularized fibula is used for the treatment of congenital bone damage, replacement of the bone segment after trauma, and in the case of a malignant tumor so that the periosteum and nutrient artery allow the graft to live and grow in the transplanted site [4, 8, 9]. The use of autografts often involves additional surgery and additional pain, and there is a frequent occurrence of morbidity at the donor site, which with limited availability is a limitation to their use. Morbidity, although low, is significant and ranges from minor to major complications, and there is a risk of injury to large blood vessels and visceral organs while taking the graft. The type of complications and their severity depends on the donor site as well as whether the graft material is taken at the same incision on the primary surgical site [2, 3, 5–8].

Allografts are much more available for orthopedic purposes. They have an osteoconductivity property, they can be well remodeled, but they are poorly osteoinductive, which can be present if they have an organic matrix. All of these properties depend on the size of the graft and the grafting site [3–6, 8]. Allografts are obtained from a bone bank containing cadaveric bones and can be found in various forms. Compared to autografts, allografts lack osteogenic properties and thus have an overall weaker bone regenerative potential, and their integration into the recipient bone over the long term may be insufficient. Allografts can induce immune response and rejection and requires caution because of the possibility of transmission of pathogens from the donor organism, and their disadvantages are also high costs and lack of availability of donors [3, 5–8]. To reduce some disadvantages and limitations by allografts, cells and proteins that can elicit an immune response can be removed, thereby also reducing the possibility of transmission of viral infection by donors. Usually, the sterilization and deactivation process of the proteins is performed before the use of the allograft, but then they lack osteoinductive factors, which in turn remain if the demineralized bone matrix is prepared [4, 8].

Xenografts are obtained from species other than humans, e.g., bovine bone, which is much used in dentistry. There are also nonbone xenograft materials such as sclera, collagen membranes, and coral-derived materials. Compared to autografts, xenografts as allografts only have osteoconductive and osteoinductive but lack osteogenic features. There is a risk of zoonotic transmission in xenografts treatment, and rejection is more likely and stronger than in the case of an allograft. Xenografts are cheaper, but the results of their application are inconsistent [4–6].

In addition to bone grafts (autograft, allograft, xenograft), newer bone substitutes are the ceramic types (calcium compounds: hydroxyapatite, tricalcium phosphate (TCP), calcium sulfate) and biological factors such as growth factors and others (bone morphogenetic proteins (BMPs), platelet-rich plasma (PRP), demineralized bone matrix (DBM)). Bone substitutes have been used for decades and have been defined as synthetic, inorganic, or organic, as well as biological origin materials, or a combination of those used to treat bone defect instead of bone [3, 4, 6]. Bone substitutes are especially used in traumatology and oncologic, spine, and prosthetic surgeries. Suitable bone substitutes should be biocompatible, not provoking an adverse inflammatory response, osteoinductive, osteoconductive, resorbable, easily molded into the bone defect, nonconductive, sterilizable, available, traceable in vivo, and at a reasonable cost [6]. The integration of bone substitutes over the long term may not be sufficient. Bone substitute materials of a synthetic nature such as calcium phosphate (CaP)-based biomaterials often behave osteoconductively only and can be remodeled. Osteoinductivity is possessed by biological factors such as bone matrix proteins or BMP-type growth factors that can be added to other bone substitutes [3, 8]. Ceramic-based bone graft substitutes include hydroxyapatite (HA), TCP, calcium sulfate, and bioglass used alone or in combination. Ceramics can be used in the form of granules, blocks, or moldable paste shape, and the occurrence of injectable cements was particularly significant because it enabled a mininvasive application [6, 7, 10]. Calcium phosphate-based bone substitutes have wide clinical use, since they are generally therapeutically effective, although they have poor mechanical properties, are less strong than bone tissue, and can be completely resorbed. The more advanced variants of HAs have biomimetic properties, since they include ions (carbonates, Mg, fluoride, Sr), so that natural HA is imitated [6]. Polymer-based bone substitutes can be degradable and nondegradable polymers and are applied alone, as co-polymers, or in combination with other materials [7, 10]. Various marine biomaterials are also used as bone substitutes, including chitosan, corals, and sponge skeleton [7]. Although biological factors generally influence good bone formation, the clinical application is not widespread due to high prices and possible adverse side effects [3]. Growth factors as bone substitutes, such as BMPs, transforming growth factor-beta (TGF-beta), platelet-derived growth factor (PDGF), and fibroblast growth factor (FGF), can be natural and recombinant and can be used alone or in combination with other materials [7]. BMPs are bone growth factors that are widely used in spine surgery and for the treatment of tibial nonunion. The efficiency of some biological factors, as is the case with the PRP and DBM, is still an open question [6, 10].

The shortcomings in the outcomes of bone healing were the impetus to seek new types of grafts and bone substitutes. On these motives, a bone tissue engineering (BTE) as a new field began to develop in the last decades of the last century, integrating multiple disciplines such as cell biology, developmental and molecular biology, biomechanics, biomaterials science, immunology, and others. With the progressive introduction of innovations and new technologies, BTE has been offering more and more solutions to reduce the disadvantages of traditional bone grafts and improve the process of healing fractures and defects by achieving better graft incorporation, osteoconductivity, osteoinductivity, and osteogenicity [5, 9–11]. Combining tissue scaffolds, growth factors, cells (especially stem cells), and gene therapies, along with three-dimensional printing and other new technological products, makes BTE a promising option. BTE has progressed over time, producing grafts with increasing ability to regenerate and repair bone [5–7, 9–12]. Cell-based treatment is emerging as a more promising approach in regenerative medicine. Cells (e.g., osteogenic or mesenchymal stem cells and others) are used to create new bone alone or are seeded onto a support matrix or scaffold to form bone tissue in vitro [6, 7, 9, 10, 13]. On these principles, engineered vascularized bone grafts can be created with some similarities to autografts [9, 10, 14]. Of particular interest in BTE is the application of mesenchymal stem cells because of their multipotency and the presence of osteogenic potential [6, 9, 10, 13, 15]. Cells can also be used as a vehicle for osteoinductive genes [6, 10]. Recent developments include ex vivo bioreactors capable at the very automated and controlled way to imitate in vivo environment producing bone with appropriate biomechanical properties before implantation [7, 9, 10, 12, 13]. To test the new features and products of BTE, as well as preclinical testing, many in vitro and in vivo methods and models have been developed with various advantages and disadvantages respectively [11, 16].

2. Sources of cells for tissue-engineered grafts

Nowadays, adult stem cells can be purified from different adult tissues and used in BTE as potential progenitors of osteogenic cells. It is reported that stem cells intended for BTE can be derived from many different tissues such as bone marrow, umbilical cord, dental pulp, as well as adipose tissue [17]. For instance, mesenchymal stem cells (MSCs) derived from bone marrow can be successfully differentiated into cells of various connective tissues [18] as well as in bone cells which give opportunity for its implementation in cell-based BTE [10, 19]. Despite its frequent use in BTE, bone marrow MSCs are reported to have some disadvantages, especially low cell quantity at isolation [20]. This is also an unfavorable characteristic for many other adult stem cells which imply in vitro cell expansion after their isolation in order to obtain sufficient quantity of cells which is mandatory for its further implementation in cell-based BTE. Morbidity and pain are also reported as accompanying side effects that are consequences of bone marrow MSC harvesting [20]. Nevertheless, MSCs are easier to isolate from accessible adipose tissue, which can be harvested with minimally harmful [21] and less painful methods. These multipotent cells derived from adipose tissue were reported by Zuk et al. [22] and suggested as a possible alternative to bone marrow MSCs [22]. Others also reported that stromal cells derived from adipose tissue rapidly proliferate and can be obtained in sufficient quantity, eliminating the need for in vitro expansion [23, 24] which is a tremendous advantage of adipose-derived stem cells (ADSCs) over other tissues that are potential sources of adult stem cells. The more recent study showed that bone morphogenic protein 2-transduced human adipose-derived MSCs had higher capacity for osteogenic differentiation than bone morphogenic protein 2-transduced MSCs from bone marrow [25]. With all this advantages, MSCs from adipose tissue are also reported to have similar potential to differentiate toward osteoblast and form bone as bone marrow MSCs [26]. Adipose tissue therefore represents a reliable source of adult stem cells intended for therapeutic purposes in BTE. In addition to this, in the past decade, we are witnessing an increase of interest for application of ADSCs in cell-based BTE.

2.1 Adipose-derived stem cells

The capacity to differentiate toward a broad spectrum of specialized cells such as bone cells, cartilage cells, muscle cells, endothelial cells, liver cells, neural cells, and others [17, 21, 27] makes ADSCs suitable generally for cell-based tissue engineering as well as for BTE. ADSCs represent a form of MSCs [28] that could be simply isolated from both subcutaneous and visceral adipose tissue that are usually sufficiently abundant in almost every individual. Nevertheless, it is reported that ADSCs derived from visceral fat have higher osteogenic potential than ADSCs from subcutaneous fat in rabbits [29] which should be taken into consideration when selecting the type of adipose tissue as starting source for ADSC isolation. Adipose tissue in humans could be obtained by liposuction or resection method that are both reported to yield similar quantity and good quality of MSCs [30]. More precisely, a direct source of ADSCs is stromal vascular fraction (SVF) which is obtained by enzymatic digestion of previously isolated fat tissue and its subsequent centrifugation [15]. There are well-described markers intended for ADSC characterization. Particularly, ADSCs are reported to have recognizable fibroblast-like, spindle-shaped morphology [22, 26], good longevity and plastic adhesion properties in in vitro condition [31], and capacity for rapid proliferation in cell culture [23, 32]. ADSCs also have characteristic expression pattern of CD cell surface markers. In general, there is an accordance in literature about the expression pattern of CD markers which should be used for ADSC characterization. For instance, Cai et al. [27] summarized that some characteristic CDs, particularly CD166, CD105, CD90, CD73, CD44, CD29, and CD13, have high expression in adipose-derived stem cells [27] which is in accordance with other reviews [33]. Also, according to Bajek et al. (2016) high expressions of CD73, CD44, CD105 and CD90 are indications mainly used for adipose-derived stem cell identification [34]. Therefore, before further steps in their application and analyses, it is very important to examine and determine expression of CDs and other markers like cell morphology in order to characterize ADSCs.

3. Bone substitutes and regulatory factors

As it is mentioned in the previous text, apart from cells, there are two more components in cell-based BTE, and those are bone substitute materials and regulatory factors. These three components together, combined in appropriate manner, makes specific construct which is an adequate alternative to bone grafts for the treatment of bone tissue defects. Bone substitutes are used as appropriate scaffolds for osteogenic cells. Chao et al. [12] described scaffold as logistic templates for guided formation of tissue [12]. Three-dimensional scaffolds that support osteogenic differentiation of the stem cells are seen as crucial components for in vitro engineering of bone construct which can be clinically usable [9]. Even more, to respond to special requirements at the defect site, engineering of the customized bone grafts was also proposed [35]. Bone substitute materials provide appropriate microenvironment for differentiation and proliferation of bone cells [36], and porosity, particle size, and material composition also play important roles [37]. At the first place, bone substitutes should be biocompatible which, among the other things, implies that they are non-toxic and non-genotoxic [38]. Biomaterials are also used to fill defects and compensate lost part of bone tissue at the defect site. Bone substitutes that belong to a group of bioactive biomaterials are capable for interaction with the biological environment and can provide conditions for cellular actions [39] which is of benefit for bone regeneration. Nowadays, many different synthetic and natural bone substitutes are reported to be in use [10, 39, 40]. Particularly, materials based on hydroxyapatite and β-tricalcium phosphate are suitable for BTE [41]. In addition, materials based on bone mineral matrix are frequently used [42–45]. Also, regulatory factors are not less important components in BTE, and at the first place, they should induce and support osteogenic differentiation, adhesion, and proliferation of implanted cells. Because of its significant properties, here the focus will be on platelet-rich plasma as a source of regulatory factors for cell-based BTE. PRP is one of the well-known natural sources of different stimulative regulatory factors [46–48]. Last decade, PRPs are constantly drawing attention of many researchers in fields of regenerative biology as well as in BTE. That is reasonable because regulatory factors from PRP is reported to enhance adhesion, differentiation, and proliferation of the cells and also enhance angiogenesis [46, 49] which may support regeneration and reparation of bone tissue. In addition, it was reported that regulatory factors from PRP can enhance osteogenic process by inducing proliferation and differentiation of MSCs [50, 51]. Nevertheless, the question about adequate and stimulating concentration of platelets in prepared PRP is of great importance, and it is still topical. The opinions about adequate concentration of platelets in PRP intended for BTE are different. There are reports that higher platelet concentrations might have an inhibitory effect [52], and on the other hand, concentrations that are lower than the physiological level is reported to be useful for bone regeneration [53]. Finally, there is a recommendation that optimal concentration of platelets in PRP intended for bone treatment should be from four to eight folds higher than the normal physiological level of platelets in the blood [46]. Another advantage of activated PRP is that it can form fibrin fibers which can couple ADSCs with bone substitute material and improve retention of all construct components [54, 55] similar to reports where fibrin was used for this purpose [56, 57]. Finally, there is a growing interest about synergistic effects of ADSCs and PRP for bone regeneration. Many studies reported promising osteogenic potential of ADSCs and PRP combination [45, 54, 55, 58] and stimulative potential of PRP that improves osteogenesis in combination with cells [50, 59]. In addition, Fernandes and Yang [48] reviewed and summarized some recently published data which implies that adipose-derived stem cells obtained from human, mouse, rat and rabbit in combination with PRP in in vitro and/or in vivo conditions are related with outcomes which are of benefit for BTE [48].

4. Approaches in application of ADSCs in cell-based BTE

4.1 One-step versus multistep approaches

Numerous literature data in the past decade are related with extensive studies about regenerative potential of adipose-derived stem cells. It is well-known that ADSCs in combination with bone substitute materials and regulatory factors possess certain osteogenic potential that can initiate and boost osteogenic process both in orthotopic and ectopic conditions. Recent studies showed that good yield of ADSCs after isolation from adipose tissue provides opportunity for its subsequent application in one-step approach in cell-based bone tissue engineering without previous in vitro expansion and differentiation. Nevertheless, standard approach in cell-based BTE usually involves in vitro pretreatment of ADSCs as an additional step before its final application in order to induce differentiation of ADSCs into osteogenic cells. Literature data showed that both approaches are promising for implementation in treatment of bone tissue defects. Our experience about osteogenic capacity of differently prepared ADSCs is mostly in accordance with other related studies. Based on our previously performed experimental studies and published results, these two approaches have quite different outcomes, and each approach has its advantages and potential to be successfully applied in treatment of bone tissue defects. Also, there is a growing number of researches that employed bioreactors for bone graft engineering.

There are well-described methods for ADSC preparation prior their application in BTE. Without purification, in vitro expansion, and osteoinduction, ADSCs contained in freshly isolated adipose-derived SVF could be prepared and applied in just one step which is described as intraoperative approach [56, 57, 60] or one-step procedure [61]. Intraoperative approach implies construct assembling during surgical procedure [13] by combining cells, bone substitutes, and regulatory factors together in one construct. One of the earlier reports by Aslan et al. [62] presented usage of noncultured human MSCs isolated from bone marrow [62]. More recently published articles demonstrated intraoperative application of freshly isolated SVF cells from human adipose tissue [56, 57] and freshly isolated adipose-derived SVF cells from mice epididymal adipose tissue in ectopic bone-forming model [55]. One-step surgical procedure is also used in oral and maxillofacial surgery for maxillary sinus floor elevation [37, 63]. All these studies suggest that previous in vitro pretreatment of ADSCs and their separation from SVF population prior their implementation in BTE is not necessary. Good yield of ADSCs enables bypassing of in vitro expansion step which goes in favor of the one-step concept in BTE. In addition, the autotransplantation of freshly isolated ADSCs for the treatment of bone tissue defects also enables avoiding problems with immune response [60] that might occur in allotransplantations and xenotransplantations. Adipose-derived SVF is reported to have great capacity for regeneration processes thanks to its heterogeneity [28] because it is composed of different cell types and growth factors [15], especially with cells that have osteogenic and angiogenic potential [37] which is of great importance for treatment of bone defects (**Figure 1**).

Also, it is reported that the entire procedure can be finished in a few hours [13, 56, 64] which reduces wait time for surgery [60] and is one of the major advantages of this approach. In addition, Jurgens et al. [61] showed that ADSCs can adhere promptly onto materials collagen type I/III and poly(L-lactide-co-caprolactone); particularly it is reported that nearly 10 minutes is sufficient time for ADSC adhesion [61] that significantly reduces time needed for construct preparation.

On the other hand, there are many well-described approaches which involve several steps for in vitro expansion and osteogenic differentiation of ADSCs before its final application [26, 45, 65]. In these approaches, by in vitro cultivation, ADSCs are additionally expanded and purified from heterogenous SVF [32] that are directly derived from adipose tissue (**Figure 1**). After that step, purified ADSCs are subjected to in vitro induction in osteogenic media to differentiate toward osteogenic cells before further application which follows in the next step. The characteristic components of osteogenic medium are dexamethasone, ascorbic acid, and β-glycerophosphate [31, 33, 66] which are frequently used for ADSC osteoinduction [67]. There are different data about the duration of in vitro osteogenic induction needed for ADSC differentiation toward osteogenic cells, but literature data mostly referred to 2 weeks [22, 33, 66, 68, 69] or between 2 and 3 weeks [21] (**Figure 2**). It was summarized that during osteogenic differentiation, ADSCs start expression of lineage-specific genes for osteogenesis such as osteocalcin, transcription factor osterix, transcription factor Runx2, bone sialoprotein, alkaline phosphatase, and others [32, 40] which might be detected by gene expression analysis [61] as confirmation of successful osteogenic differentiation of ADSCs. For instance,

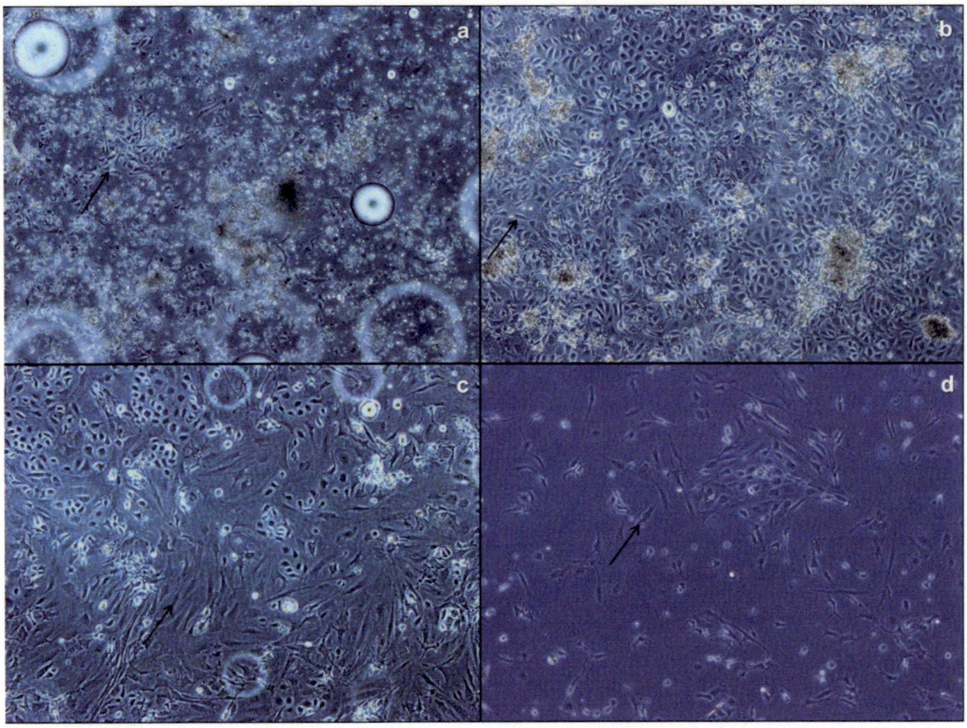

Figure 1.
Expansion and purification of ADSCs from adipose-derived SVF through in vitro cultivation. (a) Adipose-derived SVF 24 h after isolation; (b) adipose-derived SVF 72 h after isolation; (c) adipose-derived SVF 7 days after isolation; and (d) ADSCs the first day after the first passage. Black arrows show ADSCs. Magnification 100×.

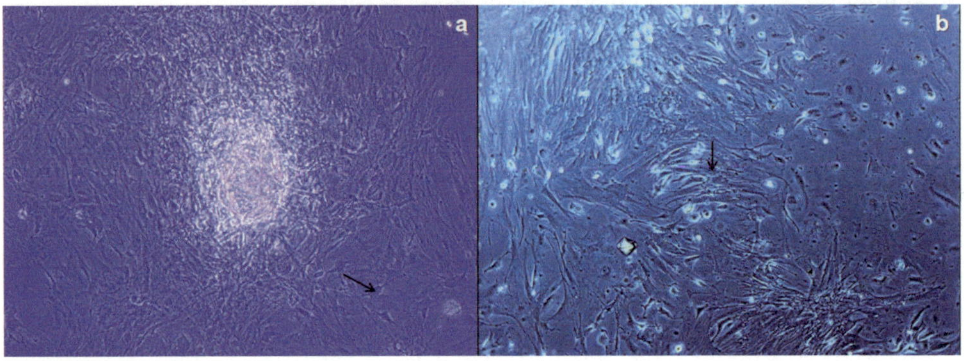

Figure 2.
In vitro osteoinduction of ADSCs. (a) ADSCs 3 days after cultivation in osteogenic media; (b) ADSCs 2 weeks after cultivation in osteogenic media. Black arrows show ADSCs. Magnification 100×.

Cvetković et al. [45] recently published that bone-related genes osteocalcin, transcription factor osterix, alkaline phosphatase, and collagen I alpha1 chain had the highest expression in in vitro osteoinduced ADSCs at 15th day of osteoinduction [45]. Also, it is reported that changes in cell morphology during osteogenic induction to a more cuboidal shape could be observed in ADSC culture [69]. The presence of mineralization signs and proliferation of the ADSCs are also reported as markers of osteogenic differentiation during in vitro osteoinduction [65, 69, 70]. Particularly, after in vitro osteogenic differentiation, mineralization of the cell matrix could be evaluated using Von Kossa and alizarin red staining [31, 66]. In the next step, when osteoinduction is confirmed, osteoinduced ADSCs are seeded on bone substitute material and supplemented with regulatory factors prior using in BTE. There are examples where prepared constructs, after ADSCs seeding on biomaterial (i.e. bone substitute material), are subjected to in vitro osteoinduction before implantation [26] which requires additional time for construct preparation and delays final application. Overall, in vitro osteoinduction is proven to be an effective method for preparation of the ADSCs, and that is confirmed in many different studies [26, 45, 65] which makes this method suitable for BTE. But methods that consider at least two steps usually few weeks for performing and additional material for preparation of ADSCs are time- and money-consuming and more complicated to perform than the one-step method.

According to literature data, both in vitro osteoinduced ADSCs and untreated freshly isolated ADSCs are capable to induce osteogenesis to some level in orthotopic as well as in ectopic conditions. However, there are differences in their capacity to initiate and maintain osteogenic process. By comparing our two recently published studies, it could be concluded that ADSCs prepared and utilized in different manners induced different expression patterns of analyzed osteogenic markers in ectopic implants [45, 55]. In one of the studies, it was shown that untreated ADSCs contained in freshly isolated SVF are capable to quickly initiate osteogenic process, but between the 4th and 8th week of implantation, decreasing bone-related gene expression was detected [55]. On the other hand, Cvetković et al. [45] reported that in vitro osteoinduced ADSCs cause steady osteogenesis with peak at the 8th week [45]. In addition, there is a study which confirmed that osteogenically differentiated human ADSCs induced forming of bone tissue after 8 weeks in ectopic condition [26]; thus the application of osteoinduced ADSCs seems to have a favorable effect on osteogenesis. In other words, all these findings indicate that freshly isolated untreated ADSCs cannot maintain osteogenesis in ectopic condition to that extent as in vitro osteoinduced ADSCs can do. Previous osteoinduction triggered differentiation of ADSCs toward osteogenic cells which had sufficient potential to start and maintain osteogenesis for a longer period [45]. It was concluded that one of the reasons why untreated ADSCs within SVF failed to maintain osteogenic process for a longer period may be because of the lack of osteogenic factors in the ectopic environment which was used as model in this study [55]. Bone tissue normally had factors such as cytokines, mechanotransduction, and closeness of osteoprogenitor cells that are reported to act stimulative in bone formation, but they are reduced in ectopic bone-forming models [71]. Therefore, these factors are characteristic only for orthotopic models which allow evaluation of osteogenic potential of examined engineered construct in real natural milieu of the bone tissue. For that purpose the frequently used orthotopic models in BTE are critical-sized defects in calvaria bone [23] and long bones [44, 72, 73] where large rodents and other mammals are suitable. In addition, it was reported that the presence of sufficient doses of osteogenic factors are needed to support osteogenic differentiation of implanted cells and bone formation in ectopic conditions [56, 64].

Deficiency of osteogenic factors in ectopic models may be bypassed to some extent by addition of stimulating factors to ADSCs such as activated PRP. The addition of activated PRP can make microenvironmental conditions similar to the natural ones that occur during bone trauma. But it is known that platelets release a major portion of regulatory factors immediately after injury [74], which might be sufficient to stimulate ADSCs immediately after its implantation but definitely not for a longer period. The manner and applied doses of PRP obviously was enough to support development and maintenance of osteogenesis guided by previously in vitro osteoinduced ADSCs [45] and was not sufficient to support maintenance of osteogenic process guided by untreated ADSCs within SVF [55]. Regarding the short period of efficient action of PRP, Fernandes and Yang [48] reported that there is a need for carrier that would deliver PRP in the manner that it can act more efficiently and release growth factors sustainably [48]. This might be the key for enhancing osteogenesis guided by freshly isolated and untreated ADSCs within SVF. Despite disadvantages of ectopic models, there are many literature data where ectopic subcutaneous implantations were conducted [42, 43, 71, 75, 76] because they allow examining the real potential of the implanted cells [64] alone and without the impact of the factors that are normally present in bone tissue. Therefore, selection of adequate animal model should depend on experimental goal, and finally it is important for interpretation and extrapolation of obtained results [1]. Nevertheless, osteogenic capacity of previously discussed combinations of differently prepared ADSCs should be evaluated in orthotopic bone-forming models because they are closer to real situations where treatment of bone defect is needed. That is especially of great importance for intraoperative (one-step) method because it is still unclear if this method ready for clinical implementation. In addition, recently a safe and feasible one-step surgical procedure for maxillary sinus floor elevation with implants consisting of calcium phosphate and freshly isolated SVF was demonstrated [63].

Preparation and utilization of freshly isolated and untreated ADSCs at the first place provides tremendous acceleration of procedure performance which is very important especially in everyday clinical practice where intraoperative method is desirable. Despite much longer period which is needed for ADSC preparation and utilization, there is no doubt that osteoinduction is a reliable method for the purposes of BTE. Overall, according to studies published so far [45, 49] that are mostly in accordance with other related studies, it could be concluded that untreated ADSCs contained in freshly isolated SVF have different potential from in vitro osteoinduced ADSCs to start and maintain osteogenic process which leads to quite different outcomes, at least in ectopic condition. Surely, each of presented approaches has its own advantages and potential to be successfully applied in treatment of bone tissue defects. We believe that both approaches could be successfully utilized in the treatment of bone tissue defects, but additional research should be conducted especially in orthotopic models in order to determine required doses of osteogenic factors needed to support osteogenic process.

4.2 ADSCs-based grafts prepared in bioreactors

We previously discuss some methods for ex vivo engineering of the grafts in in vitro static condition using cells and bone substitutes as scaffold. The advanced method for graft engineering involves the use of bioreactors. Bioreactors are defined as devices for precise monitoring and controlling of conditions which are necessary for biological and biochemical processes [77]. The controlling and monitoring of the conditions are in favor of minimalizing variability of graft production as well as standardization of the process [13] for graft engineering. Amini et al. [10] reviewed several types of bioreactors which include perfusion bioreactors, rotating bioreactors, and spinner flask bioreactors. Perfusion-based bioreactors, which are marked as mostly used, significantly stimulate osteogenic cells due to fluid flow [10]. Thus, the dynamic conditions, which bioreactors provide, are more similar to in vivo conditions which allow proliferation and differentiation of seeded cells of three-dimensional scaffolds in a much appropriate way than static in vitro conditions. There is literature evidence where human ADSCs were successfully used for engineering bone grafts in stirrer flask bioreactors [78] as well as viable bone tissue construct in perfusion bioreactor [79]. However, the engineering of the ready-to-use bone grafts using bioreactors could last for weeks, and it must be performed in several steps. Also, bioreactor devices for BTE purposes have high prizes, and the whole procedure is not economical because it requires a higher consumption of medium and other materials which reduces accessibility of this method.

5. Solving vascularization problems in bone tissue engineering by SVF and ADSCs in vitro induced into endothelial cells

5.1 The problem of insufficient vascularization in bone tissue engineering

Bone tissue is a self-renewable tissue with an excellent regeneration capacity [80]. Some bone fractures, tumors, or bone loss can cause such large bone deficiencies that cannot be healed spontaneously [80], since their size goes beyond bone self-renewing capacity [81]. In those cases, classical surgical procedures or bone tissue engineering strategies must be applied [82]. The main problem that has not yet been completely overcome is insufficient vascularization in critical-sized bone defects. Therefore, a perfect bone substitute must have excellent angiogenic features [83].

Until now, various BTE methods for resolving insufficient vascularization were performed: changing the architecture and interconnectivity of pores of the applied biomaterial [84], co-cultivation of different types of cells [85], using mechanical stimulation [86], and adding one [87] or a couple of growth factors in the implants at the same time [88]. The implants were placed into highly vascularized areas or, before the implantation procedure, seeded with cells that secrete chemoattractants for attraction of the host's cells and blood vessels with small diameter [89]. Also, microvascular fragments of adipose tissue were incorporated [90], and tissue flap procedures [91] and scaffolds made of nano- or microfibers were applied [92].

One of the possible methods to facilitate anastomosing between the bioengineered vascular structures with the ones from the surrounding tissue is the construction of prevascularized scaffolds that contain endothelial cells (ECs) [93]. ECs constitute a continuous monolayer among interstitial fluid and blood and have crucial importance in vascularization and in controlling the function of blood vessels [94]. By producing, metabolizing, and releasing numerous humoral and hormonal agents, these cells create an active antithrombotic surface in order to ease transit of plasma and cell components through the blood vessels [94]. Nevertheless, not only that ECs are important for successful developing of the functional vascular system, other cells that constitute blood vessel wall, smooth muscle cells, and perycites are also of great importance [9]. Mural precursor cells participate in vascular remodeling and contribute to better vascularization in cell cultures which is the reason why these cells are desirable as one of the cell lines in co-culture [95, 96].

An important question regarding the use of ECs, not only in BTE but in tissue engineering generally, is "which type of ECs should be used?" [97]. Sources of autologous ECs are limited [98], and mature ECs have limited proliferative capacity [99, 100]. In addition, the procedure of isolation is invasive, it is hard to collect a plentiful number of cells, and there is a possibility of contamination, infection, and change of phenotype and function of ECs during in vitro cultivation [94, 99, 101]. Also, ECs isolated from different organs manifest different phenotypes in vivo, which mean that EC types for the application in tissue engineering should not be selected randomly [102].

Bearing all this in mind, alternative methods have been developed in order to obtain more stable sources of ECs. These methods include in vitro induction of MSCs into ECs. An easily accessible tissue [103] that attracts a great attention in the last few decades is adipose tissue. Primarily cell components of adipose tissue are cells filled with lipids—adipocytes. Besides adipocytes, stromal vascular fraction of adipose tissue consists of microvascular ECs, pericytes, fibroblasts, macrophages, leukocytes, pre-adipocytes, mastocytes, and adipose-derived mesenchymal stem [104, 105]. SVF with heterogeneous cell populations can be obtained upon simple enzyme-based adipose tissue isolation procedure that includes enzymatic digestion, filtration, and centrifugation [76, 106–109]. After this procedure, SVF can be used as a source of ADSCs directly [108] or after expansion in cell culture through few passages [104] and subjecting to differentiation toward certain cell line [66, 76, 105, 109–111].

ADSCs secrete numerous angiogenesis-related mediators including vascular endothelial growth factor (VEGF), bone morphogenic proteins, placental growth factor (PGF), angiopoietin-1, hepatocyte growth factor (HGF), transforming growth factor-β, and fibroblast growth factor 2 (FGF-2) [112]. Secretion of these angiogenic factors makes ADSCs convenient for regenerative cell therapy [106]. Among the abovementioned growth factors, VEGF and BMP2 are considered to be the main factors during bone regeneration, VEGF on the vascular and BMP2 on the osteogenic side [113]. Besides soluble growth factors, ADSCs release plasma membrane-derived vesicles (MVs) that can contain some pro-angiogenic and osteogenic molecules [114] with an influence on adjacent cells. In addition, growth factors and other molecules contained within MVs (cytokines, RNAs, microRNAs) can be transported to some more distant target cells all over the body. By taking up the content of MVs, target cells use these molecules and perform certain biological activity including angiogenesis of target cells which is of crucial importance in bone tissue regeneration [115].

In order to apply SVF as a source of cells with vasculogenic capacity in bone tissue engineering, several methods have been described. These methods include application of SVFs immediately after isolation from adipose tissue as well as after in vitro induction of endothelial differentiation.

5.2 Potential of stromal vascular fraction as a source of cells with vasculogenic capacity for application in bone tissue engineering

Freshly isolated SVF contains both endothelial and skeletal progenitor cells [116]. This property was widely used to construct osteogenic and vasculogenic grafts. It has been found that three-dimensional (3D) cultures of ECs and osteoblasts (OBs) as well as osteogenic-vasculogenic constructs could be achieved by using perfusion-based bioreactor system of single cell source human SVFs in ceramic scaffolds [116]. Namely, SVFs were seeded on 3D porous ceramic scaffolds and cultivated during 5 days using bioreactor system. Eight weeks after implantation of resulting scaffolds in nude mice, formation of functional vascular network that was connected with the host's vasculature as well as ectopic bone formation was observed. Nude mice model was also used by Todorov and his colleagues [117]. This team isolated SVFs from human abdominal lipoaspirates and obtained hypertrophic cartilage (HC) pellets from bone marrow-derived stromal cells. Devitalized HC was embedded in fibrin gel and implanted with and without SVFs ectopically and in calvarial defects. Twelve weeks after implantations, vascularization and bone formation of grafts enriched with SVFs were enhanced in ectopic, subcutaneous, and in orthotopic experimental model.

The use of human SVF-derived vascular progenitor cells can speed up the engraftment of critical-sized osteogenic constructs which improves in vivo formation of the bone tissue [118]. Human SVFs have been isolated, seeded, and cultured into hydroxyapatite scaffolds. Perfusion bioreactor system was used in order to preserve the cells of $CD34^{+}/CD31^{+}$ endothelial lineage from the SVF. As a result of in vitro cultivation, 5 days after seeding, endothelial and mesenchymal progenitors from SVF constituted capillary networks that were able to anastomose with the host vasculature 7 days after implantation on an ectopic nude rat model [118].

With an aim to simulate an intraoperative procedure on an ectopic bone forming model, autologous SVFs isolated from epididymal adipose tissue of Balb/c mice and platelet-rich plasma were added to the bone mineral matrix (BMM) [108]. BMM served as a carrier for cells and growth factors. The constructs were implanted subcutaneously, and osteogenic capacity of this combination was examined. Eight weeks after implantations, these implants had significantly higher percentage of infiltrated tissue and percentage of vascularization than the control (BMM-only implants). According to osteogenesis-related gene expression analysis, implants with SVFs induced rapid onset of osteogenesis process. One of the reasons for such results probably lies in the fact that freshly isolated SVFs had upregulated expression of endothelial- and osteogenic-related genes which was proved by using real-time PCR analysis.

Non-induced ADSCs cultivated in vitro up to the third passage were mixed with allogeneic PRP taken from three healthy Wistar rats [119]. ADSCs-PRP constructs were implanted into the jaws of rats that had bisphosphonate-related osteonecrosis of the jaw. Eight weeks after the treatment, the incidence of osteonecrosis was lower, while the degree of bone turnover and number of osteoclasts were higher than the experimental groups that were not treated with ADSCs [119]. These data could be explained by the fact that PRP release numerous growth factors that can fasten both in vitro and in vivo ADSC differentiation without previous addition of any other factors inductive toward certain cell line [109]. One of the possible mechanisms of synergistic effect of ADSCs and PRP could be ascribed to the release of platelet-derived growth factor from PRP. PDGF has an impact on selectable expansion and recruitment of non-induced MSCs, as well as on proliferation and migration of progenitors of blood vessel wall cells [120]. It also triggers differentiation of MSCs into blood vessel cells [107] and enhances release of extracellular vesicles (EVs)—MVs and exosomes from ADSCs which further influence both in vitro and in vivo angiogenic process [121].

On an ectopic model, Man and associates [109] pointed out to the effect of ADSCs that is similar to the one shown in the abovementioned orthotopic model. ADSCs isolated from inguinal rabbit fat pads and mixed with PRP were loaded onto alginate microspheres. Well-developed blood vessel network and good bone mineralization were observed 3 months after subcutaneous implantations. Opposite results were obtained in another research where non-induced ADSCs were seeded on poly (D, L-lactide) scaffolds and implanted in the large rat palatal bone defect [122]. Bone formation did not occur even 12 weeks after implantations, and the defects were filled with dense fibrous tissue. The differences between the outcomes of the different studies could be attributed to the fact that adipose tissue was taken from the different localizations of the donors' body. Also, the implant preparation was done in a different manner, and different models were chosen for the implantation procedure.

Adipose tissue can also be used as a source of microvascular fragments (MVF) that can be further applied as vascularization units [123]. MVF isolated from CD-1 mice were incorporated into thermoresponsive hydrogel (TRH), cultivated, and used for filling the osteotomy gaps in the femurs of CD-1 mice. Bone healing was assessed 14 and 35 days after induction of osteotomy, while non-incorporated MVF as well as no material group served as control groups. It was found that TRH is a suitable carrier for MVF since vascularization in MVF-loaded TRH was improved in comparison to the control groups. In contrast to this finding, bone formation in this group was impaired, probably due to low levels of VEGF expression during the early stages of bone healing.

Bone substitute biomaterials based on calcium phosphate, including hydroxyapatite (HA), β-tricalcium phosphate (β-TCP), and HA/β-TCP combination, are often used in BTE due to their good biocompatibility and the absence of toxicity of their chemical compounds [124]. These materials also have such 3D features that allow immediate colonization by MSCs and extensive revascularization [125]. For those reasons, Farré-Guasch and his associates used ADSCs-containing SVF seeded on calcium-based biomaterials to treat the patients subjected to maxillary sinus floor elevation (MSFE)—a surgical procedure that in some patients must precede dental implant placement [126]. Autologous SVFs taken from patients were seeded on two types of carriers for two different groups of patients: group 1 had SVFs seeded on β-tricalcium phosphate, and group 2 had SVFs seeded on biphasic calcium phosphate, while the control group had only ceramics, without cells. Histomorphometrical analysis and immunohistochemical staining for blood vessel markers such as CD34 and alpha-smooth muscle actin revealed higher number of blood vessels and immunoexpression of blood vessel markers in both experimental than a control group. These results point out pro-angiogenic influence of SVF.

One of the recently published papers regarding pre-vascularization of various engineered tissues compares the use of ADSCs as a potential source of cells with vasculogenic capacity in combination with different types of gel-based scaffolds [127]. ADSCs were isolated from human fat tissue, cultivated, and, after second passage, molded in fibrin as well as agarose-collagen gels. After 14 days of incubation have passed, the gels were analyzed by two-photon laser scanning microscopy. Vascularization was achieved in both types of gels which were detected as branched networks of tubular vascular structures in both hydrogels. Nevertheless, volume, area, and length of vascular structures supported by ADSCs in agarose-collagen hydrogels were comparable to human dermal fibroblast control.

5.3 Potential of adipose-derived stem cells in vitro induced into ECs for application in bone tissue engineering

5.3.1 Orthotopic model

In order to increase vascularization, ADSCs induced into ECs were applied in BTE by using several models, among which orthotopic model is one of the most commonly used. Rat ADSCs in vitro induced into ECs during 8 days was used for the construction of allografts [128]. The cells were combined with sterilized and decellularized banked allografts made of calvaria from earlier sacrificed Lewis rats. Allografts were implanted into critical-sized calvarial defects in rats, and 8 weeks after the implantation, blood vessel density was increased. As a consequence, bone volume was also increased. In parallel, two other types of allografts were constructed—allografts seeded with ADSCs induced into OBs and allografts seeded with the combination of ADSCs induced into ECs and ADSCs induced into OBs. These implants had weaker vascularization and lower bone volume 8 weeks after the implantation than the ECs-only allografts.

ADSCs in vitro induced into ECs were also seeded onto poly(D, L-lactide) scaffolds and implanted into critical-sized calvarial defects of Lewis rats [110]. Scaffolds prevascularized in this manner did not caused an increase in bone formation by itself, but according to the conclusion of this team, they could possibly be used as a source of cells for accomplishing better vascularization and function of the existing OBs. On the other hand, the constructs that were constructed out of undifferentiated ADSCs or ADSCs induced into OBs had statistically greater bone volume than the implants containing ADSCs induced into ECs.

In another study, also performed on critical-sized calvarial defect model of Lewis rats, hydroxyapatite/poly(lactide-co-glycolide) [HA-PLG] was used as a biomaterial carrier, while adipose tissue was extracted from inguinal fat pads [129].

ADSCs were induced into ECs as well as into OBs. Vascularization and osteogenic process were evaluated in the following groups: (I) HA-PLG scaffolds without cells, (II) HA-PLG scaffolds seeded with non-induced ADSCs, (III) HA-PLG scaffolds seeded with ADSCs induced into ECs, and (IV) HA-PLG scaffolds seeded with ADSCs induced into OBs. The highest bone mineral density, bone regeneration, and vascular density in regenerated bone were found in group IV, although none of the found differences had statistical significance ($P > 0.05$).

In order to repair critical-sized bone defects in rat femur, ADSCs induced into ECs were used for prevascularization of the modified hierarchical mesoporous bioactive glass (MBG) scaffold with an enhanced compressive strength and then combined with ADSCs subjected to osteogenic differentiation [108]. Prevascularized MBG carrying ADSCs induced into OBs had more advanced angiogenesis both on the surface and in the interior than the non-vascularized MBG carrying ADSCs induced into OBs and MBG scaffolds that were not seeded with cells. Moreover, the group with prevascularized MBG scaffolds had the highest mineral deposition rate postoperatively. These results indicate that time-phase sequential utilization of ADSCs on MBG scaffolds is a good strategy for reparation of massive bone defects.

5.3.2 Ectopic model

Ectopic models are important in bone tissue engineering since they provide reducing external influences and side effects, thus concentrating on intrinsic potential of the applied implant components [53] and their interactions [42]. With an aim to overcome the problem of inadequate blood vessels development and consequent inability of bone tissue regeneration, the influence of ADSCs in vitro induced into ECs on vascularization and osteogenic process in ectopic osteogenic implants was examined [109]. The implants composed of ADSCs, BMM, and PRP and the ones composed of BMM and PRP were subcutaneously implanted into BALB/c mice. Endothelial-related gene expression, high percentage of vascularization, and VEGFR-2 immunoexpression show that implants enriched with ECs have increased vascularization compared to the cell-free implants. This was followed by more pronounced signs of osteogenic process in ADSCs-BMM-PRP implants than in BMM-PRP implants. By examining endothelial-related gene expression, vascular cell adhesion molecule-1 (VCAM-1) and osteopontin immunoexpression, it was also shown that the composition of implants based on biological triad (ADSCs induced into ECs, PRP and BMM) is more favorable for improving vascularization in the ectopic bone-forming model than in the BMM-only implants [76].

Uninduced ADSCs cultivated up to the 12th day after the third passage, combined with PRP and BMM and subcutaneously implanted into BALB/c mice, also have vasculogenic potential [109]. However, their vasculogenic potential is lower than that of ADSCs in vitro induced into osteogenic cells and implanted in combination with BMM and PRP. Specifically, relative gene expression analysis of endothelial gene markers *Vwf*, *Egr1*, *Flt1*, and *Vcam1* was significantly higher ($p < 0.05$) in the group that contained osteoinduced ADSCs than in the group with uninduced ADSCs for each single gene and with the exception of *Vwf* at 1 and 4 weeks after implantations, at each single observation point.

Endothelial differentiated ADSCs and osteogenic differentiated ADSCs can be simultaneously applied for the construction of ectopic osteogenic implants. A method of in vitro prevascularization applied by Zhang and his team included construction of double cell sheets (DCS) out of rabbit ADSCs previously in vitro induced into ECs and into osteogenic cells [113]. DCS were combined with coral hydroxyapatite (CHA) in four different manners. Twelve weeks after ectopic implantation into nude mice, a group that contained CHA covered with DCS such that endothelial cell sheet was inside and osteogenic cell sheet outside exhibited the most favorable results regarding vascularization and bone maturation of the graft.

5.3.3 Co-cultivation

Co-cultivation of ECs with other cell types is one of the approaches for resolving the problem of inadequate vascularization in BTE [130]. ECs were co-cultivated with different types of cells before the implantation procedure, but the most important for BTE is co-cultivation of ECs and OBs since numerous interactions between these two cell types exist during normal bone regeneration process [131, 132]. One of the mechanisms of those interactions was found by Kaigler and associates [133]. They have shown that in vitro, ECs improve osteogenic capacity of bone mesenchymal stem cells (BMSCs) during co-cultivation, in direct contact or near each other. In part, this role of ECs could be attributed to release of BMP-2. In vivo, transplanted ECs enhanced capability of transplanted BMSCs to form the bones.

The positive effect of combination of ECs and OBs was estimated in ectopically implanted HA/bTCP scaffolds. The 3D porous ceramic scaffolds were seeded with in vitro co-cultivated ADSCs induced into OBs, ADSCs induced into ECs, and $CD14^+$ osteoclast progenitors derived from human peripheral blood osteoclasts [134]. This three-dimensional organotypic culture model based on human cells was cultivated during 21 days in the perfusion bioreactor system. After cultivation, the system was implanted subcutaneously into dorsal pockets of nude mice. Eight weeks after implantation, blood vessels and bone-like tissue were formed.

In another study, co-cultivation of ADSCs induced into ECs and ADSCs induced into OBs did not have such positive effect on vascularization and osteogenic process [130]. Co-cultivation increased proliferation of this two cell types in vitro in comparison with monocultures or undifferentiated ADSCs. Nevertheless, co-cultures in a ratio 1:1 = OBs:ECs seeded on polylactic acid gas-plasma-treated scaffolds have not induced increased vascularization and signs of osteogenic process compared to the implants constituted out of non-induced ADSCs and polymer scaffolds. Unlike the co-culture group, ECs seeded on polymer scaffolds have increased vascularization, and OBs seeded on polymer scaffolds have improved osteogenesis more than a group with undifferentiated ADSCs [130].

Unlike the results of the above discussed study, ADSCs in vitro induced into OBs and ADSCs in vitro induced into ECs and seeded into self-assembling peptide RADA16-I scaffolds as co-cultures (1:1) had better osteogeneration and vascularization than the scaffolds seeded with monocultures of this type of cells or non-induced ADSCs [135]. Before seeding the cells into RADA16-I scaffolds, it has been shown that the best interaction of ADSCs induced into OBs and ADSCs induced into ECs in co-cultures was achieved when the ratio of the cells was 1:1.

The results obtained by some of the abovementioned research teams, which were worse than expected regarding a group of implants that contained previously co-cultured ECs and OBs, could lie in the ratio of the applied cell types. It has been confirmed that application of too many ECs decreases graft neovascularization probably due to increase in metabolic load and enhanced competition for nutrients [136]. The other reason for those differences can be the differences in the applied biomaterials used for the implant construction [130].

5.3.4 Arteriovenous vascular bundle

Formation of arteriovenous vascular bundle (AVB) belongs to in vivo prevascularization approaches. Incorporation of AVB into scaffolds represents a model of scaffold that have artery and vein inserted into its central part. In this way, stem cells as well as cytokines, oxygen, and nutrients can be transported, while waste products can be removed from the scaffold. Altogether, that kind of construction leads to excellent vascularization and osteogenesis within the scaffold [137].

Scaffolds with AVB were combined with rat ADSCs previously subjected to in vitro endothelial differentiation. Obtained ECs were incorporated into porous nano-hydroxyapatite-polyamide 66 (nHA-PA 66) scaffolds in vitro [111]. After that, AV bundle was inserted into ECs-based nHA-PA 66 in vivo. Also, AV bundle was inserted into nHA-PA 66 scaffolds seeded with non-induced ADSCs and into empty nHA-PA 66 scaffolds, while one experimental group had nHA-PA 66 scaffolds without inserted AV bundle and without cells. Two and four weeks after the implantation procedure, the implants were extracted from the animals and analyzed. Density of blood vessels was significantly higher, and the diameter of blood vessels was larger in ECs-based nHA-PA 66 scaffolds than that in all other groups of implants.

5.3.5 Gene therapy

Combining ex vivo gene therapy with cell transplantation techniques that include endothelial cell line is another approach for overcoming the problem of insufficient vascularization in bone. The benefit of this method was assessed by using 3D poly (lactide-co-glycolide) sintered microsphere scaffolds in a BTE approach [138]. ADSCs were isolated from human infrapatellar fat tissue, and the cells were transfected with adenovirus that encodes cDNA of VEGF and combined with endothelial ones. As a result, genetically modified ADSCs combined with ECs caused prominent growth within 3D poly (lactide-co-glycolide) scaffolds, which indicates the potential for ADSCs application in improving vascularization in BTE. Another study where gene therapy and ADSCs were combined was conducted by Peterson and associates [139]. First, ADSCs were transfected with the BMP-2 gene, then loaded on the collagen-ceramic carrier, and finally implanted in critical-sized femoral defect of nude mice. Eight weeks after implantations, histologic, radiographic, and biomechanical analyses showed that the collagen-ceramic carrier combined with ADSCs previously transfected with the BMP-2 gene caused bone formation within the defect.

Acknowledgements

The study was supported by the Ministry of Education, Science and Technological Development of the Republic of Serbia (project III41017).

Conflict of interest

The authors declare no conflict of interest.

Author details

Stevo Najman[1*], Jelena Najdanović[1] and Vladimir Cvetković[2]

1 Department of Biology and Human Genetics, Department for Cell and Tissue Engineering, Faculty of Medicine, University of Niš, Niš, Serbia

2 Department of Biology and Ecology, Faculty of Sciences and Mathematics, University of Niš, Niš, Serbia

*Address all correspondence to: stevo.najman@gmail.com; stevo.najman@medfak.ni.ac.rs

IntechOpen

© 2020 The Author(s). Licensee IntechOpen. This chapter is distributed under the terms of the Creative Commons Attribution License (http://creativecommons.org/licenses/by/3.0), which permits unrestricted use, distribution, and reproduction in any medium, provided the original work is properly cited.

References

[1] Cvetkovic V, Najman S, Rajkovic J, Zabar AL, Vasiljevic P, Djordjevic LB, et al. A comparison of the microarchitecture of lower limb long bones between some animal models and humans: A review. Veterinární Medicína. 2013;**58**(7):339-351

[2] Younger EM, Chapman MW. Morbidity at bone graft donor sites. Journal of Orthopaedic Trauma. 1989;**3**(3):192-195. DOI: 10.1097/00005131-198909000-00002

[3] Wang W, Yeung KW. Bone grafts and biomaterials substitutes for bone defect repair: A review. Bioactive Materials. 2017;**2**(4):224-247

[4] Saima S, Jan SM, Shah AF, Yousuf A, Batra M. Bone grafts and bone substitutes in dentistry. Journal of Oral Research and Review. 2016;**8**:36-38

[5] Oryan A, Alidadi S, Moshiri A, Maffulli N, et al. Bone regenerative medicine: Classic options, novel strategies, and future directions. Journal of Orthopaedic Surgery and Research. 2014;**9**:18. DOI: 10.1186/1749-799X-9-18

[6] Campana V, Milano G, Pagano E, Barba M, Cicione C, Salonna G, et al. Bone substitutes in orthopaedic surgery: From basic science to clinical practice. Journal of Materials Science. Materials in Medicine. 2014;**25**(10):2445-2461

[7] Nandi S, Roy S, Mukherjee P, Kundu B, De D, Basu D. Orthopaedic applications of bone graft & graft substitutes: A review. The Indian Journal of Medical Research. 2010;**132**:15-30

[8] Bauer TW, Muschler GF. Bone graft materials: An overview of the basic science. Clinical Orthopaedics and Related Research. 2000;**371**:10-27

[9] Fröhlich M, Grayson WL, Wan LQ, Marolt D, Drobnic M, Vunjak-Novakovic G. Tissue engineered bone grafts: Biological requirements, tissue culture and clinical relevance. Current Stem Cell Research & Therapy. 2008;**3**(4):254-264

[10] Amini AR, Laurencin CT, Nukavarapu SP. Bone tissue engineering: Recent advances and challenges. Critical Reviews in Biomedical Engineering. 2012;**40**(5):363-408. DOI: 10.1615/CritRevBiomedEng.v40.i5.10

[11] O'Keefe RJ, Mao J. Bone tissue engineering and regeneration: From discovery to the clinic-an overview. Tissue Engineering. Part B, Reviews. 2011;**17**(6):389-392. DOI: 10.1089/ten.TEB.2011.0475

[12] Chao PHG, Grayson W, Vunjak-Novakovic G. Engineering cartilage and bone using human mesenchymal stem cells. Journal of Orthopaedic Science. 2007;**12**(4):398. DOI: 10.1007/s00776-007-1147-9

[13] Jakob M, Saxer F, Scotti C, Schreiner S, Studer P, Scherberich A, et al. Perspective on the evolution of cell-based bone tissue engineering strategies. European Surgical Research. 2012;**49**(1):1-7. DOI: 10.1159/000338362

[14] Tsigkou O, Pomerantseva I, Spencer JA, Redondo PA, Hart AR, O'Doherty E, et al. Engineered vascularized bone grafts. Proceedings of the National Academy of Sciences. 2010;**107**(8):3311-3316

[15] Alabdulkarim Y, Ghalimah B, Al-Otaibi M, Al-Jallad HF, Mekhael M, Willie B, et al. Recent advances in bone regeneration: The role of adipose tissue-derived stromal vascular fraction and mesenchymal stem cells. Journal of Limb Lengthening & Reconstruction. 2017;**3**(1):4-18

[16] Buma P, Schreurs W, Verdonschot N. Skeletal tissue

engineering-from in vitro studies to large animal models. Biomaterials. 2004;**25**(9):1487-1495. DOI: 10.1016/S0142-9612(03)00492-7

[17] Seong JM, Kim B-C, Park JH, Kwon IK, Mantalaris A, Hwang YS. Stem cells in bone tissue engineering. Biomedical Materials. 2010;**5**(6):062001. DOI: 10.1088/1748-6041/5/6/062001

[18] Caplan AI. Mesenchymal stem cells: Cell-based reconstructive therapy in orthopedics. Tissue Engineering. 2005;**11**(7-8):1198-1211. DOI: 10.1089/ten.2005.11.1198

[19] Robey PG. Cell sources for bone regeneration: The good, the bad, and the ugly (but promising). Tissue Engineering Part B: Reviews. 2011;**17**(6):423-430. DOI: 10.1089/ten.teb.2011.0199

[20] Zuk PA, Zhu M, Ashjian P, De Ugarte DA, Huang JI, Mizuno H, et al. Human adipose tissue is a source of multipotent stem cells. Molecular Biology of the Cell. 2002;**13**(12):4279-4295. DOI: 10.1091/mbc.E02-02-0105

[21] Fraser JK, Wulur I, Alfonso Z, Hedrick MH. Fat tissue: An underappreciated source of stem cells for biotechnology. Trends in Biotechnology. 2006;**24**(4):150-154. DOI: 10.1016/j.tibtech.2006.01.010

[22] Zuk PA, Zhu M, Mizuno H, Huang J, Futrell JW, Katz AJ, et al. Multilineage cells from human adipose tissue: Implications for cell-based therapies. Tissue Engineering. 2001;**7**(2):211-228. DOI: 10.1089/107632701300062859

[23] Cowan CM, Shi YY, Aalami OO, Chou YF, Mari C, Thomas R, et al. Adipose-derived adult stromal cells heal critical-size mouse calvarial defects. Nature Biotechnology. 2004;**22**(5):560-567. DOI: 10.1038/nbt958

[24] Helder MN, Knippenberg M, Klein-Nulend J, Wuisman PI. Stem cells from adipose tissue allow challenging new concepts for regenerative medicine. Tissue Engineering. 2007;**13**(8):1799-1808. DOI: 10.1089/ten.2006.0165

[25] Bougioukli S, Sugiyama O, Pannell W, Ortega B, Tan MH, Tang AH, et al. Gene therapy for bone repair using human cells: Superior osteogenic potential of bone morphogenetic protein 2–transduced mesenchymal stem cells derived from adipose tissue compared to bone marrow. Human Gene Therapy. 2018;**29**(4):507-519. DOI: 10.1089/hum.2017.097

[26] Hattori H, Masuoka K, Sato M, Ishihara M, Asazuma T, Takase B, et al. Bone formation using human adipose tissue-derived stromal cells and a biodegradable scaffold. Journal of Biomedical Materials Research. Part B, Applied Biomaterials. 2006;**76**(1):230-239. DOI: 10.1002/jbm.b.30357

[27] Cai X, Su X, Li G, Wang J, Lin Y. Osteogenesis of adipose-derived stem cells. In: Lin Y, editor. Osteogenesis. Rijeka, Croatia: IntechOpen; 2012. pp. 135-152. ISBN: 978-953-51-0030-0. Available from: http://www.intechopen.com/books/osteogenesis/osteogenesis-of-adipose-derived-stem-cells

[28] Guo J, Nguyen A, Banyard DA, Fadavi D, Toranto JD, Wirth GA, et al. Stromal vascular fraction: A regenerative reality? Part 2: Mechanisms of regenerative action. Journal of Plastic, Reconstructive & Aesthetic Surgery. 2016;**69**(2):180-188

[29] Peptan IA, Hong L, Mao JJ. Comparison of osteogenic potentials of visceral and subcutaneous adipose-derived cells of rabbits. Plastic and Reconstructive Surgery. 2006;**117**(5):1462-1470. DOI: 10.1097/01.prs.0000206319.80719.74

[30] Schneider S, Unger M, van Griensven M, Balmayor ER. Adipose-derived mesenchymal stem cells from liposuction and resected fat are feasible sources for regenerative medicine. European Journal of Medical Research. 2017;**22**(1):17

[31] Barba M, Cicione C, Bernardini C, Michetti F, Lattanzi W. Adipose-derived mesenchymal cells for bone regeneration: State of the art. BioMed Research International. 2013;**2013**:416391. DOI: 10.1155/2013/416391

[32] Bourin P, Bunnell BA, Casteilla L, Dominici M, Katz AJ, March KL, et al. Stromal cells from the adipose tissue-derived stromal vascular fraction and culture expanded adipose tissue-derived stromal/stem cells: A joint statement of the International Federation for Adipose Therapeutics and Science (IFATS) and the International Society for Cellular Therapy (ISCT). Cytotherapy. 2013;**15**(6):641-648. DOI: 10.1016/j.jcyt.2013.02.006

[33] Grottkau BE, Lin Y. Osteogenesis of adipose-derived stem cells. Bone Research. 2013;**2**:133-145

[34] Bajek A, Gurtowska N, Olkowska J, Kazmierski L, Maj M, Drewa T. Adipose-derived stem cells as a tool in cell-based therapies. Archivum Immunologiae et Therapiae Experimentalis. 2016;**64**:443-454

[35] Bhumiratana S, Vunjak-Novakovic G. Concise review: Personalized human bone grafts for reconstructing head and face. Stem Cells Translational Medicine. 2012;**1**(1):64-69. DOI: 10.5966/sctm.2011-0020

[36] Zanello LP, Zhao B, Hu H, Haddon RC. Bone cell proliferation on carbon nanotubes. Nano Letters. 2006;**6**(3):562-567. DOI: 10.1021/nl051861e

[37] Farré-Guasch E, Prins H-J, Overman JR, ten Bruggenkate CM, Schulten EAJM, Helder MN, et al. Human maxillary sinus floor elevation as a model for bone regeneration enabling the application of one-step surgical procedures. Tissue Engineering. Part B, Reviews. 2013;**19**(1):69-82. DOI: 10.1089/ten.teb.2012.0404

[38] Cvetković VJ, Takić Miladinov D, Stojanović S. Genotoxicity and mutagenicity testing of biomaterials. In: Zivic F, Affatato S, Trajanovic M, Schnabelrauch M, Grujovic N, Choy KL, editors. Biomaterials in Clinical Practice: Advances in Clinical Research and Medical Devices. Springer: Cham; 2018. pp. 501-527

[39] Najdanović J, Rajković J, Najman S. Bioactive biomaterials: Potential for application in bone regenerative medicine. In: Zivic F, Affatato S, Trajanovic M, Schnabelrauch M, Grujovic N, Choy KL, editors. Biomaterials in Clinical Practice: Advances in Clinical Research and Medical Devices. Springer: Cham; 2018. pp. 333-360

[40] Beni BH, Zarei R, Esfandiari E, Valiani A. Adipose-derived stem cells and application in musculoskeletal tissue repair. Global Journal of Medicine Researches and Studies. 2013;**1**(1):11-16

[41] Jensen SS, Aaboe E, Pinholt EM, Hjørting-Hansen E, Melsen F, Ruyter IE. Tissue reaction and material characteristics of four bone substitutes. The International Journal of Oral & Maxillofacial Implants. 1996;**11**:55-66

[42] Živković JM, Najman SJ, Vukelić MĐ, Stojanović S, Aleksić MV, Stanisavljević MN, et al. Osteogenic effect of inflammatory macrophages loaded onto mineral bone substitute in subcutaneous implants. Archives of Biological Sciences. 2015;**67**(1):173-186

[43] Najdanović JG, Cvetković VJ, Stojanović S, Vukelić-Nikolić MĐ, Stanisavljević MN, Živković JM, et al. The influence of adipose-derived stem cells induced into endothelial cells on ectopic vasculogenesis and osteogenesis. Cellular and Molecular Bioengineering. 2015;**8**(4):577-590. DOI: 10.1007/s12195-015-0403-x

[44] Rajković J, Stojanović S, Đorđević LJ, Cvetković T, Najman S. Locally applied cholecalciferol and alfacalcidol act differently on healing of femur defects filled with bone mineral matrix and platelet-rich plasma in ovariectomized rats. Biotechnology and Biotechnological Equipment. 2015;**29**(5):963-969

[45] Cvetković VJ, Najdanović JG, Vukelić-Nikolić MĐ, Stojanović S, Najman SJ. Osteogenic potential of in vitro osteo-induced adipose-derived mesenchymal stem cells combined with platelet-rich plasma in an ectopic model. International Orthopaedics. 2015;**39**(11):2173-2180. DOI: 10.1007/s00264-015-2929-x

[46] Intini G. The use of platelet-rich plasma in bone reconstruction therapy. Biomaterials. 2009;**30**(28):4956-4966. DOI: 10.1016/j.biomaterials.2009.05.055

[47] Choi BH, Im CJ, Huh JY, Suh JJ, Lee SH. Effect of platelet-rich plasma on bone regeneration in autogenous bone graft. International Journal of Oral and Maxillofacial Surgery. 2004;**33**(1):56-59. DOI: 10.1054/ijom.2003.0466

[48] Fernandes G, Yang S. Application of platelet-rich plasma with stem cells in bone and periodontal tissue engineering. Bone Research. 2016;**4**:16036

[49] Rodriguez IA, Growney Kalaf EA, Bowlin GL, Sell SA. Platelet-rich plasma in bone regeneration: Engineering the delivery for improved clinical efficacy. BioMed Research International. 2014;**2014**:392398. DOI: 10.1155/2014/392398

[50] Vogel JP, Szalay K, Geiger F, Kramer M, Richter W, Kasten P. Platelet-rich plasma improves expansion of human mesenchymal stem cells and retains differentiation capacity and in vivo bone formation in calcium phosphate ceramics. Platelets. 2006;**17**(7):462-469. DOI: 10.1080/09537100600758867

[51] Kasten P, Vogel J, Beyen I, Weiss S, Niemeyer P, Leo A, et al. Effect of platelet-rich plasma on the in vitro proliferation and osteogenic differentiation of human mesenchymal stem cells on distinct calcium phosphate scaffolds: The specific surface area makes a difference. Journal of Biomaterials Applications. 2008;**23**(2):169-188. DOI: 10.1177/0885328207088269

[52] Weibrich G, Hansen T, Kleis W, Buch R, Hitzler WE. Effect of platelet concentration in platelet-rich plasma on peri-implant bone regeneration. Bone. 2004;**34**(4):665-671. DOI: 10.1016/j.bone.2003.12.010

[53] Vukelić-Nikolić MĐ, Najman SJ, Vasiljević PJ, Jevtović-Stoimenov TM, Cvetković VJ, Andrejev MN, et al. Osteogenic capacity of diluted platelet-rich plasma in ectopic bone-forming model: Benefits for bone regeneration. Journal of Cranio-Maxillofacial Surgery. 2018;**46**(11):1911-1918. DOI: 10.1016/j.jcms.2018.09.005

[54] Liu Y, Zhou Y, Feng H, Ma G-E, Ni Y. Injectable tissue-engineered bone composed of human adipose-derived stromal cells and platelet-rich plasma. Biomaterials. 2008;**29**(23):3338-3345. DOI: 10.1016/j.biomaterials.2008.04.037

[55] Najman S, Cvetković V, Najdanović J, Stojanović S, Vukelić-Nikolić M, Vučković I, et al. Ectopic osteogenic capacity of freshly

isolated adipose-derived stromal vascular fraction cells supported with platelet-rich plasma: A simulation of intraoperative procedure. Journal of Cranio-Maxillofacial Surgery. 2016;**44**(10):1750-1760. DOI: 10.1016/j.jcms.2016.08.011

[56] Müller AM, Mehrkens A, Schäfer DJ, Jaquiery C, Güven S, Lehmicke M, et al. Towards an intraoperative engineering of osteogenic and vasculogenic grafts from the stromal vascular fraction of human adipose tissue. European Cells & Materials. 2010;**19**:127-135

[57] Mehrkens A, Saxer F, Güven S, Hoffmann W, Müller AM, Jakob M, et al. Intraoperative engineering of osteogenic grafts combining freshly harvested, human adipose-derived cells and physiological doses of bone morphogenetic protein-2. European Cells & Materials. 2012;**24**:308-319

[58] Man Y, Wang P, Guo Y, Xiang L, Yang Y, Qu Y, et al. Angiogenic and osteogenic potential of platelet-rich plasma and adipose-derived stem cell laden alginate microspheres. Biomaterials. 2012;**33**(34):8802-8811. DOI: 10.1016/j.biomaterials.2012.08.054

[59] Cervelli V, De Angelis B, Lucarini L, Spallone D, Balzani A, Palla L, et al. Tissue regeneration in loss of substance on the lower limbs through use of platelet-rich plasma, stem cells from adipose tissue, and hyaluronic acid. Advances in Skin & Wound Care. 2010;**23**(6):262-272. DOI: 10.1097/01.ASW.0000363551.82058.36

[60] Coelho MB, Cabral JM, Karp JM. Intraoperative stem cell therapy. Annual Review of Biomedical Engineering. 2012;**14**:325-349. DOI: 10.1146/annurev-bioeng-071811-150041

[61] Jurgens WJ, Kroeze RJ, Bank RA, Ritt MJ, Helder MN. Rapid attachment of adipose stromal cells on resorbable polymeric scaffolds facilitates the one-step surgical procedure for cartilage and bone tissue engineering purposes. Journal of Orthopaedic Research. 2011;**29**(6):853-860. DOI: 10.1002/jor.21314

[62] Aslan H, Zilberman Y, Kandel L, Liebergall M, Oskouian RJ, Gazit D, et al. Osteogenic differentiation of noncultured immunoisolated bone marrow-derived CD105+ cells. Stem Cells. 2006;**24**(7):1728-1737. DOI: 10.1634/stemcells.2005-0546

[63] Prins H-J, Schulten EAJM, ten Bruggenkate CM, Klein-Nulend J, Helder MN. Bone regeneration using the freshly isolated autologous stromal vascular fraction of adipose tissue in combination with calcium phosphate ceramics. Stem Cells Translational Medicine. 2016;**5**(10):1362-1374. DOI: 10.5966/sctm.2015-0369

[64] Scherberich A, Müller AM, Schäfer DJ, Banfi A, Martin I. Adipose tissue-derived progenitors for engineering osteogenic and vasculogenic grafts. Journal of Cellular Physiology. 2010;**225**(2):348-353. DOI: 10.1002/jcp.22313

[65] Hicok KC, Du Laney TV, Zhou YS, Halvorsen Y-DC, Hitt DC, Cooper LF, et al. Human adipose-derived adult stem cells produce osteoid in vivo. Tissue Engineering. 2004;**10**(3-4):371-380. DOI: 10.1089/107632704323061735

[66] Stojanović S, Najman S, Korać A. Stem cells derived from lipoma and adipose tissue—similar mesenchymal phenotype but different differentiation capacity governed by distinct molecular signature. Cell. 2018;**7**(12):260. DOI: 10.3390/cells7120260

[67] Hayashi O, Katsube Y, Hirose M, Ohgushi H, Ito H. Comparison of osteogenic ability of rat mesenchymal stem cells from bone marrow,

periosteum, and adipose tissue. Calcified Tissue International. 2008;**82**(3):238-247. DOI: 10.1007/s00223-008-9112-y

[68] Halvorsen YDC, Franklin D, Bond AL, Hitt DC, Auchter C, Boskey AL, et al. Extracellular matrix mineralization and osteoblast gene expression by human adipose tissue-derived stromal cells. Tissue Engineering. 2001;7(6):729-741. DOI: 10.1089/107632701753337681

[69] Huang JI, Beanes SR, Zhu M, Lorenz HP, Hedrick MH, Benhaim P. Rat extramedullary adipose tissue as a source of osteochondrogenic progenitor cells. Plastic and Reconstructive Surgery. 2002;**109**(3):1033-1041. DOI: 10.1097/00006534-200203000-00037

[70] Im GI. Adipose stem cells and skeletal repair. Histology and Histopathology. 2013;**28**(5):557-564

[71] Scott MA, Levi B, Askarinam A, Nguyen A, Rackohn T, Ting K, et al. Brief review of models of ectopic bone formation. Stem Cells and Development. 2011;**21**(5):655-667. DOI: 10.1089/scd.2011.0517

[72] Hao W, Pang L, Jiang M, Lv R, Xiong Z, Hu YY. Skeletal repair in rabbits using a novel biomimetic composite based on adipose-derived stem cells encapsulated in collagen I gel with PLGA-β-TCP scaffold. Journal of Orthopaedic Research. 2010;**28**(2):252-257. DOI: 10.1002/jor.20969

[73] Niemeyer P, Fechner K, Milz S, Richter W, Suedkamp NP, Mehlhorn AT, et al. Comparison of mesenchymal stem cells from bone marrow and adipose tissue for bone regeneration in a critical size defect of the sheep tibia and the influence of platelet-rich plasma. Biomaterials. 2010;**31**(13):3572-3579. DOI: 10.1016/j.biomaterials.2010.01.085

[74] DeLong JM, Beitzel K, Mazzocca AD, Shepard D, Roller BL, Hanypsiak BT. Update on platelet-rich plasma. Current Orthopaedic Practice. 2011;**22**(6):514-523. DOI: 10.1097/BCO.0b013e318236bd55

[75] Goto H, Matsuyama T, Miyamoto M, Yonamine Y, Izumi Y. Platelet-rich plasma/osteoblasts complex induces bone formation via osteoblastic differentiation following subcutaneous transplantation. Journal of Periodontal Research. 2006;**41**(5):455-462. DOI: 10.1111/j.1600-0765.2006.00892.x

[76] Najdanović J, Cvetković V, Stojanović S, Vukelić-Nikolić M, Čakić-Milošević M, Živković J, et al. Effects of bone tissue engineering triad components on vascularization process: Comparative gene expression and histological evaluation in an ectopic bone-forming model. Biotechnology and Biotechnological Equipment. 2016;**30**(6):1122-1131. DOI: 10.1080/13102818.2016.1213662

[77] Martin I, Wendt D, Heberer M. The role of bioreactors in tissue engineering. Trends in Biotechnology. 2004;**22**(2):80-86

[78] Declercq HA, De Caluwé T, Krysko O, Bachert C, Cornelissen MJ. Bone grafts engineered from human adipose-derived stem cells in dynamic 3D-environments. Biomaterials. 2013;**34**(4):1004-1017

[79] Fröhlich M, Grayson WL, Marolt D, Gimble JM, Kregar-Velikonja N, Vunjak-Novakovic G. Bone grafts engineered from human adipose-derived stem cells in perfusion bioreactor culture. Tissue Engineering Parts A. 2010;**16**(1):179-189

[80] Tang D, Tare RS, Yang LY, Williams DF, Ou KL, Oreffo RO. Biofabrication of bone tissue:

Approaches, challenges and translation for bone regeneration. Biomaterials. 2016;**83**:363-382. DOI: 10.1016/J. BIOMATERIALS.2016.01.024

[81] Storti G, Scioli MG, Kim BS, Orlandi A, Cervelli V. Adipose-derived stem cells in bone tissue engineering: Useful tools with new applications. Stem Cells International. 2019;**2019**:3673857. DOI: 10.1155/2019/3673857

[82] Healy KE, Guldberg RE. Bone tissue engineering. Journal of Musculoskeletal & Neuronal Interactions. 2007;7(4): 328-330

[83] Paduano F, Marrelli M, Amantea M, Rengo C, Rengo S, Goldberg M, et al. Adipose tissue as a strategic source of mesenchymal stem cells in bone regeneration: A topical review on the most promising craniomaxillofacial applications. International Journal of Molecular Sciences. 2017;**18**(10):2140. DOI: 10.3390/ijms18102140

[84] Druecke D, Langer S, Lamme E, Pieper J, Ugarkovic M, Steinau HU, et al. Neovascularization of poly(ether ester) blockcopolymer scaffolds in vivo: Long-term investigations using intravital fluorescent microscopy. Journal of Biomedical Materials Research. Part A. 2004;**68**(1):10-18. DOI: 10.1002/ jbm.a.20016

[85] Buschmann J, Welti M, Hemmi S, Neuenschwander P, Baltes C, Giovanoli P, et al. Three-dimensional co-cultures of osteoblasts and endothelial cells in DegraPol foam: Histological and high-field magnetic resonance imaging analyses of pre-engineered capillary networks in bone grafts. Tissue Engineering. Part A. 2011;**17**(3-4):291-299. DOI: 10.1089/ten. TEA.2010.0278

[86] Von Offenberg SN, Cummins PM, Cotter EJ, Fitzpatrick PA, Birney YA, Redmond EM, et al. Cyclic strain-mediated regulation of vascular endothelial cell migration and tube formation. Biochemical and Biophysical Research Communications. 2005;**329**(2):573-582. DOI: 10.1016/j. bbrc.2005.02.013

[87] Anderson SM, Siegman SN, Segura T. The effect of vascular endothelial growth factor (VEGF) presentation within fibrin matrices on endothelial cell branching. Biomaterials. 2011;**32**:7432-7443. DOI: 10.1016/j. biomaterials.2011.06.027

[88] Sun G, Shen YI, Kusuma S, Fox-Talbot K, Steenbergen CJ, Gerecht S. Functional neovascularization of biodegradable dextran hydrogels with multiple angiogenic growth factors. Biomaterials. 2011;**32**(1):95-106. DOI: 10.1016/j.biomaterials.2010.08.091

[89] Soker S, Machado M, Atala A. Systems for therapeutic angiogenesis in tissue engineering. World Journal of Urology. 2000;**18**:10-18. DOI: 10.1007/ PL00007070

[90] Laschke MW, Kleer S, Scheuer C, Schuler S, Garcia P, Eglin D, et al. Vascularisation of porous scaffolds is improved by incorporation of adipose tissue-derived microvascular fragments. European Cells & Materials. 2012;**24**:266-277. DOI: 10.22203/eCM. v024a19

[91] Warnke PH, Springer IN, Wiltfang J, Acil Y, Eufinger H, Wehmoller M, et al. Growth and transplantation of a custom vascularised bone graft in a man. Lancet. 2004;**364**(9436):766-770. DOI: 10.1016/S0140-6736(04)16935-13

[92] Tuzlakoglu K, Bolgen N, Salgado AJ, Gomes ME, Piskin E, Reis RL. Nano- and micro-fiber combined scaffolds: A new architecture for bone tissue engineering. Journal of Materials Science. Materials in Medicine. 2005;**16**:1099-1104. DOI: 10.1007/ s10856-005-4713-8

[93] Levenberg S, Rouwkema J, Macdonald M, Garfein ES, Kohane DS, Darland DC, et al. Engineering vascularized skeletal muscle tissue. Nature Biotechnology. 2005;**23**(7):879-884. DOI: 10.1038/NBT1109

[94] Baiguera S, Ribatti D. Endothelialization approaches for viable engineered tissues. Angiogenesis. 2013;**16**:1-14. DOI: 10.1007/S10456-012-9307-8

[95] Bodnar RJ, Rodgers ME, Chen WCW, Wells A. Pericyte regulation of vascular remodeling through the CXC receptor 3. Arteriosclerosis, Thrombosis, and Vascular Biology. 2013;**33**(12):2818-2829. DOI: 10.1161/ATVBAHA.113.302012

[96] Kim J, Chung M, Kim S, Jo DH, Kim JH, Jeon NL. Engineering of a biomimetic pericyte-covered 3D microvascular network. PLoS One. 2015;**10**(7):e0133880. DOI: 10.1371/journal.pone.0133880

[97] Rademakers T, Horvath JM, van Blitterswijk CA, LaPointe VLS. Oxygen and nutrient delivery in tissue engineering: Approaches to graft vascularization. Journal of Tissue Engineering and Regenerative Medicine. 2019;**13**(10):1815-1829. DOI: 10.1002/term.2932

[98] Seifalian AM, Tiwari A, Hamilton G, Salacinski HJ. Improving the clinical patency of prosthetic vascular and coronary bypass grafts: The role of seeding and tissue engineering. Artificial Organs. 2002;**26**(4):307-320. DOI: 10.1046/j.1525-1594.2002.06841.x

[99] Unger RE, Sartoris A, Peters K, Motta A, Migliaresi C, Kunkel M, et al. Tissue-like self-assembly in cocultures of endothelial cells and osteoblasts and the formation of microcapillary-like structures on three-dimensional porous biomaterials. Biomaterials. 2007;**28**(27):3965-3976. DOI: 10.1016/j.biomaterials.2007.05.032

[100] Kim S, von Recum H. Endothelial stem cells and precursors for tissue engineering: Cell source, differentiation, selection, and application. Tissue Engineering. Part B, Reviews. 2008;**14**:133-147. DOI: 10.1089/TEB.2007.0304

[101] Boyer M, Townsend LE, Vogel L, Falk J, Reitz-Vick D, Trevor K, et al. Isolation of endothelial cells and their progenitor cells from human peripheral blood. Journal of Vascular Surgery. 2000;**31**(1):181-189. DOI: 10.1016/S0741-5214(00)70080-2

[102] Rafii S, Butler JM, Ding BS. Angiocrine functions of organ-specific endothelial cells. Nature. 2016;**529**(7586):316-325. DOI: 10.1038/nature17040

[103] Mizuno H. Adipose-derived stem cells for tissue repair and regeneration: Ten years of research and literature review. Journal of Nippon Medical School. 2009;**76**(2):56-66. DOI: 10.1272/JNMS.76.56

[104] Tapp H, Hanley EN Jr, Patt JC, Gruber HE. Adipose-derived stem cells: Characterization and current application in orthopaedic tissue repair. Experimental Biology and Medicine. 2009;**234**(1):1-9. DOI: 10.3181/0805/MR-170

[105] Lin CS, Xin ZC, Deng CH, Ning H, Lin G, Lue TF. Defining adipose tissue-derived stem cells in tissue and in culture. Histology and Histopathology. 2010;**25**(6):807-815. DOI: 10.14670/HH-25.807

[106] Schäffler A, Büchler C. Concise review: Adipose tissue-derived stromal cells-basic and clinical implications for novel cell-based therapies. Stem

Cells. 2007;**25**:818-827. DOI: 10.1634/stemcells.2006-0589

[107] Ball SG, Shuttleworth CA, Kielty CM. Platelet-derived growth factor receptors regulate mesenchymal stem cell fate: Implications for neovascularization. Expert Opinion on Biological Therapy. 2010;**10**:57-71. DOI: 10.1517/14712590903379510

[108] Du J, Xie P, Lin S, Wu Y, Zeng D, Li Y, et al. Time-phase sequential utilization of adipose-derived mesenchymal stem cells on mesoporous bioactive glass for restoration of critical size bone defects. ACS Applied Materials & Interfaces. 2018;**10**(34):28340-28350. DOI: 10.1021/acsami.8b08563

[109] Najdanović J, Cvetković V, Vukelić-Nikolić M, Stojanović S, Živković J, Najman S. Vasculogenic potential of adipose-derived mesenchymal stem cells in vitro induced into osteoblasts applied with platelet-rich plasma in an ectopic osteogenic model. Acta Medica Medianae. 2019;**58**(4):57-65. DOI: 10.5633/amm.2019.0408

[110] Sahar DE, Walker JA, Wang HT, Stephenson SM, Shah AR, Krishnegowda NK, et al. Effect of endothelial differentiated adipose-derived stem cells on vascularity and osteogenesis in poly(D,L-lactide) scaffolds in vivo. The Journal of Craniofacial Surgery. 2012;**23**(3):913-918. DOI: 10.1097/SCS.0b013e31824e5cd8

[111] Yang P, Huang X, Shen J, Wang C, Dang X, Mankin H, et al. Development of a new pre-vascularized tissue-engineered construct using pre-differentiated rADSCs, arteriovenous vascular bundle and porous nanohydroxyapatide—polyamide 66 scaffold. BMC Musculoskeletal Disorders. 2013;**14**:318. DOI: 10.1186/1471-2474-14-318

[112] Planat-Benard V, Silvestre JS, Cousin B, André M, Nibbelink M, Tamarat R, et al. Plasticity of human adipose lineage cells toward endothelial cells: Physiological and therapeutic perspectives. Circulation. 2004;**109**(5):656-663. DOI: 10.1161/01.CIR.0000114522.38265.61

[113] Zhang H, Zhou Y, Zhang W, Wang K, Xu L, Ma H, et al. Construction of vascularized tissue-engineered bone with a double-cell sheet complex. Acta Biomaterialia. 2018;**77**:212-227. DOI: 10.1016/j.actbio.2018.07.024

[114] Marędziak M, Marycz K, Lewandowski D, Siudzińska A, Śmieszek A. Static magnetic field enhances synthesis and secretion of membrane-derived microvesicles (MVs) rich in VEGF and BMP-2 in equine adipose-derived stromal cells (EqASCs)-a new approach in veterinary regenerative medicine. In Vitro Cellular & Developmental Biology. Animal. 2015;**51**(3):230-240. DOI: 10.1007/s11626-014-9828-0

[115] Kang T, Jones TM, Naddell C, Bacanamwo M, Calvert JW, Thompson WE, et al. Adipose-derived stem cells induce angiogenesis via microvesicle transport of miRNA-31. Stem Cells Translational Medicine. 2016;**5**(4):440-450. DOI: 10.5966/sctm.2015-0177

[116] Scherberich A, Galli R, Jaquiery C, Farhadi J, Martin I. Three-dimensional perfusion culture of human adipose tissue-derived endothelial and osteoblastic progenitors generates osteogenic constructs with intrinsic vascularization capacity. Stem Cells. 2007;**25**(7):1823-1829. DOI: 10.1634/STEMCELLS.2007-0124

[117] Todorov A, Kreutz M, Haumer A, Scotti C, Barbero A, Bourgine PE, et al. Fat-derived stromal vascular

fraction cells enhance the bone-forming capacity of devitalized engineered hypertrophic cartilage matrix. Stem Cells Translational Medicine. 2016;**5**(12):1684-1694. DOI: 10.5966/SCTM.2016-0006

[118] Güven S, Mehrkens A, Saxer F, Schaefer DJ, Martinetti R, Martin I, et al. Engineering of large osteogenic grafts with rapid engraftment capacity using mesenchymal and endothelial progenitors from human adipose tissue. Biomaterials. 2011;**32**(25):5801-5809. DOI: 10.1016/j.biomaterials.2011.04.064

[119] Barba-Recreo P, Del Castillo Pardo de Vera JL, Georgiev-Hristov T, Ruiz Bravo-Burguillos E, Abarrategi A, Burgueño M, et al. Adipose-derived stem cells and platelet-rich plasma for preventive treatment of bisphosphonate-related osteonecrosis of the jaw in a murine model. Journal of Cranio-Maxillo-Facial Surgery. 2015;**43**:1161-1168. DOI: 10.1016/J.JCMS.2015.04.026

[120] Hellström M, Kalén M, Lindahl P, Abramsson A, Betsholtz C. Role of PDGF-B and PDGFR-beta in recruitment of vascular smooth muscle cells and pericytes during embryonic blood vessel formation in the mouse. Development. 1999;**126**(14):3047-3055

[121] Lopatina T, Bruno S, Tetta C, Kalinina N, Porta M, Camussi G. Platelet-derived growth factor regulates the secretion of extracellular vesicles by adipose mesenchymal stem cells and enhances their angiogenic potential. Cell Communication and Signaling. 2014;**12**:26. DOI: 10.1186/1478-811X-12-26

[122] Conejero JA, Lee JA, Parrett BM, Terry M, Wear-Maggitti K, Grant RT, et al. Repair of palatal bone defects using osteogenically differentiated fat-derived stem cells. Plastic and Reconstructive Surgery. 2006;**117**:857-863. DOI: 10.1097/01.prs.0000204566.13979.c1

[123] Orth M, Altmeyer MAB, Scheuer C, Braun BJ, Holstein JH, Eglin D, et al. Effects of locally applied adipose tissue-derived microvascular fragments by thermoresponsive hydrogel on bone healing. Acta Biomaterialia. 2018;**77**:201-211. DOI: 10.1016/j.actbio.2018.07.029

[124] Al-Sanabani JS, Madfa AA, Al-Sanabani FA. Application of calcium phosphate materials in dentistry. International Journal of Biomaterials. 2013;**2013**:876132. DOI: 10.1155/2013/876132

[125] Li Y, Jiang T, Zheng L, Zhao J. Osteogenic differentiation of mesenchymal stem cells (MSCs) induced by three calcium phosphate ceramic (CaP) powders: A comparative study. Materials Science & Engineering. C, Materials for Biological Applications. 2017;**80**:296-300. DOI: 10.1016/j.msec.2017.05.145

[126] Farré-Guasch E, Bravenboer N, Helder MN, Schulten EAJM, Ten Bruggenkate CM, Klein-Nulend J. Blood vessel formation and bone regeneration potential of the stromal vascular fraction seeded on a calcium phosphate scaffold in the human maxillary sinus floor elevation model. Materials (Basel). 2018;**11**(1):161. DOI: 10.3390/ma11010161

[127] Kniebs C, Kreimendahl F, Köpf M, Fischer H, Jockenhoevel S, Thiebes AL. Influence of different cell types and sources on pre-vascularisation in fibrin and agarose–collagen gels. Organogenesis. 2020;**16**(1):14-26. DOI: 10.1080/15476278.2019.1697597

[128] Cornejo A, Sahar DE, Stephenson SM, Chang S, Nguyen S, Guda T, et al. Effect of adipose

tissue-derived osteogenic and endothelial cells on bone allograft osteogenesis and vascularization in critical-sized calvarial defects. Tissue Engineering. Part A. 2012;**18**(15-16):1552-1561. DOI: 10.1089/ten.tea.2011.0515

[129] Orbay H, Busse B, Leach JK, Sahar DE. The effects of adipose-derived stem cells differentiated into endothelial cells and osteoblasts on healing of critical size calvarial defects. The Journal of Craniofacial Surgery. 2017;**28**(7):1874-1879. DOI: 10.1097/SCS.0000000000003910

[130] Shah AR, Cornejo A, Guda T, Sahar DE, Stephenson SM, Chang S, et al. Differentiated adipose-derived stem cell cocultures for bone regeneration in polymer scaffolds in vivo. The Journal of Craniofacial Surgery. 2014;**25**(4):1504-1509. DOI: 10.1097/SCS.0000000000000755

[131] Stahl A, Wenger A, Weber H, Stark GB, Augustin HG, Finkenzeller G. Bi-directional cell contact-dependent regulation of gene expression between endothelial cells and osteoblasts in a three-dimensional spheroidal coculture model. Biochemical and Biophysical Research Communications. 2004;**322**(2):684-692. DOI: 10.1016/j.bbrc.2004.07.175

[132] Clarkin CE, Emery RJ, Pitsillides AA, Wheeler-Jones CP. Evaluation of VEGF-mediated signaling in primary human cells reveals a paracrine action for VEGF in osteoblast-mediated crosstalk to endothelial cells. Journal of Cellular Physiology. 2008;**214**(2):537-544. DOI: 10.1002/jcp.21234

[133] Kaigler D, Krebsbach PH, West ER, Horger K, Huang YC, Mooney DJ. Endothelial cell modulation of bone marrow stromal cell osteogenic potential. The FASEB Journal. 2005;**19**(6):665-667. DOI: 10.1096/fj.04-2529fje

[134] Papadimitropoulos A, Scherberich A, Guven S, Theilgaard N, Crooijmans HJ, Santini F, et al. A 3D in vitro bone organ model using human progenitor cells. European Cells & Materials. 2011;**21**:445-458. DOI: 10.22203/ecm.v021a33

[135] Yang H, Hong N, Liu H, Wang J, Li Y, Wu S. Differentiated adipose-derived stem cell cocultures for bone regeneration in RADA16-I in vitro. Journal of Cellular Physiology. 2018;**233**(12):9458-9472. DOI: 10.1002/jcp.26838

[136] Paik KJ, Zielins ER, Atashroo DA, Maan ZN, Duscher D, Luan A, et al. Studies in fat grafting: Part V. Cell-assisted lipotransfer to enhance fat graft retention is dose dependent. Plastic and Reconstructive Surgery. 2015;**136**(1):67-75. DOI: 10.1097/PRS.0000000000001367

[137] Huang RL, Kobayashi E, Liu K, Li Q. Bone graft prefabrication following the in vivo bioreactor principle. EBioMedicine. 2016;**12**:43-54. DOI: 10.1016/j.ebiom.2016.09.016

[138] Jabbarzadeh E, Starnes T, Khan YM, Jiang T, Wirtel AJ, Deng M, et al. Induction of angiogenesis in tissue-engineered scaffolds designed for bone repair: A combined gene therapy-cell transplantation approach. Proceedings of the National Academy of Sciences of the United States of America. 2008;**105**(32):11099-11104. DOI: 10.1073/pnas.0800069105

[139] Peterson B, Zhang J, Iglesias R, Kabo M, Hedrick M, Benhaim P, et al. Healing of critically sized femoral defects, using genetically modified mesenchymal stem cells from human adipose tissue. Tissue Engineering. 2005;**11**(1-2):120-129. DOI: 10.1089/ten.2005.11.120

Chapter 12

MicroRNAs as Next Generation Therapeutics in Osteoporosis

Taruneet Kaur, Rajeev Kapila and Suman Kapila

Abstract

Bone is an active tissue that works as a tissue and an organ as well. It is constituted of cells and blood vessels by nearly 10% of its volume, while the rest 90% is majorly contributed by extracellular portion. Bone is a living structure stably undertaking continual remodeling between bone formation and bone resorption, where bone-forming cells (osteoblasts) and bone-resorbing cells (osteoclasts) exhibit a crucial role. The differentiation process of osteoblasts and osteoclasts takes place in a balanced manner under normal conditions. This intricate balance is chiefly sustained by biochemical signaling cascades, facilitating accurate bone homeostasis in the body. Loss of balance/misregulated signaling in the bone development or disruption may lead to pathological conditions such as osteoporosis, arthritis, etc. Among several regulators for bone-signaling pathways, microRNAs have appeared as an imperative control of gene expression at the level of post-transcription while addressing the genes that control bone remodeling with appropriate responses in the pathogenesis and perhaps the management of bone diseases. Further, microRNAs control the proliferation and differentiation of osteoblasts and osteoclasts, which finally influence the bone formation. Hence, there is a great possibility in exploiting microRNAs as putative therapeutic targets for the medical relief of bone associated disorders, including osteoporosis.

Keywords: bone formation, signaling pathways, osteoporosis, microRNAs, therapeutics

1. Introduction

Bone is a tough and dynamic tissue that provides shape to our body while protecting the organs [1]. Bone formation is chiefly regulated by the precise biochemical signaling pathways that maintain the action of the bone cells viz. osteoblasts and osteoclasts [2]. These bone cells act in a balanced and stable fashion in the normal functioning of the bone. Disruptions in this intricate balance results in absurd bone functions with the consequent occurrence of bone associated disorders. Osteoporosis is one such well-recognized bone disease that is patented by the decreased bone mineral density and loss of connectivity in the bone trabeculae [3]. Osteoporosis has been documented to elicit approximately 8.9 million fractures annually, targeting around 200 million osteoporotic women across the globe [4, 5]. As per the International Osteoporosis Foundation, osteoporosis results in 1.5 million fractures per year in the USA while in Europe, more than 3.5 million osteoporotic fractures have been reported each year [6, 7]. Besides, in

IntechOpen

India approximately 61 million people are stated as diseased osteoporotic patients [8, 9]. Therefore, management of osteoporosis is the urgent need of the hour for providing relief to the masses and hence refining the quality of life. Apart from numerous therapeutic measures available for the treatment, osteoporosis is still largely undertreated and seeks improved strategies that are associated with fewer side effects.

MicroRNA (miRNA) antagonism might be a new therapeutic approach for the check of osteoporosis. miRNAs are small RNAs (21–23 nucleotides) that act as post-transcriptional regulators of gene expression [10]. In a broader sense, miRNAs execute their functions either by degrading the gene (mRNAs) or by repressing the translation of the protein for the respective gene [11]. miRNA mediated targeting of expression for the genes that are involved in bone remodeling and regeneration is a novel and specific mode of therapeutic strategy. Various miRNAs control the proliferation and differentiation potential of osteoblasts and osteoclasts that ultimately regulates the bone formation [12]. There are numerous studies that report the prominence of miRNA functions and miRNA-based antagonism in the maintenance of bone homeostasis [13]. While acting on the mRNAs, miRNAs can stimulate as well inhibit the activity of osteoblasts and osteoclasts in the bone remodeling [14]. miRNAs are able to obstruct the excessive bone loss during osteoporosis and encourages the bone formation [15]. In short, miRNAs are anticipated to serve as putative gene therapy targets for the treatment of bone-related injuries [16]. Hence the present chapter details the role and efficacy of miRNA in the management of osteoporosis. Finally, we describe the mechanism by which miRNAs can regulate the gene expression in bone formation and resorption.

2. Bone

Bone is an active connective tissue that behaves like an organ as well [1]. The most fundamental function of the bone is to offer support and shape to the body [17]. Other than that, bone also serves endocrine functions and assists in hematopoiesis [18]. Broadly, the structure of bone is categorized into two types, namely cancellous or cortical bone. Cortical/compact type comprises of 80% of the bone skeleton, whereas cancellous/spongy makes up to 20% [19]. Cortical bone forms the dense outer linings of the strong bones, and spongy bone is present at the ends of the long bones [20]. Bone is associated with dynamic character and undertakes continual remodeling, wherein the aged bone is resorbed, and new bone is continually ossified [21]. The bone resorptive episode takes around 10 days to complete, whereas the formation of bone persists for a period of 3 months [22].

2.1 Components of bone

Two vital components of the bone composition are matrix and cells [23]. Matrix is further consists of organic part (30%) and inorganic part/minerals (70%) [23]. Around 90% of the bone organic matrix is made of collagen type 1 and rest 10% includes proteins such as osteocalcin, osteopontin, osteonectin, etc. [19]. In addition, bone is a storehouse for minerals, especially calcium and phosphorous, that makes the hydroxyapatite element of the bone. Hydroxyapatite provides framework and strength to the bone. Furthermore, bone is comprised of four basic cell types, viz. osteoblasts, osteoclasts, osteocytes and bone lining cells [24]. Osteoblasts are bone-forming cells that arise from mesenchymal stem cells. Several growth (FGF) and transcription factors (Runx2, Osterix) are responsible for the differentiation of mesenchymal cells to the osteoblastic lineage [25]. Osteoclasts are bone-resorbing cells that originate from hematopoietic monocyte-macrophage lineage, which differentiates via the assistance of the receptor activator of nuclear factor-κB ligand (RANK ligand) and Macrophage colony-stimulating factor (M-CSF) [26]. Osteoclasts are the biggest (in size) of all other cell types of the bone. Osteocytes constitute 95% of the cells in the mature skeleton [1]. These are the mineralized differentiated osteoblast cells that regulate the process of bone remodeling. Bone lining cells are a type of flat osteoblastic cells that sheet the quiescent bone surfaces [27]. They favor to safeguard the bone, maintain the bone fluids and form a barrier between the bone and bone marrow.

3. Physiological bone regeneration

Bone modeling is a specialized process wherein old bones are removed from one location and replaced by new bone at a distinct location. This process defines the ultimate shape and size of the skeleton [28]. While bone remodeling is a characteristic process in the mature skeleton that is marked by constant bone restoration via a frequent exchange of aged bone with the fresh one at the same site. The process results in the comprehensive regeneration of mature skeleton in an adult every 10 years [29]. The body tries to sustain the balance between bone formation and elimination during the process of bone remodeling. It takes place in discrete sites called basic multicellular units (BMU). The process initiates by activation phase where an initiating signal (e.g., mechanical strain on the bone, fracture healing, etc.) flags the requirement of the remodeling process [30]. After the activation, the commencement of the resorptive phase occurs, wherein osteoclasts depletes bone by proteolytic degradation and acidification. Osteoblasts travel to the eroded space and begin the ossification after the stimulation of transcription factors that encourages the bone formation [31]. Ossified bone is subsequently mineralized and eventually remodeling cycle ends.

4. Biochemical signaling pathways that regulate the bone formation

Bone formation is controlled by numerous elements including transcription factors, hormones, growth factors, oxidative processes, mechanical loading, stress, bone fractures and aging [32]. Osteoblasts and osteoclasts are able to read these external stimulants and propagate the biochemical signals via various signaling cascades. The biological response of the selected signaling pathways results either in bone formation or disruption. Some of the crucial pathways operating in the osteoblasts and osteoclasts are described as follows:

4.1 Wnt/β-catenin pathway

The Wnt signaling pathway has an enormous vital role in the bone development and maintenance of bone homeostasis [33]. Wnt is a secreted protein ligand that binds to a receptor complex of Frizzled (Fz) and low-density lipoprotein receptor-related proteins (LRP). There are two modes of functioning for the Wnt proteins, i.e., canonical and non-canonical pathways, wherein the canonical pathway has a more specific role to play in the bone development. In the canonical pathway (**Figure 1**), the interaction of Wnt to the receptor complex hinders the functioning of axin, glycogen synthase kinase 3β (GSK-3β) and adenomatous polyposis coli (APC) protein. This primes the accumulation of β-catenin in the cytoplasm, further β-catenin travels down to the nucleus and ultimately stimulates lymphoid-enhancer-binding factor/T-cell-specific transcription factors (LEF/TCF). This results in the transcriptional activation for the genes that participate in bone formation and regeneration. While the absence of Wnt signal leads to phosphorylation of the cytosolic β-catenin and its subsequent ubiquitin-mediated degradation [34]. The degradation of the β-catenin finally turns off the downstream activation of the osteogenic genes. Accurate Wnt signaling is a pre-requisite for adequate bone mass in the body while mutation of the Wnt signaling components results in fractures and bone injuries [35].

4.2 BMP-Smad pathway

Bone morphogenetic protein (BMP) holds a well-known and fundamental role in the bone development [36]. BMP signaling is initiated through the interaction of BMPs with the BMP-receptors (type I and type II). This binding stimulates the

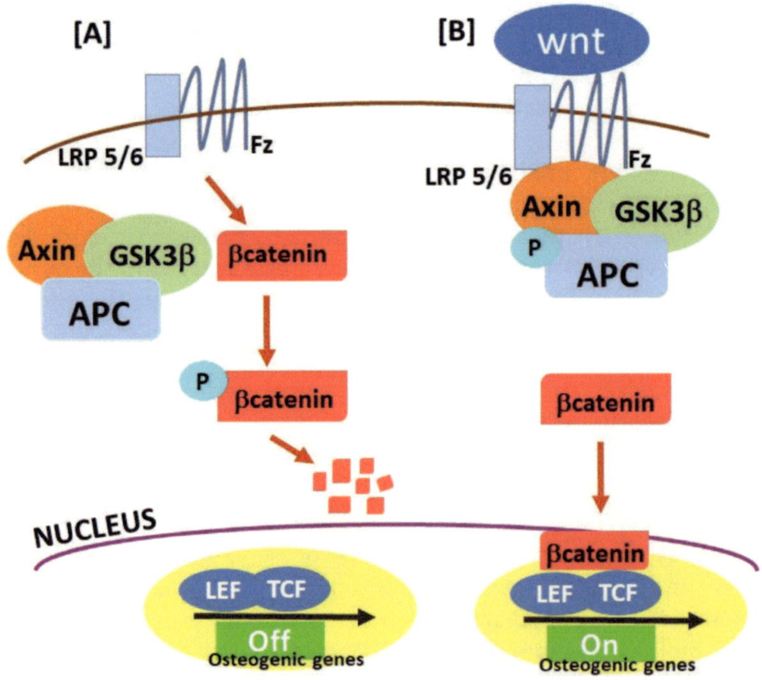

Figure 1.
Wnt/β-catenin (canonical) signaling pathway in the osteoblasts. [A] In the absence of Wnt protein, the degradation complex Axin, GSK-3β and APC protein phosphorylates the β-catenin and results in the ubiquitin-mediated degradation of β-catenin. This turns off the transcription machinery for the osteogenic genes and hence transcription for the genes involved in osteogenic differentiation is hampered resulting in defective bone formation. [B] Wnt ligand interacts with the receptor complex of Fz and LRP that restricted the action of Axin, GSK-3β, and APC protein and hence permitted the transport of β-catenin to the nucleus. β-catenin combines with LEF/TCF transcription factors in the nucleus, thereby potentiating the transcription for the osteogenic genes.

process of phosphorylation in the receptors that leads to recruitment and activation of Smad proteins, i.e., Smad 1, 5, 8 and Smad4. Smad proteins act as transcriptional regulators in the nucleus and ultimately induce the expression of the genes responsible for osteoblastogenesis (**Figure 2**) [37, 38]. There are a total of 14 members in the BMP family, out of which BMP-2,4,5,6,7 and 9 are reported to have high bone formation ability [37].

4.3 RANKL mediated signaling

RANKL-based pathway is an essential signaling cascade for the osteoclast differentiation. RANKL binds to its receptor RANK (present on the osteoclast precursors) and recruits TNF receptor-associated factor (TRAF) adaptor proteins to the conserved TRAF domain present at the cytoplasmic domain of the RANK [39, 40]. TRAF transduces the signal to downstream proteins viz. nuclear factor kappa B (NF-κB), extracellular signal-regulated kinase (ERK), c-Jun N-terminal kinase (JNK), and Nuclear Factor Of Activated T Cells 1 (NFATc1) (**Figure 3**) [41, 42]. NF-κB is an important regulator for the osteoclast differentiation. It is mainly responsible for the inflammation-based osteolysis and bone resorption [43].

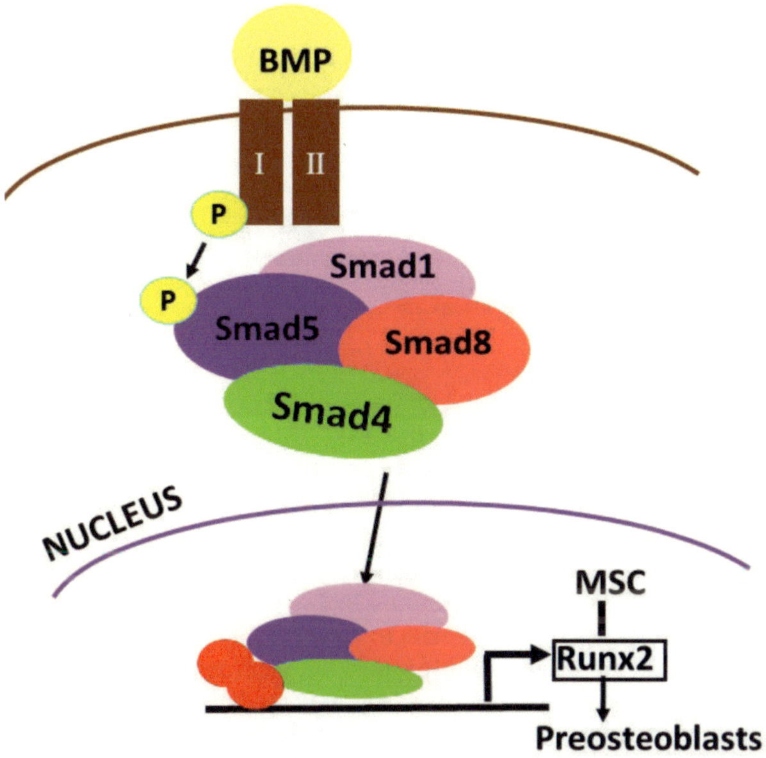

Figure 2.
Bmp-Smad signaling pathway in the osteoblasts. BMP ligand binds to receptor complex viz. type I (BMPRI) and type II receptor (BMPRII). Type II receptor which is a serine/threonine kinase in nature phosphorylates and stimulates type I receptor. Upon activation, type I receptor causes phosphorylation of the downstream proteins—receptor activated Smads (R-Smads), Smad 1/5/8. Further, R-Smads complexes with co-Smad, Smad4 and hence the complex transports to the nucleus. In the nucleus, Smad complex interacts with coactivators and finally results in the transcription of osteogenic gene viz. Runx2. Runx2 is a master transcription factor for the bone development. It aids in the differentiation of mesenchymal stem cells (MSC) to the osteogenic lineage.

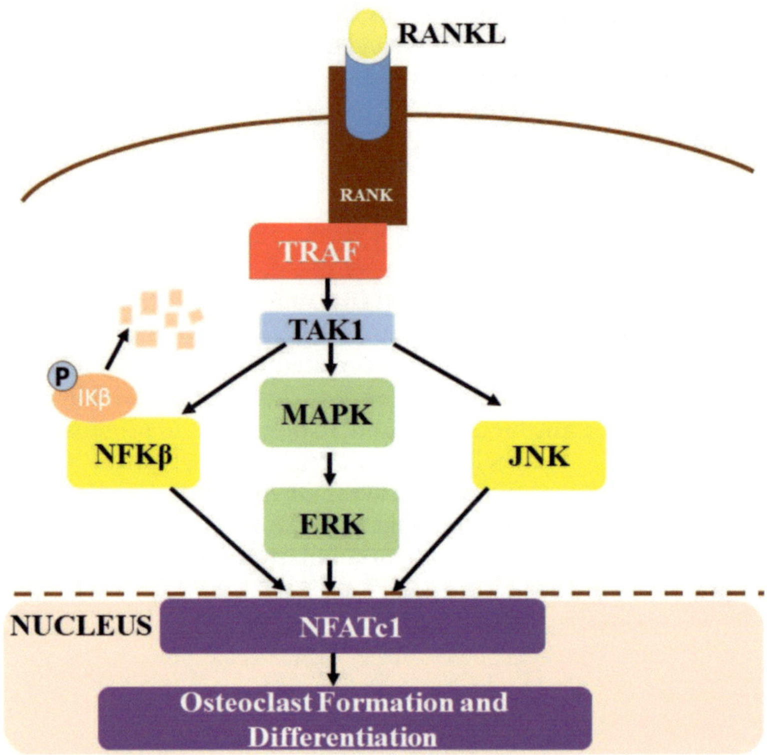

Figure 3.
RANKL-RANK signaling pathway in the osteoclasts. RANKL (present on the surface of osteoblasts) interacts with RANK receptor (on the surface of osteoclasts). RANK does not possess any kinase activity and hence recruits TRAF proteins to the cytoplasmic region of the receptor. This further transduces the signal to downstream components and activates. (1) TAK1 (member of mitogen activated kinase family, MAPK), promotes the ERK dependent activation of NFATc1. (2) NFK-β, after the phosphorylation based degradation of inhibitor of NFK-β (IKβ). (3) Other downstream proteins viz. JNK that leads to transcriptional activation of NFATc1 and additional factors resulting in the osteoclastogenesis.

5. Osteoporosis

Osteoporosis is regarded as a silent bone disorder. Though it is silent and associated with least symptoms, it seeks the most attention. It is reported that osteoporosis targets every third woman and every fifth man beyond 50 years of their ages [44]. Osteoporosis is a pathological condition in which bone mineral density is severely diminished with weakened bone microarchitecture [45]. Bones at the areas specific to hip, wrist and spine are highly vulnerable for the osteoporotic fractures. The occurrence ratio in female to male for the osteoporosis is 1:6 with 61% of fractures befalling in the women [46]. Besides, postmenopausal women have a greater tendency towards osteoporosis [47]. It is predicted that there would be around 6 million victims having osteoporosis by the year 2050 [48]. Osteoporosis is categorized into two major types mentioned as follows:

5.1 Primary osteoporosis

Primary osteoporosis is the most usual type of osteoporosis. It has two sub-categories: Type-I osteoporosis/postmenopausal osteoporosis, is a well-recognized bone issue in the postmenopausal women that is chiefly instigated by estrogen deficit due to menopause, while type-II osteoporosis/age-related osteoporosis is mainly caused as a result of aging in women and men both [49]. In Type-I primary osteoporosis, bone loss hastens in the first 5 years of menopause and then slowly becomes constant. Estrogen executes the fundamental role in the bone development. It stimulates pro-collagen synthesis in the osteoblasts while acting against the bone resorbing cytokines [50, 51]. Estrogen is also capable of supporting osteoblast differentiation [52]. Moreover, estrogen deficiency induces the production of reactive oxygen species that results in increased osteoclast differentiation [53]. Thus, a shortage of estrogen after menopause is one prime cause of osteoporosis majorly in women. In the case of type II primary osteoporosis, age is the main cause that leads to fractures. With growing age, availability of minerals decreases, oxidants production increases while the body becomes less active and does not absorb calcium and vitamin D efficiently that overall thins out the density of bone and reduces the strength [54].

5.2 Secondary osteoporosis

Bone disorders which are secondary impediments of other health-related issues, e.g., adverse effects of drugs interventions, fluctuations in the cycle of physical activities, etc. are acknowledged under the category of secondary Osteoporosis [49]. Glucocorticosteroids and anticonvulsant-based interventions are majorly reported in the cases of secondary osteoporosis [55]. Several other disorders, e.g., endocrinopathies, which have the tendency to reduce the bone mass and interfere with normal bone formation, are also capable of inducing secondary osteoporosis. This form of osteoporosis is found in both pre/post- menopausal women and men [55].

6. Current therapeutic measures for osteoporosis

With recent advances in technology and knowledge, many therapeutic strategies are available for the management of osteoporosis (**Table 1**). Broadly, treatment measures against osteoporosis are classified under two classes: anti-resorptive and anabolic. Anti-resorptive agents work to reduce the rate of bone dissolution while anabolic agents attempt to boost bone formation and development.

Drug	Administration dose of the drug	Mechanism/effect	Harmful effects
Anti-resorptive strategies			
1. Bisphosphonates			
Alendronate	5 mg, 10 mg	Inhibits osteoclastogenesis by binding to minerals of the bone matrix	Severe joint and bone pain, serious allergic reactions, and osteonecrosis
Zoledronic acid	5 mg/ml	Diminishes osteoclast mediated bone disruption, also treats hypercalcemic conditions	Kidney-related issues, seizure, intense dizziness, and trouble while breathing
2. Estrogen modulators			
Raloxifene	60 mg	Mimics estrogen like effects in the bone that decreases bone resorption and enhances bone density	Risk of breast cancer, venous thromboembolism, and leg cramps

Drug	Administration dose of the drug	Mechanism/effect	Harmful effects
3. RANKL antagonist			
Denosumab	60 mg/ml	It is a human monoclonal antibody against RANKL that prevents the formation and maturation of osteoclasts	Shortness of breathing cycle, warm skin with pus, pain while urinating, and night sweats
Anabolic strategies			
1. Parathyroid hormone (PTH)			
Teriparatide	250 mcg/ml	It is a recombinant part of PTH, that stimulates the osteoblastogenesis with augmented bone mineral density	Heartbeat rate is increased, severe dizziness, allergies, itching and swelling of face, tongue, faintness, and osteosarcoma
Abaloparatide	2000 mcg/ml	Same as Teriparatide	Hypercalciuria, palpitations, and spinning sensation
2. Calcitonin	200 IU/ml	Encourages bone formation, reduces calcium levels in the plasma, increases net bone mass	Light-headed sensation, flushing, nausea, and vomiting

Table 1.
Different anti-osteoporotic therapeutic measures currently available in the market [56, 57].

7. New therapeutic drug targets for osteoporosis

Apart from tremendous progress in the therapeutic measures currently available for the check of osteoporosis, the disease still lacks complete eradication and immediate effective relief. The side effects, e.g., in bisphosphonate-based treatment, adverse effects like femoral fractures and jaw osteonecrosis, etc. are often observed. Moreover, instances of osteosarcoma are also reported in the anabolic therapies like parathyroid infusions [56, 58]. Hence, the hunt for the novel drugs that are specific in action is still continued. In the past few years, promising research on the topics related to functional genomics and system biology has emerged as a powerful remedial tool. Within this regard, RNAi (RNA interference) can serve as a new approach of therapeutics in combating bone associated injuries. miRNA-based gene antagonism is one such influential arena in the RNAi technology. miRNAs can interact well with genes or proteins involved in the process of osteogenic differentiation and mineralization.

7.1 MicroRNAs (miRNAs)

miRNAs, a category of small non-coding RNAs, are basically 21–23 nucleotides in length. They regulate the gene expression by interacting and degrading the complementary mRNA counterparts. Additionally, they also control the expression at the protein level via the mode of translational repression of the selected proteins. For the suppression of gene, miRNAs mediate mRNA degradation, mRNA decay, insulation in P bodies and mRNA deadenylation [59]. At the protein level, miRNAs act via inhibiting the initiation or elongation steps of the translation. miRNA might also cause ribosome drops and degradation of the nascent protein chain [59]. miRNAs were discovered in the year of 1990 as regulators of gene expression for the developmental processes in the Caenorhabditis elegans [60]. Interestingly, it has been stated that miRNA targets one-third of the genes in the human genome [61]. miRNAs are also found in extracellular fluids apart from the cells. Further, they are regarded as highly conserved elements among plant and animal kingdoms. In the context of nomenclature for the miRNAs, the preface "miR" is succeeded by a number that represents the order of naming, i.e. among miR-150 and miR-180, 150 represents the fact that it is discovered before 180 was found and named [62].

7.2 Biogenesis of miRNA

The miRNA synthesis can be briefly summarized in the following points (**Figure 4**) [63]:

a. The miRNAs genes are generally transcribed by RNA Polymerase II as pri-miRNA (primary-miRNA) in the animals.

b. A pri-miRNA may encompass one to seven miRNA precursors.

c. Enzymes Drosha and Pasha present in a microprocessor complex cleave the long pri-miRNA to shorter pre-miRNA with 2 nucleotide overhangs at 3′ end and 5′ phosphates.

d. Finally, a nucleocytoplasmic shuttle protein viz. exportin translocates the pre-miRNA to the cytoplasm.

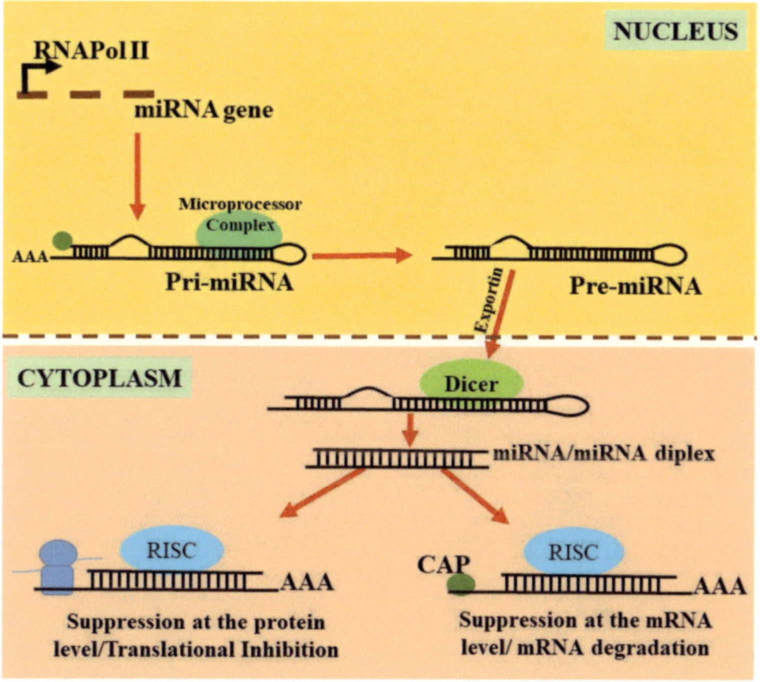

Figure 4.
Synthesis pathway for the miRNA. miRNA gene is synthesized by RNA polymerase II in the form of a primary transcript (Pri-miRNA). Pri-miRNA is acted upon by microprocessor complex (Drosha and Pasha) resulting in the formation of pre-miRNA. From the nucleus, pre-miRNA is transported to the cytoplasm by the shuttle protein exportin. In the cytoplasm, dicer targets the pre-miRNA and splices it to miRNA-miRNA duplex. The dicer cleavage is linked with the unwinding of the duplex and only one strand is selected to be incorporated into the RISC complex. In the RISC complex, miRNA executes its action either on mRNA via mRNA degradation or at the protein level by translational repression.

e. RNase III enzyme called Dicer slices the pre-miRNA into miRNA-miRNA duplex in the cytoplasm.

f. The Dicer mediated cleavage is usually associated with the unwinding of miRNA duplex wherein one miRNA strand (guide strand) is selected to be incorporated in the RISC (RNA induced silencing complex), and the other miRNA strand (passenger strand) is frequently degraded. The RISC contains Dicer, miRNA, argonaute and other accessory proteins.

g. Argonaute proteins generally interact with the mature miRNA and prepare it in the correct orientation for the subsequent binding with mRNA.

h. Perfect base pairing between the miRNA and cognate mRNA leads to degradation of the target mRNA while imperfect or partial complementarity usually results in the suppression at the protein level.

8. miRNA regulation in osteoblast proliferation

Most often, miRNA binds to 3′UTR regions of the genes and executes its action. miRNAs are generally regarded as post-transcriptional regulators that check the process of proliferation, apoptosis, differentiation and development [64]. Several miRNAs are documented to regulate the process of osteogenic proliferation, such as excessive expression of miR-221 and miR-215 in the mouse osteoblast cells encourages the proliferative capacity of the cells [65, 66]. Likewise, downregulation of miR-185 results in the declined osteoblast proliferation [67]. Besides, increased expression of miR-495 in osteoblasts results in diminished proliferation and stimulated apoptosis in the cells [68].

9. miRNA regulation in osteoblast differentiation

Differentiation of the osteoblast cells is an essential facet for the development of the adult skeleton. Most importantly, miRNAs have great potential to act against

miRNA	Target gene	Targeted signaling pathway	Reference
miR-433-3p	DKK1	Wnt/β-catenin	[69]
miR-208a-3p	ACVR1	BMP	[70]
miR-1187	BMPR2	BMP2	[71]
miR-29a	Histone deacetylase 4	β-catenin	[72]
miR-590-5p	Smad7	BMP-Smad-Runx2	[73]
miR-450b	BMP-3	BMP	[74]
miR-135	Smad5	BMP-Smad	[75]
miR-34c	Notch1	Delta-Notch	[76]
miR-224	Smad4	BMP-Smad	[77]
miR-21	HIF-1α	PTEN/PI3K/Akt	[78]

Table 2.
Role of miRNAs in the osteogenic differentiation by acting on various components in the bone signaling pathways.

or in favor of the genes that are involved in the process of bone differentiation (**Table 2**). miRNA usually targets genes that are participating in the osteo-signaling resulting in the bone differentiation.

10. miRNA regulation in bone resorption

miRNAs not only regulates the osteoblastogenesis but also sustains the bone disruptive processes by acting on the genes or proteins partaking in the signaling pathways that are functional inside the osteoclast (**Table 3**). Understanding the miRNA mediated regulation of osteoclastic differentiation will highlight the mechanism behind the differentiation process for the osteoclasts in the bone [84]. Initiating signal (binding of RANKL to the receptors) stimulates various downstream pathways (PI3K, NFK-β, MAPK) that on activation of distinct transcription factors (c-Fos, NFATc1, PU.1) control the osteoclast differentiation [84].

miRNA	Target	Effect	Reference
miR-503	RANK	Represses osteoclast formation in PBMC	[79]
miR-141	Calcr	Suppresses osteoclast differentiation, increases bone mineral density	[80]
miR-29a	RANKL and CXCL12	Decreases osteoclast formation and controls osteoporosis	[81]
miR-124	Nfatc1	Represses osteoclast differentiation	[82]
miR-155	MITF	Suppression of the osteoclastogenesis	[83]
miR-21	FasL PDCD4	Hinders the apoptosis of osteoclasts	[84]
miR-148a	MAFB	Encourages osteoclasts development	[84]
miR-125a	TRAF6	Restricts the formation of osteoclasts	[84]

PBMC, peripheral blood mononuclear cells; Calcr, calcitonin receptor; CXCL12, C-X-C motif chemokine 12; MITF, microphthalmia-associated transcription factor; PDCD4, programmed cell death protein 4; MAFB, MAF BZIP transcription factor B.

Table 3.
Representation of a few examples where miRNAs have played a vital role in the bone resorption.

11. miRNAs as therapeutics

Both the overexpression and inhibition of miRNA can be exploited for the development of potential therapeutics. miRNA sponges, Anti-miRNAs and miRNA masks are few strategies for the suppression of intracellular miRNAs. Anti-miRNAs are the miRNA inhibitors which are constructed as complementary to miRNA sequences. They prohibit the binding of miRNAs to the mRNA targets and relieve the gene suppression phenotype. Anti-miRNAs are specific in action as they are custom synthesized as entirely complementary to naturally existing miRNAs [85]. While, delivery of miRNA is achieved with the help of miRNA mimics, that imitates the sequence and action of miRNAs in the in vitro or in vivo systems. Furthermore, miRNA work as both oncogenes and tumor suppressors, thus contributes to the pathogenesis of several cancerous diseases. MiR-21 founds to be highly upregulated during breast tumors while the levels of miR-196a are significantly increased in the pancreatic cancers [86, 87]. Role of miRNAs is also evidently noticed in many other diseases viz. liver diseases, cardiac dysfunctions, renal failures, neurodegenerative diseases, etc. [88].

11.1 miRNA-based therapeutics in osteoporosis

During osteoporosis, the balance between bone formation and bone elimination is disrupted [89]. Bone dissolution dominates the bone formation and thereby results in the weakened matrix and compromised bone strength. miRNA attempts to correct the imbalance and preserves the bone homeostasis towards bone development during the process of remodeling. miRNAs suppress the genes or proteins involved in the biological signaling pathway and hence aid the pathway to proceed in accurate and normal fashion [90]. This normalization of the pathway further facilitates the optimum differentiation of the mesenchymal stem cells to the osteoblastic lineage. In the past few years, several investigations have emerged which conveys the role of miRNAs in the prognosis and treatment of osteoporosis (**Table 4**).

miRNA	Treatment: gain/ loss of function of the miRNA	Disease (osteoporotic models)	Effect	Reference
miR-148a	Loss of function using AntagomiR-148a	OVX mice	Diminished bone resorption and enhanced bone mass	[91]
miR-103a	AntagomiR-103a	Hindlimb unloaded mice	Neutralized the loss of bone, better bone mass	[92]
miR-31a-5p	AnatgomiR-31a-5p	Aged rats (Injections at the bone marrow cavity in the femur)	Reduced osteoclastogenesis and increased osteoblastogenesis	[93]
miR-1187	Anti-miR-1187	Ovariectomized BALB/c mice	Improved bone microarchitecture	[71]
miR-214	miR-214 sponges	OVX rat with femoral metaphysis critical size defect	Healing of critical size defect	[94]
miR-451a	Gain of function using miR-451a mimic	OVX mice	Improved bone strength and increased bone mineralization	[95]
miR-7b	miR-7b mimic	OVX mice	Augmented bone vascularization and bone volume	[96]
miR-199a-5p	miR-199a-5p agomiR	Sprague-Dawley rats	Better bone regeneration in the tibia-defects	[97]

Table 4.
Representation of the current studies where miRNAs are used as therapeutics in the treatment of osteoporosis.

12. miRNAs as biomarkers

Circulatory miRNAs that are available in the extracellular fluids, e.g., serum, plasma, tears, etc., are potent to be utilized as essential biomarkers in the bone associated issues. Circulatory miRNAs are generally secreted in the form of exosomes or microvesicles, and thus they are guarded against the action of nucleases. Blood plasma miRNAs have been reported as biomarkers in the diagnosis of Non-small-cell lung carcinoma stage I and II [98]. Further, miRNAs present in the human saliva have also been described as biomarkers during the menstrual cycle in women [99]. Serum biomarkers from the osteoporotic patients representing precise pathological condition may serve as crucial diagnostic tools in the clinical practice. Studies in the past years have depicted the relevance of extracellular miRNAs in the plasma or serum samples from the osteoporotic patients relative to healthy controls. miRNAs viz. hsa-miR-122-5p and hsa-miR-4516 have been documented as putative markers in the diagnosis of osteoporosis [100]. Similarly, in another study, miR-21, miR-23a, miR-24, miR-93 and miR-100 are highly upregulated in the serum of osteoporotic patients [101]. Even in the investigation of postmenopausal osteoporosis, miR-422 has been regarded as an essential biomarker gene [102]. Based on several validated studies, it can precisely be concluded that miRNAs may act as useful potential biomarkers in the examination of distinct medical implications, including osteoporosis.

13. miRNA as potential new generation drugs

miRNAs are emerging as promising drugs in the pharmaceutical market. They are endogenous and hence associated with less harmful events for the body. Employing miRNAs as therapeutic targets have one key benefit that nucleotide content of the miRNAs can be easily modified by chemicals for the improved pharmacokinetics and pharmacodynamics of the potential miRNA-based drugs. Besides, miRNA has the capability of targeting multiple genes at a time. Moreover, nowadays chemical locked nucleic acid modifications are present for addressing the issues related to the susceptibility of miRNAs to the intracellular nucleases. Likewise, phosphorothioate alteration is another way of improving the efficacy of miRNAs in the in vivo systems [103]. Recently FDA approved drug, Onpattro against polyneuropathy marks the foundation of RNAi technology-based medicines in the commercial space. **Table 5** describes a few miRNA-based therapeutic compounds that are on the success path of drug development at the preclinical and clinical stages [104, 105].

miRNA	Drug format	Disease	Stage of clinical trial
miR-122	miR-122 Antisense inhibitor	HCV	Phase II
RG-012	Anti-miR-21	Alport syndrome	At the initiating stage of the phase II trial
miR-3	Mimic replacement	Cancers including hepatocellular	Phase I
Let-7	Mimic Replacement	Cancer	Preclinical
miR-103/105	miR-inhibitor	Insulin resistance	Preclinical
miR-10b	miR-10b inhibitor	Glioblastoma	Preclinical

Table 5.
List of few miRNAs which are presently in the development.

14. Conclusion

In healthy body conditions, miRNAs are expected to assist in the maintenance of a regulated balance between the osteoblast-based bone-forming activity and osteoclast dependent bone-resorbing activity. This balance is dependent on the action of miRNAs on the biochemical signaling pathways operating inside the bone. While, during pathologies, the aberrant expression of the miRNAs due to misregulated bone signaling comes into existence. The upregulated or downregulated miRNAs during osteoporosis may serve as biomarkers or gene therapy targets respectively in the management of bone associated injuries including osteoporosis. As miRNAs are expressed in tissue specific manner, therefore miRNA-based biomarkers can differentiate between variable bone-related medical conditions, i.e. defects in bone fragility, reduction in bone mass density, osteoclast malfunctioning, etc. In addition, miRNA bears pleiotropic nature that favors controlling the diseases that have no efficient treatments as yet. Advances in the number of reports regarding miRNA therapeutics in osteoporosis display massive translational utility of miRNAs in the clinical practices. miRNAs are naturally occurring and expected to pose nil or few side effects to the body. The access of the first miRNA mediated therapy against hepatitis C virus infection (HCV) in the clinical phase has fulfilled the hopes for the success of miRNAs as potential therapeutic agents in the drug market. To conclude, miRNAs can undoubtedly be addressed as new generation drugs for the efficient and effective check of osteoporosis.

Conflict of interest

The authors declare no conflict of interest.

Author details

Taruneet Kaur, Rajeev Kapila and Suman Kapila*
Animal Biochemistry Department, ICAR-National Dairy Research Institute, Karnal, India

*Address all correspondence to: skapila69@gmail.com

IntechOpen

© 2020 The Author(s). Licensee IntechOpen. This chapter is distributed under the terms of the Creative Commons Attribution License (http://creativecommons.org/licenses/by/3.0), which permits unrestricted use, distribution, and reproduction in any medium, provided the original work is properly cited.

References

[1] Florencio-Silva R, Sasso GR, Sasso-Cerri E, Simões MJ, Cerri PS. Biology of bone tissue: Structure, function, and factors that influence bone cells. BioMed Research International. 2015;**2015**:1-17

[2] Hayrapetyan A, Jansen JA, van den Beucken JJ. Signaling pathways involved in osteogenesis and their application for bone regenerative medicine. Tissue Engineering Part B: Reviews. 2014;**21**(1):75-87

[3] Sözen T, Özışık L, Başaran NÇ. An overview and management of osteoporosis. European Journal of Rheumatology. 2017;**4**(1):46

[4] Kanis JA, Melton LJ III, Christiansen C, Johnston CC, Khaltaev N. The diagnosis of osteoporosis. Journal of Bone and Mineral Research. 1994;**9**(8):1137-1141

[5] Johnell O, Kanis JA. An estimate of the worldwide prevalence and disability associated with osteoporotic fractures. Osteoporosis International. 2006;**17**(12):1726-1733

[6] Rosen CJ. Postmenopausal osteoporosis. The New England Journal of Medicine. 2005;**353**(6):595-603

[7] Hernlund E, Svedbom A, Ivergård M, Compston J, Cooper C, Stenmark J, et al. Osteoporosis in the European Union: Medical management, epidemiology and economic burden. Archives of Osteoporosis. 2013;**8**(1-2):136

[8] Malhotra N, Mithal A. Osteoporosis in Indians. The Indian Journal of Medical Research. 2008;**127**(3):263-268

[9] Sharma D, Rao S. Osteoporosis epidemiology review and panacea osteoporosis evaluation study. Journal of the Indian Medical Association. 2000;**98**(10):655, 658-655, 659

[10] Obernosterer G, Leuschner PJ, Alenius M, Martinez J. Post-transcriptional regulation of microRNA expression. RNA. 2006;**12**(7):1161-1167

[11] Huntzinger E, Izaurralde E. Gene silencing by microRNAs: Contributions of translational repression and mRNA decay. Nature Reviews. Genetics. 2011;**12**(2):99

[12] Lian JB, Stein GS, Van Wijnen AJ, Stein JL, Hassan MQ, Gaur T, et al. MicroRNA control of bone formation and homeostasis. Nature Reviews. Endocrinology. 2012;**8**(4):212

[13] Sun M, Zhou X, Chen L, Huang S, Leung V, Wu N, et al. The regulatory roles of microRNAs in bone remodeling and perspectives as biomarkers in osteoporosis. BioMed Research International. 2016;**2016**:1652417

[14] Ell B, Kang Y. MicroRNAs as regulators of bone homeostasis and bone metastasis. BoneKEy Reports. 2014;**3**:549

[15] Ge DW, Wang WW, Chen HT, Yang L, Cao XJ. Functions of microRNAs in osteoporosis. European Review for Medical and Pharmacological Sciences. 2017;**21**(21):4784-4789

[16] Dong J, Cui X, Jiang Z, Sun J. MicroRNA-23a modulates tumor necrosis factor-alpha-induced osteoblasts apoptosis by directly targeting fas. Journal of Cellular Biochemistry. 2013;**114**(12):2738-2745

[17] Su N, Yang J, Xie Y, Du X, Chen H, Zhou H, et al. Bone function, dysfunction and its role in diseases including critical illness. International Journal of Biological Sciences. 2019;**15**(4):776

[18] Guntur A, Rosen C. Bone as an endocrine organ. Endocrine Practice. 2012;**18**(5):758-762

[19] Downey PA, Siegel MI. Bone biology and the clinical implications for osteoporosis. Physical Therapy. 2006;**86**(1):77-91

[20] Arana-Chavez VE, Soares AM, Katchburian E. Junctions between early developing osteoblasts of rat calvaria as revealed by freeze-fracture and ultrathin section electron microscopy. Archives of Histology and Cytology. 1995;**58**(3):285-292

[21] Crockett JC, Rogers MJ, Coxon FP, Hocking LJ, Helfrich MH. Bone remodelling at a glance. Journal of Cell Science. 2011;**124**(7):991-998

[22] Hienz SA, Paliwal S, Ivanovski S. Mechanisms of bone resorption in periodontitis. Journal of Immunology Research. 2015;**2015**:615486

[23] Olszta MJ, Cheng X, Jee SS, Kumar R, Kim YY, Kaufman MJ, et al. Bone structure and formation: A new perspective. Materials Science & Engineering R: Reports. 2007;**58**(3-5):77-116

[24] Marks SC Jr, Popoff SN. Bone cell biology: The regulation of development, structure, and function in the skeleton. The American Journal of Anatomy. 1988;**183**(1):1-44

[25] Zhang J, Niu C, Ye L, Huang H, He X, Tong WG, et al. Identification of the haematopoietic stem cell niche and control of the niche size. Nature. 2003;**425**(6960):836

[26] Udagawa N, Takahashi N, Akatsu T, Tanaka H, Sasaki T, Nishihara T, et al. Origin of osteoclasts: Mature monocytes and macrophages are capable of differentiating into osteoclasts under a suitable microenvironment prepared by bone marrow-derived stromal cells. Proceedings of the National Academy of Sciences. 1990;**87**(18):7260-7264

[27] Talmage RV. Morphological and physiological considerations in a new concept of calcium transport in bone. The American Journal of Anatomy. 1970;**129**(4):467-476

[28] Hadjidakis DJ, Androulakis II. Bone remodeling, Annals of the New York Academy of Sciences. Decubitus. 2006;**1092**(1):385-396

[29] Manolagas SC. Birth and death of bone cells: Basic regulatory mechanisms and implications for the pathogenesis and treatment of osteoporosis. Endocrine Reviews. 2000;**21**(2):115-137

[30] Raggatt LJ, Partridge NC. Cellular and molecular mechanisms of bone remodeling. The Journal of Biological Chemistry. 2010;**285**(33):25103-25108

[31] Matsuo K, Irie N. Osteoclast–osteoblast communication. Archives of Biochemistry and Biophysics. 2008;**473**(2):201-209

[32] Javed A, Chen H, Ghori FY. Genetic and transcriptional control of bone formation. Oral and Maxillofacial Surgery Clinics. 2010;**22**(3):283-293

[33] Xu H, Duan J, Ning D, Li J, Liu R, Yang R, et al. Role of Wnt signaling in fracture healing. BMB Reports. 2014;**47**(12):666

[34] Bonewald LF, Johnson ML. Osteocytes, mechanosensing and Wnt signaling. Bone. 2008;**42**(4):606-615

[35] Pinzone JJ, Hall BM, Thudi NK, Vonau M, Qiang YW, Rosol TJ, et al. The role of Dickkopf-1 in bone development, homeostasis, and disease. Blood: The Journal of the American Society of Hematology. 2009;**113**(3):517-525

[36] Wang RN, Green J, Wang Z, Deng Y, Qiao M, Peabody M, et al. Bone morphogenetic protein (BMP) signaling in development and human diseases. Genes & diseases. 2014;**1**(1):87-105

[37] Chen G, Deng C, Li YP. TGF-β and BMP signaling in osteoblast

differentiation and bone formation. International Journal of Biological Sciences. 2012;**8**(2):272

[38] Wu M, Chen G, Li YP. TGF-β and BMP signaling in osteoblast, skeletal development, and bone formation, homeostasis and disease. Bone Research. 2016;**4**:16009

[39] Walsh MC, Choi Y. Biology of the TRANCE axis. Cytokine & Growth Factor Reviews. 2003;**14**(3-4):251-263

[40] Darnay BG, Haridas V, Ni J, Moore PA, Aggarwal BB. Characterization of the intracellular domain of receptor activator of NF-κB (RANK) interaction with tumor necrosis factor receptor-associated factors and activation of NF-κB and c-Jun N-terminal kinase. The Journal of Biological Chemistry. 1998;**273**(32):20551-20555

[41] Wong BR, Josien R, Lee SY, Vologodskaia M, Steinman RM, Choi Y. The TRAF family of signal transducers mediates NF-κB activation by the TRANCE receptor. The Journal of Biological Chemistry. 1998;**273**(43):28355-28359

[42] Takayanagi H, Kim S, Koga T, Nishina H, Isshiki M, Yoshida H, et al. Induction and activation of the transcription factor NFATc1 (NFAT2) integrate RANKL signaling in terminal differentiation of osteoclasts. Developmental Cell. 2002;**3**(6):889-901

[43] Abu-Amer Y. NF-κB signaling and bone resorption. Osteoporosis International. 2013;**24**(9):2377-2386

[44] Sözen T, Özışık L, Başaran NÇ. An overview and management of osteoporosis. European Journal of Rheumatology. 2017;**4**(1):46

[45] Leslie WD, Adler RA, Fuleihan GE, Hodsman A, Kendler DL, McClung M, et al. Application of the 1994 WHO classification to populations other than postmenopausal Caucasian women: The 2005 ISCD official positions. Journal of Clinical Densitometry. 2006;**9**(1):22-30

[46] Johnell O, Kanis JA. An estimate of the worldwide prevalence and disability associated with osteoporotic fractures. Osteoporosis International. 2006;**17**(12):1726-1733

[47] Tella SH, Gallagher JC. Prevention and treatment of postmenopausal osteoporosis. The Journal of Steroid Biochemistry and Molecular Biology. 2014;**142**:155-170

[48] Cauley JA. Public health impact of osteoporosis. The Journals of Gerontology. Series A, Biological Sciences and Medical Sciences. 2013;**68**(10):1243-1251

[49] Feng X, McDonald JM. Disorders of bone remodeling. Annual Review of Pathology: Mechanisms of Disease. 2011;**6**:121-145

[50] Chidi-Ogbolu N, Baar K. Effect of estrogen on musculoskeletal performance and injury risk. Frontiers in Physiology. 2018;**9**:1834

[51] Riggs BL. The mechanisms of estrogen regulation of bone resorption. The Journal of Clinical Investigation. 2000;**106**(10):1203-1204

[52] Okazaki RY, Inoue D, Shibata M, Saika M, Kido S, Ooka H, et al. Estrogen promotes early osteoblast differentiation and inhibits adipocyte differentiation in mouse bone marrow stromal cell lines that express estrogen receptor (ER) α or β. Endocrinology. 2002;**143**(6):2349-2356

[53] Cenci S, Weitzmann MN, Roggia C, Namba N, Novack D, Woodring J, et al. Estrogen deficiency induces bone loss by enhancing T-cell production of TNF-α. The Journal of Clinical Investigation. 2000;**106**(10):1229-1237

[54] Lobo V, Patil A, Phatak A, Chandra N. Free radicals, antioxidants and functional foods: Impact on human health. Pharmacognosy Reviews. 2010;**4**(8):118

[55] Mirza F, Canalis E. Secondary osteoporosis: Pathophysiology and management. European Journal of Endocrinology/European Federation of Endocrine Societies. 2015;**173**(3):R131

[56] Tu KN, Lie JD, Wan CK, Cameron M, Austel AG, Nguyen JK, et al. Osteoporosis: A review of treatment options. Pharmacy and Therapeutics. 2018;**43**(2):92

[57] Gennari L, Rotatori S, Bianciardi S, Gonnelli S, Nuti R, Merlotti D. Appropriate models for novel osteoporosis drug discovery and future perspectives. Expert Opinion on Drug Discovery. 2015;**10**(11):1201-1216

[58] Gennari L, Rotatori S, Bianciardi S, Gonnelli S, Nuti R, Merlotti D. Appropriate models for novel osteoporosis drug discovery and future perspectives. Expert Opinion on Drug Discovery. 2015;**10**(11):1201-1216

[59] Morozova N, Zinovyev A, Nonne N, Pritchard LL, Gorban AN, Harel-Bellan A. Kinetic signatures of microRNA modes of action. RNA. 2012;**18**(9):1635-1655

[60] Miska EA, Alvarez-Saavedra E, Abbott AL, Lau NC, Hellman AB, McGonagle SM, et al. Most Caenorhabditis elegans microRNAs are individually not essential for development or viability. PLoS Genetics. 2007;**3**(12):e215

[61] Davis BN, Hata A. Regulation of MicroRNA biogenesis: A miRiad of mechanisms. Cell Communication and Signaling: CCS. 2009;**7**(1):18

[62] Fromm B, Billipp T, Peck LE, Johansen M, Tarver JE, King BL, et al. A uniform system for the annotation of vertebrate microRNA genes and the evolution of the human microRNAome. Annual Review of Genetics. 2015;**49**:213-242

[63] Li Z, Rana TM. Molecular mechanisms of RNA-triggered gene silencing machineries. Accounts of Chemical Research. 2012;**45**(7):1122-1131

[64] Catalanotto C, Cogoni C, Zardo G. MicroRNA in control of gene expression: An overview of nuclear functions. International Journal of Molecular Sciences. 2016;**17**(10):1712

[65] Zheng X, Dai J, Zhang H, Ge Z. MicroRNA-221 promotes cell proliferation, migration, and differentiation by regulation of ZFPM2 in osteoblasts. Brazilian Journal of Medical and Biological Research. 2018;**51**(12):e7574

[66] Chen CH, Lu HT, Tsuang YH, Kuo YJ. MicroRNA-215 promotes proliferation and differentiation of osteoblasts by regulation of c-fos. International Journal of Clinical and Experimental Pathology. 2017;**10**(6):6536-6543

[67] Yao CJ, Lv Y, Zhang CJ, Jin JX, Xu LH, Jiang J, et al. MicroRNA-185 inhibits the growth and proliferation of osteoblasts in fracture healing by targeting PTH gene through down-regulating Wnt/β-catenin axis: In an animal experiment. Biochemical and Biophysical Research Communications. 2018;**501**(1):55-63

[68] Tian Z, Zhou H, Xu Y, Bai J. MicroRNA-495 inhibits new bone regeneration via targeting high mobility group AT-Hook 2 (HMGA2). Medical Science Monitor: International Medical Journal of Experimental and Clinical Research. 2017;**23**:4689

[69] Tang X, Lin J, Wang G, Lu J. MicroRNA-433-3p promotes osteoblast

differentiation through targeting DKK1 expression. PLoS One. 2017;**12**(6):e0179860

[70] Arfat Y, Basra MA, Shahzad M, Majeed K, Mahmood N, Munir H. miR-208a-3p suppresses osteoblast differentiation and inhibits bone formation by targeting ACVR1. Molecular Therapy—Nucleic Acids. 2018;**11**:323-336

[71] John AA, Prakash R, Kureel J, Singh D. Identification of novel microRNA inhibiting actin cytoskeletal rearrangement thereby suppressing osteoblast differentiation. Journal of Molecular Medicine. 2018;**96**(5):427-444

[72] Ko JY, Chuang PC, Chen MW, Ke HC, Wu SL, Chang YH, et al. MicroRNA-29a ameliorates glucocorticoid-induced suppression of osteoblast differentiation by regulating β-catenin acetylation. Bone. 2013;**57**(2):468-475

[73] Vishal M, Vimalraj S, Ajeetha R, Gokulnath M, Keerthana R, He Z, et al. MicroRNA-590-5p stabilizes Runx2 by targeting Smad7 during osteoblast differentiation. Journal of Cellular Physiology. 2017;**232**(2):371-380

[74] Fan L, Fan J, Liu Y, Li T, Xu H, Yang Y, et al. miR-450b promotes osteogenic differentiation in vitro and enhances bone formation in vivo by targeting BMP3. Stem Cells and Development. 2018;**27**(9):600-611

[75] Dallas SL, Prideaux M, Bonewald LF. The osteocyte: An endocrine cell… and more. Endocrine Reviews. 2013;**34**(5):658-690

[76] Bae Y, Yang T, Zeng HC, Campeau PM, Chen Y, Bertin T, et al. miRNA-34c regulates Notch signaling during bone development. Human Molecular Genetics. 2012;**21**(13):2991-3000

[77] Luo Y, Cao X, Chen J, Gu J, Zhao J, Sun J. MicroRNA-224 suppresses osteoblast differentiation by inhibiting SMAD4. Journal of Cellular Physiology. 2018;**233**(10):6929-6937

[78] Yang C, Liu X, Zhao K, Zhu Y, Hu B, Zhou Y, et al. Ning Y. miRNA-21 promotes osteogenesis via the PTEN/PI3K/Akt/HIF-1α pathway and enhances bone regeneration in critical size defects. Stem Cell Research & Therapy. 2019;**10**(1):65

[79] Chen C, Cheng P, Xie H, Zhou HD, Wu XP, Liao EY, et al. MiR-503 regulates osteoclastogenesis via targeting RANK. Journal of Bone and Mineral Research. 2014;**29**(2):338-347

[80] Yang S, Zhang W, Cai M, Zhang Y, Jin F, Yan S, et al. Suppression of bone Resorption by miR-141 in aged rhesus monkeys. Journal of Bone and Mineral Research. 2018;**33**(10):1799-1812

[81] Lian WS, Ko JY, Chen YS, Ke HJ, Hsieh CK, Kuo CW, et al. MicroRNA-29a represses osteoclast formation and protects against osteoporosis by regulating PCAF-mediated RANKL and CXCL12. Cell Death & Disease. 2019;**10**(10):1-4

[82] Hrdlicka HC, Lee SK, Delany AM. MicroRNAs are critical regulators of osteoclast differentiation. Current Molecular Biology Reports. 2019;**5**(1):65-74

[83] Lozano C, Duroux-Richard I, Firat H, Schordan E, Apparailly F. MicroRNAs: key regulators to understand osteoclast differentiation? Frontiers in Immunology. 2019;**10**:375

[84] Tang P, Xiong Q, Ge W, Zhang L. The role of microRNAs in osteoclasts and osteoporosis. RNA Biology. 2014;**11**(11):1355-1363

[85] Mendell JT, Olson EN. MicroRNAs in stress signaling and human disease. Cell. 2012;**148**(6):1172-1187

[86] Si ML, Zhu S, Wu H, Lu Z, Wu F, Mo YY. miR-21-mediated tumor growth. Oncogene. 2007;**26**(19):2799

[87] Szafranska AE, Davison TS, John J, Cannon T, Sipos B, Maghnouj A, et al. MicroRNA expression alterations are linked to tumorigenesis and non-neoplastic processes in pancreatic ductal adenocarcinoma. Oncogene. 2007;**26**(30):4442

[88] Walayat A, Yang M, Xiao D. Therapeutic Implication of miRNA in human disease. In: Antisense Therapy. Rijeka: IntechOpen; 2018

[89] Andersen TL, Abdelgawad ME, Kristensen HB, Hauge EM, Rolighed L, Bollerslev J, et al. Understanding coupling between bone resorption and formation: Are reversal cells the missing link? The American Journal of Pathology. 2013;**183**(1):235-246

[90] Sun M, Zhou X, Chen L, Huang S, Leung V, Wu N, et al. The regulatory roles of microRNAs in bone remodeling and perspectives as biomarkers in osteoporosis. BioMed Research International. 2016;**2016**:1652417

[91] Cheng P, Chen C, He HB, Hu R, Zhou HD, Xie H, et al. miR-148a regulates osteoclastogenesis by targeting V-maf musculoaponeurotic fibrosarcoma oncogene homolog B. Journal of Bone and Mineral Research. 2013;**28**(5):1180-1190

[92] Zuo B, Zhu J, Li J, Wang C, Zhao X, Cai G, et al. microRNA-103a functions as a mechanosensitive microRNA to inhibit bone formation through targeting Runx2. Journal of Bone and Mineral Research. 2015;**30**(2):330-345

[93] Xu R, Shen X, Si Y, Fu Y, Zhu W, Xiao T, et al. Micro RNA-31a-5p from aging BMSC s links bone formation and resorption in the aged bone marrow microenvironment. Aging Cell. 2018;**17**(4):e12794

[94] Li KC, Chang YH, Yeh CL, Hu YC. Healing of osteoporotic bone defects by baculovirus-engineered bone marrow-derived MSCs expressing MicroRNA sponges. Biomaterials. 2016;**74**:155-166

[95] Karvande A, Kushwaha P, Ahmad N, Adhikary S, Kothari P, Tripathi AK, et al. Glucose dependent miR-451a expression contributes to parathyroid hormone mediated osteoblast differentiation. Bone. 2018;**117**:98-115

[96] Dou C, Ding N, Luo F, Hou T, Cao Z, Bai Y, et al. Graphene-based microRNA transfection blocks preosteoclast fusion to increase bone formation and vascularization. Advanced Science. 2018;**5**(2):1700578

[97] Chen X, Gu S, Chen BF, Shen WL, Yin Z, Xu GW, et al. Nanoparticle delivery of stable miR-199a-5p agomir improves the osteogenesis of human mesenchymal stem cells via the HIF1a pathway. Biomaterials. 2015;**53**:239-250

[98] Zhang H, Mao F, Shen T, Luo Q, Ding Z, Qian L, et al. Plasma miR-145, miR-20a, miR-21 and miR-223 as novel biomarkers for screening early-stage non-small cell lung cancer. Oncology Letters. 2017;**13**(2):669-676

[99] Rekker K, Saare M, Roost AM, Salumets A, Peters M. Circulating microRNA profile throughout the menstrual cycle. PLoS One. 2013;**8**(11):e81166

[100] Mandourah AY, Ranganath L, Barraclough R, Vinjamuri S, Hof RV, Hamill S, et al. Circulating microRNAs as potential diagnostic biomarkers for osteoporosis. Scientific Reports. 2018;**8**(1):8421

[101] Seeliger C, Karpinski K, Haug AT, Vester H, Schmitt A, Bauer JS, et al. Five freely circulating miRNAs and bone tissue miRNAs are associated with osteoporotic fractures. Journal

of Bone and Mineral Research. 2014;**29**(8):1718-1728

[102] Cao Z, Moore BT, Wang Y, Peng XH, Lappe JM, Recker RR, et al. MiR-422a as a potential cellular microRNA biomarker for postmenopausal osteoporosis. PLoS One. 2014;**9**(5):e97098

[103] Lennox KA, Behlke MA. Chemical modification and design of anti-miRNA oligonucleotides. Gene Therapy. 2011;**18**(12):1111

[104] Li Z, Rana TM. Therapeutic targeting of microRNAs: Current status and future challenges. Nature Reviews. Drug Discovery. 2014;**13**(8):622-638

[105] Chakraborty C, Sharma AR, Sharma G, Doss CG, Lee SS. Therapeutic miRNA and siRNA: Moving from bench to clinic as next generation medicine. Molecular Therapy—Nucleic Acids. 2017;**8**:132-143